Health, Quality of Life and Sport Rehabilitation

Health, Quality of Life and Sport Rehabilitation

Editors

Redha Taiar
Mario Bernardo-Filho
Ana Cristina Rodrigues Lacerda

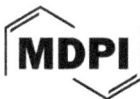

Basel • Beijing • Wuhan • Barcelona • Belgrade • Novi Sad • Cluj • Manchester

Editors

Redha Taiar
University of Reims
Champagne-Ardenne
Reims
France

Mario Bernardo-Filho
Rio de Janeiro State
University (UERJ)
Rio de Janeiro
Brazil

Ana Cristina Rodrigues
Lacerda
Federal University of
Jequitinhonha and Mucuri
Valleys (UFVJM)
Diamantina
Brazil

Editorial Office
MDPI
St. Alban-Anlage 66
4052 Basel, Switzerland

This is a reprint of articles from the Special Issue published online in the open access journal *Journal of Clinical Medicine* (ISSN 2077-0383) (available at: https://www.mdpi.com/journal/jcm/special_issues/Sport_Rehabilitation).

For citation purposes, cite each article independently as indicated on the article page online and as indicated below:

Lastname, A.A.; Lastname, B.B. Article Title. *Journal Name* **Year**, *Volume Number*, Page Range.

ISBN 978-3-0365-9744-7 (Hbk)
ISBN 978-3-0365-9745-4 (PDF)
doi.org/10.3390/books978-3-0365-9745-4

© 2023 by the authors. Articles in this book are Open Access and distributed under the Creative Commons Attribution (CC BY) license. The book as a whole is distributed by MDPI under the terms and conditions of the Creative Commons Attribution-NonCommercial-NoDerivs (CC BY-NC-ND) license.

Contents

Amparo Oliver, Trinidad Sentandreu-Mañó, José M. Tomás, Irene Fernández and Patricia Sancho
Quality of Life in European Older Adults of SHARE Wave 7: Comparing the Old and the Oldest-Old
Reprinted from: *J. Clin. Med.* **2021**, *10*, 2850, doi:10.3390/jcm10132850 1

Marco Gervasi, Elena Barbieri, Italo Capparucci, Giosuè Annibalini, Davide Sisti, Stefano Amatori, et al.
Treatment of Achilles Tendinopathy in Recreational Runners with Peritendinous Hyaluronic Acid Injections: A Viscoelastometric, Functional, and Biochemical Pilot Study
Reprinted from: *J. Clin. Med.* **2021**, *10*, 1397, doi:10.3390/jcm10071397 13

Razvan Anghel, Cristina Andreea Adam, Dragos Traian Marius Marcu, Ovidiu Mitu and Florin Mitu
Cardiac Rehabilitation in Patients with Peripheral Artery Disease—A Literature Review in COVID-19 Era
Reprinted from: *J. Clin. Med.* **2022**, *11*, 416, doi:10.3390/jcm11020416 25

Dan Alexandru Szabo, Nicolae Neagu, Silvia Teodorescu, Corina Predescu, Ioan Sabin Sopa and Loredana Panait
TECAR Therapy Associated with High-Intensity Laser Therapy (Hilt) and Manual Therapy in the Treatment of Muscle Disorders: A Literature Review on the Theorised Effects Supporting Their Use
Reprinted from: *J. Clin. Med.* **2022**, *11*, 6149, doi:10.3390/jcm11206149 45

Sae Maruyama, Chie Sekine, Mayuu Shagawa, Hirotake Yokota, Ryo Hirabayashi, Ryoya Togashi, et al.
Menstrual Cycle Changes Joint Laxity in Females—Differences between Eumenorrhea and Oligomenorrhea
Reprinted from: *J. Clin. Med.* **2022**, *11*, 3222, doi:10.3390/jcm11113222 65

Markus Regauer, Gordon Mackay, Owen Nelson, Wolfgang Böcker and Christian Ehrnthaller
Evidence-Based Surgical Treatment Algorithm for Unstable Syndesmotic Injuries
Reprinted from: *J. Clin. Med.* **2022**, *11*, 331, doi:10.3390/jcm11020331 79

Luana Rocha Paulo, Ana Cristina Rodrigues Lacerda, Fábio Luiz Mendonça Martins, José Sebastião Cunha Fernandes, Leonardo Sette Vieira, Cristiano Queiroz Guimarães, et al.
Can a Single Trial of a Thoracolumbar Myofascial Release Technique Reduce Pain and Disability in Chronic Low Back Pain? A Randomized Balanced Crossover Study
Reprinted from: *J. Clin. Med.* **2021**, *10*, 2006, doi:10.3390/jcm10092006 103

Anna Piotrowska, Wanda Pilch, Łukasz Tota, Marcin Maciejczyk, Dariusz Mucha, Monika Bigosińska, et al.
Local Vibration Reduces Muscle Damage after Prolonged Exercise in Men
Reprinted from: *J. Clin. Med.* **2021**, *10*, 5461, doi:10.3390/jcm10225461 115

Norollah Javdaneh, Tadeusz Ambroży, Amir Hossein Barati, Esmaeil Mozafaripour and Łukasz Rydzik
Focus on the Scapular Region in the Rehabilitation of Chronic Neck Pain Is Effective in Improving the Symptoms: A Randomized Controlled Trial
Reprinted from: *J. Clin. Med.* **2021**, *10*, 3495, doi:10.3390/jcm10163495 127

Leonardo Augusto Costa Teixeira, Jousielle Marcia dos Santos, Adriana Netto Parentoni, Liliana Pereira Lima, Tamiris Campos Duarte, Franciane Pereira Brant, et al.
Adiponectin Is a Contributing Factor of Low Appendicular Lean Mass in Older Community-Dwelling Women: A Cross-Sectional Study
Reprinted from: *J. Clin. Med.* **2022**, *11*, 7175, doi:10.3390/jcm11237175 . . . . **141**

Paweł Wiśniowski, Maciej Cieśliński, Martyna Jarocka, Przemysław Seweryn Kasiak, Bartłomiej Makaruk, Wojciech Pawliczek, et al.
The Effect of Pressotherapy on Performance and Recovery in the Management of Delayed Onset Muscle Soreness: A Systematic Review and Meta-Analysis
Reprinted from: *J. Clin. Med.* **2022**, *11*, 2077, doi:10.3390/jcm11082077 . . . . **153**

Dolores Escrivá, Jordi Caplliure-Llopis, Inmaculada Benet, Gonzalo Mariscal, Juan Vicente Mampel and Carlos Barrios
Differences in Adiposity Profile and Body Fat Distribution between Forwards and Backs in Sub-Elite Spanish Female Rugby Union Players
Reprinted from: *J. Clin. Med.* **2021**, *10*, 5713, doi:10.3390/jcm10235713 . . . . **173**

Marco Bravi, Chiara Fossati, Arrigo Giombini, Andrea Macaluso, José Kawazoe Lazzoli, Fabio Santacaterina, et al.
Criteria for Return-to-Play (RTP) after Rotator Cuff Surgery: A Systematic Review of Literature
Reprinted from: *J. Clin. Med.* **2022**, *11*, 2244, doi:10.3390/jcm11082244 . . . . **187**

Yuge Tian and Zhenguo Shi
Effects of Physical Activity on Daily Physical Function in Chinese Middle-Aged and Older Adults: A Longitudinal Study from CHARLS
Reprinted from: *J. Clin. Med.* **2022**, *11*, 6514, doi:10.3390/jcm11216514 . . . . **199**

Juan Lopez-Barreiro, Pablo Hernandez-Lucas, Jose Luis Garcia-Soidan and Vicente Romo-Perez
Effects of an Eccentric Training Protocol Using Gliding Discs on Balance and Lower Body Strength in Healthy Adults
Reprinted from: *J. Clin. Med.* **2021**, *10*, 5965, doi:10.3390/jcm10245965 . . . . **211**

Magdalena Plandowska, Agnieszka Kędra, Przemysław Kędra and Dariusz Czaprowski
Trunk Alignment in Physically Active Young Males with Low Back Pain
Reprinted from: *J. Clin. Med.* **2022**, *11*, 4206, doi:10.3390/jcm11144206 . . . . **221**

Anna Hadamus, Tomasz Jankowski, Karolina Wiaderna, Aneta Bugalska, Wojciech Marszałek, Michalina Błażkiewicz, et al.
Effectiveness of Warm-Up Exercises with Tissue Flossing in Increasing Muscle Strength
Reprinted from: *J. Clin. Med.* **2022**, *11*, 6054, doi:10.3390/jcm11206054 . . . . **231**

Renato Fleury Cardoso, Ana Cristina Rodrigues Lacerda, Vanessa Pereira Lima, Lucas Fróis Fernandes de Oliveira, Sofia Fróis Fernandes de Oliveira, Rafaela Paula Araújo, et al.
Efficacy of Acupuncture on Quality of Life, Functional Performance, Dyspnea, and Pulmonary Function in Patients with Chronic Obstructive Pulmonary Disease: Protocol for a Randomized Clinical Trial
Reprinted from: *J. Clin. Med.* **2022**, *11*, 3048, doi:10.3390/jcm11113048 . . . . **245**

Roberto Ucero-Lozano, Raúl Pérez-Llanes, José Antonio López-Pina and Rubén Cuesta-Barriuso
Approach to Knee Arthropathy through 180-Degree Immersive VR Movement Visualization in Adult Patients with Severe Hemophilia: A Pilot Study
Reprinted from: *J. Clin. Med.* **2022**, *11*, 6216, doi:10.3390/jcm11206216 . . . . **257**

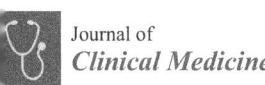

Article

Quality of Life in European Older Adults of SHARE Wave 7: Comparing the Old and the Oldest-Old

Amparo Oliver [1], Trinidad Sentandreu-Mañó [2,*], José M. Tomás [1], Irene Fernández [1] and Patricia Sancho [3]

1. Department of Methodology for the Behavioral Sciences, University of Valencia, 46010 Valencia, Spain; amparo.oliver@uv.es (A.O.); jose.m.tomas@uv.es (J.M.T.); irene.fernandez@uv.es (I.F.)
2. Department of Physiotherapy, University of Valencia, 46010 Valencia, Spain
3. Department of Educational and Developmental Psychology, University of Valencia, 46010 Valencia, Spain; patricia.sancho@uv.es
* Correspondence: trinidad.sentandreu@uv.es; Tel.: +34-963-864-007

Abstract: CASP-12 (Control, Autonomy, Self-realization, and Pleasure scale) is one of the most common internationally used measures for quality of life in older adults, although its structure is not clearly established. Current research aims to test the factor structure of the CASP-12, so as to provide evidence on reliability and external validity, and to test for measurement invariance across age groups. Data from 61,355 Europeans ($\geq$60 years old) from the Survey of Health, Ageing and Retirement in Europe wave 7 were used. CASP-12, EURO-D (European depression scale), self-perceived health, and life satisfaction measurements were included. Reliability and validity coefficients, competing confirmatory factor models, and standard measurement invariance routine were estimated. A second-order factor model with the original factor structure was retained. The scale showed adequate reliability coefficients except for the autonomy dimension. The correlation coefficients for external validity were all statistically significant. Finally, CASP-12 is scalar invariant across age. We conclude that the best-fitting factor structure retained allows using CASP-12 either by factors, or as an overall score, depending on the research interests. Findings related to CASP-12 measurement invariance encourage its use in the oldest-old too. When comparing the dimensions across age groups, as people age, autonomy slightly increases and the rest of the dimensions decline.

Keywords: quality of life; older adults; oldest-old; measurement invariance; SHARE European Survey

1. Introduction

Quality of life (QoL) has frequently been operationalized as an economic or health-related indicator, but this narrow measurement has been criticized [1]. What these authors argue, following several sociological authors (Anthony Giddens, Ulrich Beck, and Zygmunt Bauman), is that in current societies, at least in the so-called advanced ones, QoL is no longer determined by economic survival and/or health problems and diseases. These authors argue that 'the contemporary phase of modernity (or postmodernity) is one where the personal is central and the construction of identity the ever-present task for everybody' (p. 240) [1]. This person-centered and subjective approach is not new and was also held by the World Health Organization's Quality of Life assessment group, which stated a widely accepted approach of QoL: 'QoL assesses individuals' perception of their position in life in the context of the culture and value systems in which they live and in relation to their goals, expectations, standards and concerns' (p. 1403) [2].

That said, regarding QoL in the general population is even more obvious for the older population. Older adults' QoL is of paramount interest for gerontologists, but it lacks a sufficiently agreed-upon definition, as well as theoretically grounded models for its measurement [3]. Due to the lack of theoretically grounded measures of QoL, indicators of health status have been used as proxies [4]. This has given rise to many instruments used in clinical and medical settings acknowledged as 'health-related QoL' [3]. Indeed, there are many authors who claim that the main problem for measuring QoL in old age is that it remains undertheorized and poorly defined [5–7].

One attempt to overcome this state of affairs was the development of the Control Autonomy, Self-realization and Pleasure-19 (CASP-19) scale [3]. This scale is theoretically driven by the 'needs satisfaction' approach to measure QoL in early old age. It is based on Maslow's Hierarchy of Needs [8]. This model includes four dimensions: Control Autonomy, Self-realization and Pleasure. Following Wiggins et al. [9], Control and Autonomy are previous conditions to feel able to participate in society, while the extent to which these feelings can be realized is shown in the self-realization and pleasure dimensions. The dimension of pleasure is also extremely aligned with the theories on subjective well-being [10]. The CASP-19 is composed of 19 items tapping these four theoretical dimensions with four response categories. This version of the scale has been used in many local, regional, national and international studies [9,11]: the English Longitudinal Study of Ageing (ELSA); the British Household Panel Survey (BHPS); the Boyd-Orr survey; the Health, Alcohol and Psychosocial factors in Eastern Europe (HAPIEE) Study; the American Health and Retirement Survey; the Korean longitudinal Study of Ageing (KLoSA); the Irish Longitudinal Study of Ageing; the GAZEL Study; and the CONSTANCE study among others.

Wiggins et al. [9] were the first ones to assess the factor structure and other psychometric properties of the CASP-19. The theoretical four-factor structure, either with a second-order factor or only first-order factors, did not achieve a good model fit, and a shortened 12-item version was proposed. These authors additionally proposed collapsing control and autonomy into a single factor. Since then, several studies have analyzed the psychometric properties of the CASP-19. Results of these validations suggest that the four-factor structure (either with or without a second-order factor) is compromised, while solutions collapsing control and autonomy, and self-realization and pleasure obtained better fit, while results also showed reliability of autonomy to be deficient [12–15]. Most of these studies included the shortened 12-item version and concluded that its psychometric characteristics were better [9,15].

Indeed, the version employed across the different waves of the Survey of Health Ageing and Retirement in Europe (SHARE) is that composed of 12 items. This version of the instrument, the CASP-12, has also been validated in several studies. For example, Borrat-Besson et al. [16] analyzed all countries in SHARE Wave 4 and found that the theoretical four-factor structure of the CASP did not fit the data well. Instead, they proposed a two-factor structure (control/autonomy and self-realization/pleasure) and a further reduction to 10 items. Along the same lines, a study by Towers et al. [17] also found ill fit for the four theoretical domains and performed an Exploratory Factor Analysis (EFA) that found a three-dimensional structure: control, independence and global QoL, additionally deleting another item. Kerry [18], employing Item Response Theory (IRT) models, found a bifactor model with a strong global factor of QoL to better represent CASP-12 scores, with data from SHARE Wave 6.

Nevertheless, other studies have found good fit for the four-factor theoretical structure in the CASP-12. For example, Hamren et al. [19] found a good fit for the four-factor structure and good reliability in older Ethiopians, although they had to delete one item. Pérez-Rojo et al. [11] tested several Confirmatory Factor Analysis (CFA) models in Spanish dwelling older adults (one, three and four first-order factors and a second-order factor model including four first-order factors). The best-fitting model had four first-order factors but two items of autonomy had low loadings, and reliability of the autonomy dimension was poor. Finally, Rodríguez-Blázquez et al. [20] used Portuguese participants in the sixth wave of SHARE to test for the four-factor structure in CASP-12 scale and found good fit again with low reliability estimates of the autonomy and pleasure dimensions.

In sum, setting the factor structure of a scale is critical in order to study its psychometric properties, and this structure has not been clearly established for the CASP-12. Since this scale is being widely used in a good number of international studies, the aim of this study is threefold: (a) to test the factor structure of the CASP-12 in the data from SHARE Wave 7; (b) to establish reliability and external validity of the dimensions found; and (c) to test for measurement invariance of three age groups (60–75 years old, 76–85 years old, and 86+ years old) since the original CASP scale was designed for 'early' older adults and not for the oldest-old.

2. Methods

2.1. Sample and Procedure

This study was carried out using data from the SHARE wave 7 [21,22]. SHARE is a longitudinal study focused on the study of European populations aged 50 and older. Data were gathered using probability-based sampling, further details of which can be found in Bergmann et al. [23].

The data included a total of 61,355 Europeans aged 60 years old or older from the 7th wave of SHARE (including Israel). Of the sample, 55.9% was female and the remaining 44.1% was male. The mean age was 71.87 years (Standard Deviation, SD = 8.23). Most were either living with their spouse (67.2%) or had become widowed (18.6%), while the rest had registered partnership (1.1%), lived separated from their spouse (1.1%), had never married (4.5%), or were divorced (7.4%). Mean years of education was 10.68 (SD = 4.28).

2.2. Instruments

The CASP-12 scale is a modification of the original CASP-19 [3]. The scale was designed to tap four dimensions of QoL: control, autonomy, self-realization, and pleasure. Answers are given in a Likert scale with four points, from 'never' to 'often'. Higher scores indicate a higher position on each dimension.

The European depression scale (EURO-D) [24] summarizes depression symptoms from various instruments on late-life depression used in different European countries. The scale comprises 12 items with dichotomously coded responses (absence vs. presence): depressed mood, pessimism, suicidal tendencies, guilt, sleep problems, loss of interest, irritability, loss of appetite, fatigue, concentration problems, enjoyment, and tearfulness. A scale score of 4 or higher could be considered as 'case of depression' and a scale score below 4 as 'not depressed' [25].

The self-perceived health measure rates present general health on a 5-point Likert scale between 'excellent' and 'poor'. It is based on the 36-item Short-Form Health Survey (SF-36) [26] and uses the question 'Would you say your health is ... ?'

Life satisfaction was measured with a single indicator asking about the respondents' degree of satisfaction with their life, ranging from 1 (least satisfied) to 10 (most satisfied).

2.3. Statistical Analyses

SPSS 26 was used for calculating descriptive statistics of the variables under study, Cronbach's alpha coefficients, corrected item-total correlations, and correlations among the dimensions in the CASP-12 and external criteria. Additionally, an R function [27] was used for alpha coefficients confidence intervals. The factor structure was tested using a series of competing Confirmatory Factor Analyses (CFA), estimated with Weighted Least Squares Mean and Variance corrected (WLSMV) in Mplus 8.4 [28]. This method of estimation was selected because the variables are ordinal and not multivariate normal [29,30]. Model fit was assessed with the most widely employed fit indexes. Specifically, we used the chi-square statistic; the Comparative Fit Index (CFI); the Root Mean Square Error of Approximation (RMSEA), with a 90% Confidence Interval (CI); and the Standardized Root Mean Square Residual (SRMR). The adopted criteria for accepting a model were those in Hu and Bentler [31] and Marsh et al. [32]: a CFI of at least 0.90, together with a RMSEA and SRMR less than 0.08, indicate adequate fit, while a CFI of at least 0.95 and RMSEA and SRMR below 0.08 indicate excellent fit. The Composite Reliability Index (CRI) for each of the scale's dimensions was calculated using standardized factor loadings in the best-fitting CFA.

Finally, a standard measurement invariance routine was estimated including the testing of three CFAs: configural invariance model, weak or metric invariance model, and strong or scalar invariance model [33]. The configural model estimates the four-factor model in the three age groups at the same time, with separate estimates for each group. The fit indexes of this configural model are used as the baseline fit. The metric or weak invariance model sets factor loadings to be equal across groups. The scalar or strong invariance model further constraints items' thresholds in the intercepts to equality. The models in this sequence are nested, and therefore they may be compared with chi-square differences (in the case of WLSMV estimation, the DIFFTEST). Non-significant chi-square differences suggest multi-group equivalence or invariance. However, this test is extremely powerful in detecting trivial differences, especially with relatively large samples [34,35]. Therefore, a modeling approach has been advocated which employs CFI differences <0.01 as cut-off criteria to accept the more parsimonious model [34]. If a more parsimonious model evinces adequate levels of practical fit, then the imposed constraints are considered a reasonable approximation for modeling the data, and invariance at that level is declared.

3. Results

3.1. Factor Structure

Several competing CFAs were estimated. These competing models come from the structures that were supported in previous validations of the CASP-12. Specifically, the CFAs tested were:

(1) One-factor model, found in Kerry [18].
(2) Two-factor model (control/autonomy and self-realization/pleasure), supported, for example, by Borrat-Besson et al. [16].
(3) Three-factor model (control/autonomy, self-realization, and pleasure), found, for example, in Stoner et al. [15].
(4) Four-factor model (control, autonomy, self-realization, and pleasure), theoretically proposed during the scale development.
(5) Four-factor model with a second-order factor (QoL), also based on the theory underlying the scale development.

The goodness-of-fit indexes for all tested models are presented in Table 1. The best-fitting model is that originally thought for the scale. That is, the four correlated factors model. Nevertheless, the fit of the second-order factor model is also very good, and extremely similar to the fit of the four correlated factors model. Given that the second-order model is more parsimonious and opens the possibility of using the scale with the dimensions or as a general factor, depending on research interests, this second-order model will be retained.

Table 1. Goodness-of-fit indexes for the five CFAs and the measurement invariance routine.

Model	χ^2	df	p	RMSEA	90%CI	CFI	SRMR	$\Delta\chi^2$	df	p	ΔCFI
One-factor model	48,906.4	54	<0.001	0.123	0.123–0.124	0.903	0.062	-	-	-	-
Two-factor model	28,867.4	53	<0.001	0.096	0.095–0.097	0.943	0.048	-	-	-	-
Three-factor model	21,564.1	51	<0.001	0.084	0.083–0.085	0.957	0.044	-	-	-	-
Four-factor model	16,443.1	48	<0.001	0.076	0.075–0.077	0.968	0.038	-	-	-	-
Second-order model	19,963.1	50	<0.001	0.082	0.081–0.083	0.961	0.043	-	-	-	-

Table 1. Cont.

Model	χ^2	df	p	RMSEA	90%CI	CFI	SRMR	$\Delta\chi^2$	df	p	ΔCFI
Measurement invariance											
Configural	14,656.3	144	<0.001	0.071	0.070–0.072	0.969	0.037	-	-	-	-
Metric	13,461.7	160	<0.001	0.065	0.064–0.066	0.972	0.038	887.2	16	<0.001	0.003
Scalar	19,973.2	200	<0.001	0.071	0.070–0.072	0.958	0.041	7233.4	40	<0.001	0.014
Modified scalar	17,266.5	198	<0.001	0.066	0.065–0.067	0.964	0.040	4607.9	38	<0.001	0.008

Note. CFA = Confirmatory Factor Analyses; χ^2 = chi-square statistic; df = degrees of freedom; p = probability; RMSEA = Root Mean Square Error of Approximation; 90%CI = 90% Confidence Interval; CFI = Comparative Fit Index; SRMR = Standardized Root Mean Square Residual; $\Delta\chi^2$ = differences in chi-square; ΔCFI = differences in Comparative Fit Indexes.

Standardized parameter estimates are presented in Figure 1. Although all the factor loadings, both in the first-order factors and the second-order factor, were statistically significant ($p < 0.01$), the second item in the autonomy dimension had a relatively low factor loading in this dimension. This item has repeatedly been found to be problematic in the literature. Its content is 'Family responsibilities prevent me from doing what I want to do'.

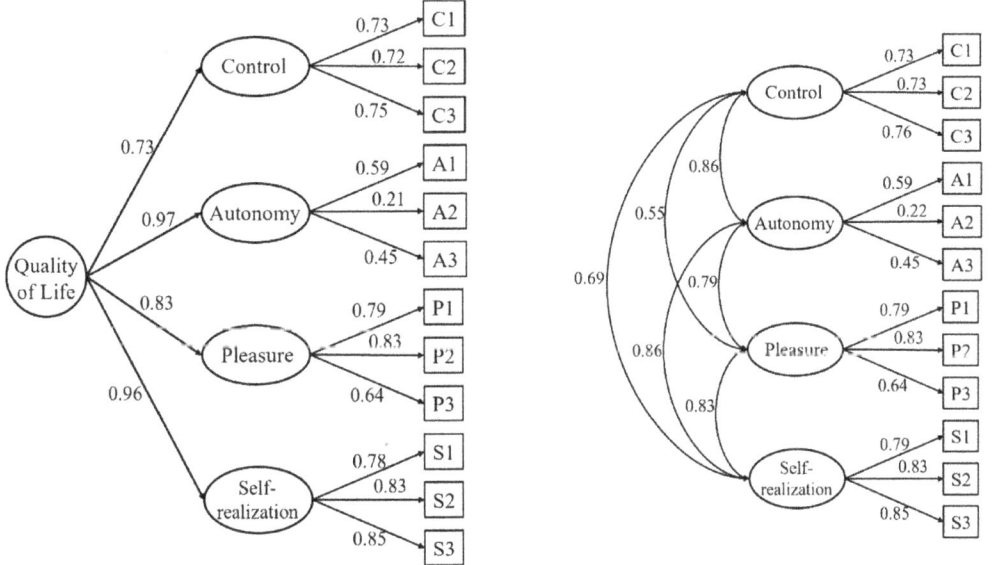

Figure 1. Standardized factor loadings for the retained model. Note: all estimates $p < 0.01$.

3.2. Internal Consistency

For the overall scale and the four first-order factors, both the alpha coefficient and the CRI were estimated. The alpha for the global measure of QoL was 0.833 (95% CI (0.831–0.834)), and the CRI was also very high (CRI = 0.932). Regarding the reliabilities of the four dimensions, all of them were adequate except the estimates of autonomy. In the case of control, the alpha was 0.709 (95% CI (0.705–0.712)) with a CRI = 0.784. Self-realization had an alpha of 0.816 (95% CI (0.813–0.818)) and a CRI of 0.865. Pleasure's estimates of reliability were adequate: alpha = 0.695 (95% CI (0.691–0.698)), and CRI = 0.801. The two estimates of reliability, alpha and CRI, were inadequate for the autonomy dimension: alpha = 0.351 (95% CI (0.342–0.359)), and CRI = 0.394.

Table 2 presents basic descriptive statistics for the 12 items in the scale, means and standard deviations. It also shows the corrected item-total correlations.

Table 2. Means, standard deviations (SD), and corrected item-total correlations (r_{it}) for the 12 items in the CASP measure (Control, Autonomy, Self-realization and Pleasure).

Item	Mean	SD	r_{it}
Control 1	2.53	1.04	0.48
Control 2	2.79	0.99	0.58
Control 3	3.14	0.95	0.52
Autonomy 1	3.18	0.89	0.13
Autonomy 2	3.09	0.96	0.20
Autonomy 3	2.61	1.10	0.28
Pleasure 1	3.47	0.77	0.29
Pleasure 2	3.47	0.79	0.32
Pleasure 3	3.37	0.76	0.20
Self-realization 1	3.06	0.87	0.39
Self-realization 2	3.03	0.89	0.48
Self-realization 3	2.98	0.91	0.48

3.3. External Validity

The correlation coefficients are displayed in Table 3, with all being statistically significant ($p < 0.001$). As a global score for QoL, CASP-12 is positively and similarly highly related to satisfaction with life and self-perceived health, and negatively correlated with depression. The highest positive association with CASP-12 dimensions is found with life satisfaction. As expected, all CASP dimensions negatively correlate with depression, as measured by EURO-D, with the pleasure dimension (-0.498, $p < 0.001$) being the one with the strongest association.

Table 3. Correlations among CASP dimensions, CASP-12 and criteria (all statistically significant $p < 0.001$).

	(1)	(2)	(3)	(4)	(5)	(6)	(7)
(1) Control	1						
(2) Autonomy	0.442	1					
(3) Self-realization	0.365	0.334	1				
(4) Pleasure	0.528	0.391	0.609	1			
(5) CASP-12	0.789	0.694	0.732	0.836	1		
(6) Life satisfaction	0.406	0.366	0.472	0.510	0.573	1	
(7) Depression	−0.442	−0.257	−0.422	−0.498	−0.524	−0.416	1
(8) Self-perceived health	0.405	0.233	0.304	0.494	0.479	0.361	−0.439

3.4. Measurement Invariance

Given that the original scale (CASP-19) was developed to be used in early old age, and first validated for older adults in the age range of 65 to 75 years, we consider it important to test for measurement invariance outside this age range. Therefore, a measurement invariance routine across age groups was tested. Age was divided into three groups: 60–75, or early old adults; 76–85, or old adults; and 86+, or oldest-old.

Goodness-of-fit indexes and chi-square differences for the invariance routine are shown in Table 1. DIFFTESTS (chi-square differences) were all statistically significant, but as already mentioned, due to the power of this test, that was expected. Therefore, CFI differences will be used to establish invariance. The configural model fitted the data well and established the baseline fit. When factor loadings were constrained to be equal across groups (metric invariance), model fit improved, and therefore the CASP-12 could be considered to be metric invariant. Furthermore, when all thresholds were fixed to be equal across groups (scalar invariance), fit slightly worsened (CFI difference = 0.014).

Attending to Modification Indexes, one constraint, threshold for item 4, was released, and a modified scalar-invariant model was tested. This model again reached very good fit with no statistically significant differences. Therefore, except for item 4's threshold, the CASP-12 can also be considered scalar invariant.

Once scalar invariance was established, latent mean differences could be calculated. Table 4 offers these latent differences, their statistical significance, and Cohen's d as an estimator of the effect size. The reference group is the age group 60–75. As can be seen in Table 4, all differences between the reference group and group 2 (76–85) and group 3 (86+) were statistically significant, with effect sizes being small to moderate. The pattern of differences is clear. As people age, control, self-realization and pleasure decline, while autonomy slightly increases.

Table 4. Latent mean differences and effect size estimators.

Factor	Group 2 vs. 1			Group 3 vs. 1		
	$\overline{X}$ Difference	p	Cohen's d	$\overline{X}$ Difference	p	Cohen's d
Control	−0.514	<0.001	0.471	−0.950	<0.001	0.811
Autonomy	0.196	<0.001	0.234	0.668	<0.001	0.655
Self-realization	−0.628	<0.001	0.498	−1.111	<0.001	0.478
Pleasure	−0.365	<0.001	0.290	−0.598	<0.001	0.857

4. Discussion

It is nowadays accepted that measuring the extent to which needs are fulfilled provides a measure of QoL richer than an overall personal assessment (such as life satisfaction), allowing for comparisons between people's different QoL scores [1]. Once the indubitable interest of approaching QoL's measurement from a contemporary, more sociological, perspective is established, a measure such as the CASP-12 produces more interest. This measure includes eudaimonic and hedonic components, and it has been widely used in international studies [9,11]. In particular, it has been selected as the measure of QoL for protocols in different international longitudinal surveys, and the evidence on its psychometric properties points out that it outperforms the CASP-19 [9,15].

Despite its extended use and its clear four-dimension conceptualization, its factor structure has been controversial since the beginning; different studies in different populations have found different structures [16 18]. Therefore, analyzing the large and new database of the SHARE longitudinal study may aid in shedding light onto the factor structure of the CASP-12, at least in older populations.

For the sake of completeness, all factor structures with empirical (and/or theoretical) support in the literature have been tested: one-factor model [18]; two-factor model based on control/autonomy and self-realization/pleasure [16]; three-factor model with control/autonomy, self-realization, and pleasure [15]; four-factor model (control, autonomy, self-realization, and pleasure) as theoretically proposed during the scale development; and finally a four-factor model with a second-order factor (QoL). According to the underlying theory, control and autonomy are two domains that constitute prerequisites for being able to participate in society, and the extent to which these feelings of freedom are fulfilled is captured by the self-realization and pleasure dimensions [9].

Regarding the best-fitting factor structure, a second-order solution with four subscales was retained. On the one hand, the studies by Stoner et al. [15] and Wiggins et al. [9] both found this solution to better represent the data, even when compared to the 19-item version. On the other hand, among those studies contemplating the 12-item version only, a variety of solutions have been suggested: one-factor model of QoL [18], two-factor model of control/autonomy and self-realization/pleasure [16], three-factor model of control independence and global QoL [17], and four-factor model of control, autonomy, self-realization and pleasure [11,19,20]. However, work by Borrat-Besson et al. [16] and

Towers et al. [17] recommended deletion of two and one items, respectively. This was also the case for Hamren et al. [19]. For their part, Pérez-Rojo et al.'s [11] results suggested that both four first- and second-order factor solutions fitted the data well. Nevertheless, in these models, item 5 and item 6 presented low factor loadings: 0.35 and 0.35 in the autonomy dimension of both models. Rodríguez-Blázquez et al. [20] also found diminished factor loadings of items 5 (0.25) and 6 (0.31) in the autonomy dimension. Our study found a similar low loading of item 5 (referred to as A2 in Figure 1, 0.22) and a moderate factor loading of item 6 (referred to as A3 in Figure 1, 0.45).

Reliability for the CASP-12 in this research was adequate for the overall scale as well as for control, self-realization and pleasure, but the autonomy dimension's alpha and CRI were quite low. These results are similar to other studies. For the overall CASP-12, reliability measured by alpha was 0.83, ranging from 0.35 (autonomy) to 0.82 (self-realization) for the domains, very similar to Rodríguez-Blázquez et al. [20], who reported values for overall CASP-12 of 0.78 with values between 0.37 (autonomy) and 0.73 (self-realization) for the dimensions. This same pattern of findings was found by Pérez-Rojo et al. [11], with an alpha value of 0.86 for the overall scale, and alpha estimates between 0.39 and 0.82 for the four dimensions. Across all revised studies, the reliability of the autonomy domain was the weakest one [9,16,36]. The autonomy domain refers to self-determination and the absence of unwanted interference from others. It is an inner endorsement of one's actions, the sense that they emanate from oneself and are one's own [37]. In our study (and others), problems of reliability within this dimension came from its first item ('I can do the things that I want to do').

Given that the CASP was originally designed for 'early' older adults, the age of the samples could contribute to the differences in factor structure obtained so far. Previous research carried out with the CASP-12 SHARE version has included people aged 50 and older and sometimes included a small proportion of people below 50 years old [16]. Therefore, a relevant contribution of this work is the formal test of measurement invariance across age groups (60–75 years old, 76–85 years old, and 86+ years old). Results showed that CASP-12 could be considered scalar invariant only with the exception of one threshold for item 4 ('I can do the things that you want to do'). Baltes and Smith [38] pointed out the important distinction between the third and fourth ages, the latter being what is commonly referred to as the 'oldest-old'. This age bracket is gaining more and more attention, which should come as no surprise, given that it is growing at a proportionately higher rate than the younger brackets. In fact, the proportion of people aged 80 or over based on United Nations Population Division [39] is growing twice as quickly as the 60 and older bracket.

Generally speaking, population studies in developed countries show that measures of wellbeing (such as life satisfaction) remain steady throughout life [38], perhaps with minor fluctuations [40]. However, the 'oldest-old' (people over the age of 80) do seem to notice a pronounced decline in life satisfaction [41–43]. Anyway, many studies with old people have found a slight drop in life satisfaction with age [44,45].

Previous CASP-12 validation studies used samples with a wide range of age [17,18,20] not paying attention to potential age group differences, both in structure and mean levels. Regarding factor structure, this research points out that the scale is psychometrically sound across ages. Regarding mean differences, we found evidence that QoL decreases over time, and this decrease is greater in the oldest-old [46–48]. In a longitudinal study using CASP-12 and latent growth models, Ward et al. [49] found that QoL decreased non-linearly with age. However, this was not true for autonomy. We have no clear explanation for this result, but we may anticipate some tentative reasons. First, this is the dimension with the lowest reliability. Second, two items of autonomy are very specific about why autonomy is lacking: because of family responsibilities and/or shortage of money. These difficulties for autonomy may be present at different times in life, but less present in very old age.

When compared to previous evidence on external validity, the correlations between the CASP-12 and the EURO-D (depression) supported previous research on the negative relation between QoL and depression [50,51]. Additionally, Portellano-Ortiz et al. [52], using data from SHARE Wave 5, found moderate or strong relations with depression ($r = -0.59$) in all European countries, and, albeit using an indicator of physical rather than self-perceived health (very good, good, fair, poor), similar results were found for the association between QoL and health (0.51 vs. 0.48). Similarly, CASP-12 total scores from the Portuguese sample of the 6th wave of SHARE correlated -0.57 with depression, 0.52 with life satisfaction and similar correlation (0.47) with self-perceived health [20]. For the domains, while in the 6th wave in Portugal, the pleasure factor showed the lowest correlation with the external variables; the current research using wave 7 and including all Europeans showed the autonomy dimension to have the lowest one. These differences could be affected by the exceptionally low reliability found in Portugal for the pleasure dimension ($\alpha = 0.34$) in wave 6 [14].

All in all, this study provides evidence of CASP-12's construct validity for data coming from the 7th wave of SHARE, while also acknowledging some issues related to the autonomy dimension, such as low factor loadings which simultaneously lead to diminished estimated reliability. This study also fills the gap in the literature regarding CASP-12's adequacy for use in oldest-old adults, given that it was initially designed for 'early'" older adults. Future research should aim to study the scale's psychometric characteristics across regions, as QoL may be culture-dependent.

Author Contributions: Conceptualization, A.O. and J.M.T.; methodology, A.O., J.M.T. and P.S.; formal analysis, A.O. and J.M.T.; investigation, A.O., T.S.-M., J.M.T., I.F. and P.S.; resources, A.O. and I.F.; writing—original draft preparation, A.O. and J.M.T.; writing—review and editing, T.S.-M.; I.F. and P.S., project administration, A.O. and J.M.T.; funding acquisition, A.O. and J.M.T. All authors have read and agreed to the published version of the manuscript.

Funding: This work is part of the project RTI2018-093321-B-100 funded by FEDER/Ministerio de Ciencia e Innovación—Agencia Estatal de Investigación, Spain.

Institutional Review Board Statement: The Ethical Approval for gathering of the data used in this study was obtained by the SHARE project and it can be publicly consulted at: http://www.share-project.org/fileadmin/pdf_documentation/MPG_Ethics_Council_SHARE_overall_approval_29.05.2020__en_.pdf. Accessed on 23 May 2021.

Informed Consent Statement: Not applicable.

Data Availability Statement: The SHARE data are distributed by SHARE-ERIC (Survey of Health, Ageing and Retirement in Europe—European Research Infrastructure Consortium) to registered users through the SHARE Research Data Center. The SHARE Research Data Center (FDZ-SHARE) complies with the Criteria of the German Council for Social and Economic Data for providing access to microdata. Börsch-Supan, A. (2020). Survey of Health, Ageing and Retirement in Europe (SHARE) Wave 7. Release version: 7.1.1. SHARE-ERIC. Data set. DOI: 10.6103/SHARE.w7.711.

Acknowledgments: Irene Fernández was awarded a predoctoral contract within the program 'Grants for pre-doctoral contracts for doctors' training 2019' from the Ministry of Science and Innovation (PRE2019-089021). The SHARE data collection was primarily funded by the European Commission through FP5 (QLK6-CT-2001-00360), FP6 (SHARE-I3: RII-CT-2006-062193, COMPARE: CIT5-CT-2005-028857, SHARELIFE: CIT4-CT-2006-028812) and FP7 (SHARE-PREP: N211909, SHARE-LEAP: N227822, SHARE M4: N261982). Additional funding from the German Ministry of Education and Research, the Max Planck Society for the Advancement of Science, the U.S. National Institute on Aging (U01_AG09740-13S2, P01_AG005842, P01_AG08291, P30_AG12815, R21_AG025169, Y1-AG-4553-01, IAG_BSR06-11, OGHA_04-064, HHSN271201300071C) and from various national funding sources is gratefully acknowledged (see www.share-project.org, accessed on 23 May 2021).

Conflicts of Interest: The authors declare no conflict of interest.

References

1. Higgs, P.; Hyde, M.; Wiggins, R.; Blane, D. Researching quality of life in early old age: The importance of the sociological dimension. *Soc. Policy Adm.* **2003**, *37*, 239–252. [CrossRef]
2. WHOQOL Group. The World Health Organization quality of life assessment (WHOQOL): Position paper from the World Health Organization. *Soc. Sci. Med.* **1995**, *41*, 1403–1409. [CrossRef]

3. Hyde, M.; Wiggins, R.D.; Higgs, P.; Blane, D.B. A measure of quality of life in early old age: The theory, development and properties of a needs satisfaction model (CASP-19). *Aging Ment. Health* **2003**, *7*, 186–194. [CrossRef]
4. Bowling, A. *Measuring Health. A Review of Quality of Life Measurement Scales*, 2nd ed.; Open University Press: Milton Keynes, UK, 1997.
5. De Leval, N. Quality of life and depression: Symmetry concepts? *Qual. Life Res.* **1999**, *8*, 283–291. [CrossRef] [PubMed]
6. Mozes, B.; Maor, Y.; Shnueli, A. Do we know what global ratings of health related quality of life measure? *Qual. Life Res.* **1999**, *8*, 269–273. [CrossRef] [PubMed]
7. Smith, A.E. Quality of life: A review. *Educ. Ageing* **2000**, *15*, 419–435.
8. Maslow, A.H. *Toward a Psychology of Being*, 2nd ed.; Van Nostrand Reinhold: New York, NY, USA, 1968.
9. Wiggins, R.D.; Netuveli, G.; Hyde, M.; Higgs, P.; Blane, D. The evaluation of a self-enumerated scale of quality of life (CASP-19) in the context of research on ageing: A combination of exploratory and confirmatory. *Soc. Indic. Res.* **2008**, *89*, 61–77. [CrossRef]
10. Eid, M.; Diener, E. Global judgements of subjective well-being: Situational variability and long term stability. *Soc. Indic. Res.* **2004**, *65*, 245–277. [CrossRef]
11. Pérez-Rojo, G.; Martín, N.; Noriega, C.; López, J. Psychometric properties of the CASP-12 in a Spanish older community dwelling sample. *Aging Ment. Health* **2018**, *22*, 700–708. [CrossRef]
12. Heravi-Karimooi, M.; Rejeh, N.; Garshasbi, A.; Montazeri, A.; Bandari, R. Psychometric properties of the Persian version of the quality of life in early old age (CASP-19). *Iran. J. Psychiatry Behav. Sci.* **2018**, *12*, e8378. [CrossRef]
13. Kim, G.R.; Netuveli, G.; Blane, D.; Peasy, A.; Malyutina, S.; Simonova, G.; Kubinova, R.; Pajak, A.; Croezen, S.; Bobak, M.; et al. Psychometric properties and confirmatory factor analysis of the CASP-19, a measure of quality of life in early old age: The HAPIEE study. *Aging Ment. Health* **2015**, *19*, 595–609. [CrossRef] [PubMed]
14. Neri, A.L.; Borin, F.S.A.; Batistoni, A.A.T.; Cachioni, M.; Rabelo, D.F.; Fontes, A.P.; Yassuda, M.S. New semantic-cultural validation and psychometric study of the CASP-19 scale in adult and elderly Brazilians. *Cad. Saude Publica* **2018**, *34*, e00181417. [CrossRef] [PubMed]
15. Stoner, C.R.; Orrell, M.; Spector, A. The psychometric properties of the Control, Autonomy, Self-realisation and Pleasure Scale (CASP-19) for older adults with dementia. *Aging Ment. Health* **2019**, *23*, 643–649. [CrossRef] [PubMed]
16. Borrat-Besson, C.; Ryser, V.A.; Gonçalves, J. *An Evaluation of the CASP-12 Scale Used in the Survey of Ageing and Retirement in Europe (SHARE) to Measure Quality of Life Among People Aged 50+*; FORS Working Paper Series: Paper 2015–4; FORS: Lausanne, Switzerland, 2015.
17. Towers, A.; Yeung, P.; Stevenson, B.; Stephens, C.; Alpass, F. Quality of life in indigenous and non-indigenous older adults: Assessing the CASP-12 factor structure and identifying a brief CASP-3. *Qual. Life Res.* **2015**, *24*, 193–203. [CrossRef]
18. Kerry, M.J. Bifactor model of the CASP-12's general factor for measuring quality of life in older patients. *J. Patient Rep. Outcomes* **2018**, *2*, 1–57. [CrossRef]
19. Hamren, K.; Chungkham, H.S.; Hyde, M. Religion, spirituality, social support and quality of life: Measurement and predictors CASP-12(v2) amongst other Ethiopians living in Addis Ababa. *Aging Ment. Health* **2015**, *19*, 610–621. [CrossRef]
20. Rodríguez-Blázquez, C.; Ribeiro, O.; Ayala, A.; Teixeira, L.; Araujo, L.; Forjaz, M.J. Psychometric properties of the CASP-12 scale in Portugal: An analysis using SHARE data. *Int. J. Environ. Res. Public Health* **2020**, *17*, 6610. [CrossRef]
21. Börsch-Supan, A. *Survey of Health, Ageing and Retirement in Europe (SHARE). Wave 7*, Release version 7.1.1; SHARE-ERIC: Munich, Germany, 2020. [CrossRef]
22. Börsch-Supan, A.; Brandt, M.; Hunkler, C.; Kneip, T.; Korbmacher, J.; Malter, F.; Schaan, B.; Stuck, S.; Zuber, S.; SHARE Central Coordination Team. Data Resource Profile: The Survey of Health, Ageing and Retirement in Europe (SHARE). *Int. J. Epidemiol.* **2013**, *42*, 992–1001. [CrossRef]
23. Bergmann, M.; Scherpenzeel, A.; Börsch-Supan, A. (Eds.) *SHARE Wave 7 Methodology: Panel Innovations and Life Histories*; MEA, Max Planck Institute for Social Law and Social Policy: Munich, Germany, 2019.
24. Prince, M.J.; Reischies, F.; Beekman, A.T.F.; Fuhrer, R.; Jonker, C.; Kivela, S.L.; Lawlor, B.A.; Lobo, A.; Magnusson, H.; Fichter, M.; et al. Development of the EURO-D scale—A European Union initiative to compare symptoms of depression in 14 European centres. *Br. J. Psychiatry* **1999**, *174*, 330–338. [CrossRef]
25. Mehrbrodt, T.; Gruber, S.; Wagner, M. *Scales and Multi-Item Indicators*; Center for the Economics of Aging (MEA): Munich, Germany, 2019.
26. Ware, J.E.; Gandek, B. Overview of the SF-36 health survey and the international quality of life assessment (IQOLA) project. *J. Clin. Epidemiol.* **1998**, *51*, 903–912. [CrossRef]
27. Diedenhofen, B.; Musch, S. Cocron: A web interface and R package for the statistical comparison of Cronbach's alpha coefficients. *Int. J. Internet Sci.* **2016**, *11*, 51–60.
28. Muthén, L.K.; Muthén, B.O. *Mplus User's Guide*, 8th ed.; Muthén & Muthén: Los Angeles, CA, USA, 2017.
29. Finney, S.J.; DiStefano, C. Nonnormal and categorical data in structural equation modeling. In *Structural Equation Modeling: A Second Course*; Hancock, G.R., Mueller, R.O., Eds.; IAP Information Age Publishing: Charlotte, NC, USA, 2013; pp. 439–492.
30. Li, C.H. Confirmatory factor analysis with ordinal data: Comparing robust maximum likelihood and diagonally weighted least squares. *Behav. Res. Methods* **2016**, *48*, 936–949. [CrossRef] [PubMed]
31. Hu, L.T.; Bentler, P.M. Cutoff criteria for fit indexes in covariance structure analysis: Conventional criteria versus new alternatives. *Struct. Equ. Model.* **1999**, *6*, 1–55. [CrossRef]

32. Marsh, H.W.; Hau, K.T.; Wen, Z. In search of golden rules: Comment on hypothesis-testing approaches to setting cutoff values for fit indexes and dangers in overgeneralizing Hu and Bentler's (1999) findings. *Struct Equ. Model.* **2004**, *11*, 320–341. [CrossRef]
33. Van de Schoot, R.; Lugtig, P.; Hox, J. A checklist for testing measurement invariance. *Eur. J. Dev. Psychol.* **2012**, *9*, 486–492. [CrossRef]
34. Cheung, G.W.; Rensvold, R.B. Evaluating goodness-of-fit indexes for testing measurement invariance. *Struct Equ. Model.* **2002**, *9*, 233–255. [CrossRef]
35. Little, T.D. Mean and covariance structures (MACS) analyses of cross-cultural data: Practical and theoretical issues. *Multivar. Behav. Res.* **1997**, *32*, 53–76. [CrossRef]
36. Sim, J.; Bartlam, B.; Bernard, M. The CASP-19 as a measure of quality of life in old age: Evaluation of its use in a retirement community. *Qual. Life Res.* **2011**, *20*, 997–1004. [CrossRef]
37. Deci, E.L.; Ryan, R.M. The support of autonomy and the control of behavior. *J. Pers Soc. Psychol.* **1987**, *57*, 1024–1037. [CrossRef]
38. Baltes, P.B.; Smith, J. New frontiers in the future of aging: From successful aging of the young old to the dilemmas of the fourth age. *Gerontology* **2003**, *49*, 123–135. [CrossRef]
39. United Nations Population Division. *World Population Ageing 1950–2050*; United Nations, Department of Economic and Social Affairs, Population Division: New York, NY, USA, 2002.
40. Angelini, V.; Cavapozzi, D.; Corazzini, L.; Paccagnella, O. Age, health and life satisfaction among older Europeans. *Soc. Indic. Res.* **2012**, *105*, 293–308. [CrossRef] [PubMed]
41. Gutiérrez, M.; Tomás, J.M.; Sancho, P.; Galiana, L.; Francisco, E. Perception of quality of life in an elderly Angolan sample. *Rev. Psicol. Soc.* **2014**, *29*, 346–370. [CrossRef]
42. Gwozdz, W.; Sousa-Poza, A. Ageing, health and life satisfaction of the oldest old: An analysis for Germany. *Soc. Indic. Res.* **2010**, *97*, 397–417. [CrossRef]
43. Smith, J.; Borchelt, M.; Maier, H.; Jopp, D. Health and well-being in the young old and oldest old. *J. Soc. Issues* **2002**, *58*, 715–732. [CrossRef]
44. Berg, A.I.; Hoffman, L.; Hassing, L.B.; McClearn, G.E.; Johansson, B. What matters, and what matters most, for change in life satisfaction in the oldest-old? A study over 6 years among individuals 80+. *Aging Ment. Health* **2009**, *13*, 191–201. [CrossRef]
45. Enkvist, Å.; Ekström, H.; Elmståhl, S. What factors affect life satisfaction (LS) among the oldest-old? *Arch. Gerontol. Geriatr.* **2012**, *54*, 140–145. [CrossRef]
46. McCrory, C.; Leahy, S.; Mcgarrigle, C. What factors are associated with change in older people's quality of life? In *The over 50s in a Changing Ireland. Economic Circumstances, Health and Well-Being*; Nolan, A., O'Regan, C., Dooley, C., Wallace, D., Hever, A., Cronin, H., Hudson, E., Kenny, R.A., Eds.; The Irish Longitudinal Study on Ageing: Dublin, Ireland, 2014; pp. 153–186. Available online: https://tilda.tcd.ie/publications/reports/pdf/w2-key-findings-report/Wave2-Key-Findings-Report.pdf (accessed on 23 May 2021).
47. Tampubolon, G. Delineating the third age: Joint models of older people's quality of life and attrition in Britain 2002–2010. *Aging Ment. Health* **2015**, *19*, 576–583. [CrossRef]
48. Zaninotto, P.; Falaschetti, E.; Sacker, A. Age trajectories of quality of life among older adults: Results from the English longitudinal study of Ageing. *Qual. Life Res.* **2009**, *18*, 1301–1309. [CrossRef]
49. Ward, M.; McGarridge, C.A.; Kenny, R.A. More than health: Quality of life trajectories among older adults—Findings from The Irish Longitudinal Study of Ageing (TILDA). *Qual. Life Res.* **2019**, *28*, 429–439. [CrossRef]
50. Ponte, C.; Almeida, V.; Fernandes, L. Suicidal ideation, depression and quality of life in the elderly: Study in a gerontopsychiatric consultation. *Span. J. Psychol.* **2014**, *17*, E14. [CrossRef] [PubMed]
51. Unalan, D.; Gocer, S.; Basturk, M.; Baydur, H.; Ozturk, A. Coincidence of low social support and high depressive score on quality of life in elderly. *Eur. Geriatr. Med.* **2015**, *6*, 319–324. [CrossRef]
52. Portellano-Ortiz, C.; Garre-Olmo, J.; Calvó-Perxas, L.; Conde-Sala, J.L. Depression and variables associated with quality of life in people over 65 in Spain and Europe. Data from SHARE 2013. *Eur. J. Psychiatry* **2018**, *32*, 122–131. [CrossRef]

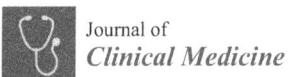

Article

Treatment of Achilles Tendinopathy in Recreational Runners with Peritendinous Hyaluronic Acid Injections: A Viscoelastometric, Functional, and Biochemical Pilot Study

Marco Gervasi [1,*], Elena Barbieri [1,2], Italo Capparucci [1], Giosuè Annibalini [1], Davide Sisti [1], Stefano Amatori [1], Vittoria Carrabs [1], Giacomo Valli [1], Sabrina Donati Zeppa [1], Marco Bruno Luigi Rocchi [1], Vilberto Stocchi [1] and Piero Sestili [1]

1. Department of Biomolecular Sciences, University Urbino Carlo Bo, via A. Saffi 2, 61029 Urbino, Italy; elena.barbieri@uniurb.it (E.B.); italo.capparucci@libero.it (I.C.); giosue.annibalini@uniurb.it (G.A.); davide.sisti@uniurb.it (D.S.); s.amatori1@campus.uniurb.it (S.A.); vittoria.carrabs@uniurb.it (V.C.); giacomo.valli@uniurb.it (G.V.); sabrina.zeppa@uniurb.it (S.D.Z.); marco.rocchi@uniurb.it (M.B.L.R.); vilberto.stocchi@uniurb.it (V.S.); piero.sestili@uniurb.it (P.S.)
2. Interuniversity Institute of Myology (IIM), 06121 Perugia, Italy
* Correspondence: marco.gervasi@uniurb.it; Tel.: +39-072-230-3013

Abstract: Background: Achilles tendinopathy (AT) affects ca. 10 million recreational runners in Europe; the practice of hyaluronic acid (HA) infiltration is being increasingly adopted. The aim of this pilot study was to monitor the effects of a three-local time-spaced injections regimen of HA in the treatment of AT in middle-aged runners combining for the first time viscoelastometric, biochemical, and functional methodologies with routine clinical examinations. Methods: Eight male runners (Age 49.3 ± 3.9), diagnosed for unilateral AT, were given three ultrasound (US) guided peritendinous HA injections at the baseline (T0) and every fifteenth day with a follow-up on the forty-fifth day (T1, T2, and T3). At all-time points patients were assessed for viscoelastic tone and stiffness, maximal voluntary isometric contraction (MVIC), and pain level (Likert scale 0–5). The peritendinous effusions of the injured tendon were collected at T0 and T2 to quantify the volume variations and the IL-1β and MMP-3 levels. Results: At T0 MVIC and pain score were significantly lower and higher, respectively, in injured tendons. The volume, IL-1β and MMP-3 levels decreased in the course of treatment and the clinical endpoints ameliorated over time. Tone, stiffness, and functional performance also varied significantly at T2 and T3, as compared to T0 Conclusions: The sequential peritendinous injections of HA were effective in the amelioration of the clinical symptoms, as well as of the functional and viscoelastic state associated with AT. The determination of the viscoelastometric state may help to precisely evaluate the healing process in AT patients.

Keywords: tendinopathy; Achilles tendon; hyaluronic acid; viscoelastic properties; isometric contraction; matrix metalloproteinase 3; interleukin-1beta

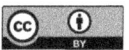

1. Introduction

Tendinopathies are degenerative musculoskeletal conditions occurring across the age spectrum. It accounts for up to 30% of general practice musculoskeletal consultations, mostly in active and sporting people [1]. Notably, overuse tendon injury is a condition where a tendon has been repeatedly strained until it is unable to withstand further loading, at which point damage occurs, and it is claimed to account for 30–50% of all sports-related injuries [2].

Achilles tendons are the most common site of injuries accounting for 6–17% of all sports-related injuries [2]. Achilles tendinopathies (AT) represent serious injuries for athletes of all levels, often causing (up to 5%) the end of a career in professional sports [3]. In runners, the Achilles tendon musculotendinous unit, consisting of the fusion of the gastrocnemius and soleus tendons, provides the primary propulsive force for locomotion. During running, the Achilles tendon load reaches six to eight times the bodyweight, a load close to the ultimate strength of the tendon [4]. Training errors, including a sudden increase in training volume and/or intensity, changing of terrain or shoe, or an excess in interval training, are the most common causes of Achilles tendon damage of runners [5].

The term "Achilles tendinitis" implies an inflammatory pathologic process within the tendon itself. There are many terms given for the same type of pathologic entity denoting inflammation of the paratenon, such as tenosynovitis, tenovaginitis, peritendinitis, or paratenonitis. Furthermore, various pathologic conditions sometimes coexist (for example, paratenonitis with tendinosis). However, in all cases, the tendinopathy is a failed healing response, with degeneration and haphazard proliferation of tenocytes, disruption of collagen fibers, and subsequent increase in the non-collagenous matrix [6]. In these processes, it has been reported that pro-inflammatory cytokines play a major role [7]. In particular, the interleukin-1 beta (IL-1β) regulates inflammatory mediators and matrix metalloproteinases (MMPs) which degrade the extracellular matrix (ECM) and contribute to the development of tendinopathy and even tendon rupture [8].

The first suspicion of AT is based on history and clinical examination of the patient [9]. Patients commonly experience morning stiffness after a period of inactivity, followed by a gradual onset of pain during activity; in severe cases, pain occurs also at rest [9]. Diagnosis can be integrated by magnetic resonance imaging (MRI) or Ultrasound imaging (USI). Nowadays, it is also possible to monitor a number of mechanical and functional parameters, which may not only integrate clinical assessments, but also add novel and valuable information on the progression of AT and the efficacy of treatments. USI has been used to evaluate the thickness and cross-sectional area (CSA) in musculoskeletal conditions including AT. In particular several studies, [10–13] demonstrated that the etiology of AT is multifactorial, showing changes in the thickness and CSA of the tendons and of intrinsic and extrinsic foot muscles. These alterations are of paramount importance, as it will be discussed, in the sports medicine management of athletes. To this regard, a novel approach based on handheld myotonometer, a non-invasive digital palpation device, has the capability to precisely determine quantitative differences in viscoelastometric parameters, specifically the transverse stiffness and tone of Achilles tendon [14]. These parameters reflect the tendon structural state, which conceivably varies as a result of AT. Indeed, it has been demonstrated that the symptomatic AT tissue is softer (more compliant) in the painful region [15]; moreover, Finnamore et al. [16] found a lower stiffness in AT as compared with the healthy tendon in recreational runners. These findings suggest that the AT pathological events impact on structural/viscoelastic properties of the tendon. Another functional parameter that can be monitored in AT is the maximum voluntary isometric contraction (MVIC) of the ankle plantar flexion; indeed, people with AT may display reduced maximal plantar flexor torque due to the tenderness and the reduced ability of the tendon to transfer forces to the joint and/or to the onset/presence of pain [17].

The standard pharmacological treatment of AT typically involves systemic nonsteroidal anti-inflammatory drugs (NSAIDs) without or with local corticosteroid injections [18], whose frequent and repeated use may however increase the risk of tendon rupture [19].

Despite very few studies on AT in humans, among the therapeutic options for tendinopathies peritendinous hyaluronic acid (HA) injection is gaining increasing importance as a reliable option for the management of this disease. Under homeostatic conditions, HA is a high molecular mass polymer that is naturally found in most of the tissues, particularly in the ECM of soft connective tissues and synovial fluids of vertebrates. HA regulates important physiological processes related to tissue integrity [20]: it possesses unique viscoelastic properties, is an ideal biological lubricant and also exerts analgesic, anti-inflammatory, and anti-adhesive effects [21]. Recently, clinical trials showed the efficacy and safety of treatment with a cycle of three low molecular weight HA peritendinous injection (one per week, 2 mL, 500–730 kDa) on pain reduction in patients affected by lateral elbow, Achilles, or patellar tendinopathy [22,23]. Another recent study, although on a different human tendinopathy setting (long head of biceps tendinopathy), also showed that high molecular weight (3000 kDa) HA treatments decrease the inflammatory marker levels in the peritendinous effusion and ameliorate tendinopathy-associated symptoms [24].

That being the case, we hypothesize that the sequential tendon infiltration of HA can reduce the inflammation and improve the clinical and functional parameters. Hence, this pilot study aimed to better evaluate the efficacy of treatment with a cycle of three peritendinous injections of 2–1000 kDa HA (one each 15-day, 2 mL, RegenFlex T&M, Regenyal Laboratories SRL, Italy) on clinical, viscoelastometric, functional, and biochemical determinations, in middle-aged recreational runners affected of unilateral AT.

2. Materials and Methods

We performed a pilot study carried out in a real-life clinical setting on recreational runners diagnosed with unilateral AT and to whom the specialist physician prescribed three local injections of HA every fifteen days with a follow-up visit to the forty-fifth day. After approval from the institutional ethical committee on 26 November 2018, the study was carried out according to the Helsinki Declaration for research with human volunteers. All patients were enrolled from 10 May 2019 to 30 June 2019 and signed an informed consent form to participate.

2.1. Participants

Eight male patients were enrolled (age 49.3 ± 3.9; weight 81.1 ± 15.0 kg; height 173.3 ± 10.3 cm; BMI 27.1 ± 5.0 kg/m^2). The inclusion criteria were an experience of at least 4 years in recreational running; pain with tendinopathic features and peritendinous effusion on US imaging before HA treatments.

The exclusion criteria were suspected tendon rupture or insertional tendinopathy, general, severe inflammatory-based illnesses (diabetes mellitus, rheumatoid arthritis, peripheral neuropathy), known sensitivity to HA, smokers, and patients with BMI $\geq$ 35. Subjects taking supplements (i.e., chondroitin sulphate or methylsulfonylmethane) or medications, including steroidal and nonsteroidal anti-inflammatory drugs per os or per infiltration in the target tendon within the last 3 months were also excluded.

Patients were allowed to walk immediately after the infiltration, but were advised to refrain from running and any other type of moderate/vigorous activity for three to four days after the first injection and at least within forty-eight hours following the second and the third injections. Moreover, any kind of physiotherapy or rehabilitation exercises were not permitted as well as the use of any type of orthosis for the entire study duration.

2.2. Experimental Design

Viscoelatometric and functional parameters were chosen to obtain qualitative and quantitative information on the progression of AT and the efficacy of treatments. All patients were given three (US) guided peritendinous injections (every fifteenth day) of HA (molecular weight, MW): a blend of 2 to 1000 KDa, 2 mL (RegenFlex T&M, Regenyal Laboratories SRL, Italy) according to the methodology described by Frizziero et al. [23]. US evaluations were performed by an experienced ecographist in the clinic center and no anesthetic or rescue drug was used after injections. The patients underwent the examinations lying prone with the foot hanging freely over the edge of the examination table to inspect the Achilles tendon. Tendinopathy with peritendinous effusion was confirmed using US imaging and a sonographic transducer. A 1.5-inch needle was visualized in the long axis of the transducer and, with US control, was advanced. Once the needle tip was seen within the peritendinous effusion, the effusion was aspirated and collected for further analysis as described in Wu et al. [24], Chiodo et al. [25], and Peters et al. [26]. HA was injected into the peritendinous area using real-time US monitoring (T0). Thirty days after the first HA injection (T2), the AT peritendinous effusion was confirmed, aspirated, and collected again for further analysis. A clinical evaluation of tendinopathy based on redness, warmth, swelling, tenderness, and crepitus during movement, peritendinous effusion was performed at any clinical visit and adverse events were assessed for safety. No adverse effect was observed. The contralateral non-painful tendon was also examined as an intra-patient comparison. Before each HA injection at the specific time points (T0, T1, T2, and T3), MVIC parameters and the level of the patient's pain were respectively assessed (Figure 1).

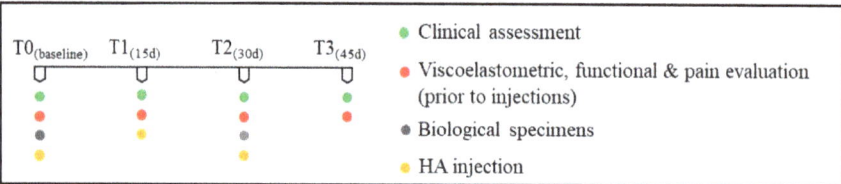

Figure 1. Experimental design.

2.3. Clinical and Functional Assessments

On the first day of visit (T0), weight and height were measured, and the body mass index was calculated; the clinical examination and magnetic resonance imaging (MRI) were performed to confirm the diagnosis or to exclude severe tendon lesions. The criteria for a diagnosis of tendinopathy were primarily based on patient history and physical examination based on Royal London Hospital Test [9]: in this test, the medical staff elicits local tenderness by palpating the tendon with the ankle in neutral position or slightly plantar flexed. The tenderness significantly decreased or became totally painless when the ankle was dorsiflexed. With the ankle in maximum dorsiflexion and in maximum plantar flexion, the portion of the tendon originally found to be tender was palpated again. Results were classified as presence or absence of tenderness on dorsiflexion. In asymptomatic tendons, the test was performed selecting an area in the tendon 3 cm proximal to its calcaneal insertion when the ankle was held in neutral as described by Maffulli et al. [9].

In order to determine the viscoelastic state of the tendon, a handheld myotonometer (MyotonPro; Myoton Ltd., Tallinn, Estonia) capable of measuring the quantitative mechanical parameters of the Achilles tendon in vivo was used. This device has good to excellent test-retest reliability and has been established in previous studies in muscles and tendons [21,22]. The assessments were carried out by an expert in the use of myotonometer technology. Participants were asked to lay prone on a couch; both injured and healthy tendon of each participant were then assayed positioning the probe of the device (3 mm in diameter) along the tendon, at 8 cm from the plantar aspect of the heel up to the proximal component of the musculotendinous junction [21]. Tendons' tone and stiffness were measured at the relaxed state. The probe of the device, preloaded at 0.18 N, applied brief (15 ms) low force (0.4 N) mechanical impulses, inducing damped natural oscillations of the underlying tendon. These oscillations were recorded by an accelerometer connected to a friction measurement mechanism in the device. The device then simultaneously calculated the resting tone [frequency of oscillation (Hz)] and stiffness (N/m) parameters. A set of 10 mechanical impulses at one-second intervals was carried out and the mean of each set of 10 was used for analysis. To determine the MVIC participants performed three repetitions of a MVIC of a plantar flexion according to the similar procedure applied by Kelly et al. [23]. Subjects were asked to lay down over a couch in the prone position. Upper and lower back, as well as the popliteal fossa were anchored to the couch with some straps. Another band was wrapped at the metatarsal level, connected to a ring and a carabiner; the band was covered and tape-fixed on the foot to avoid accidental movements and the ankle was maintained at 0 degrees neutral (see Figure 2).

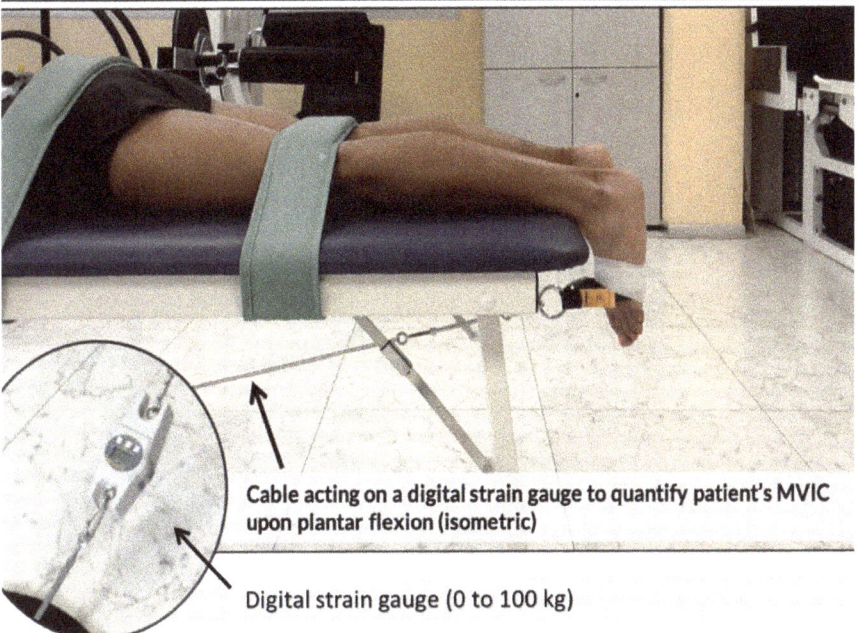

Figure 2. Subject positioning for isometric gastrocnemius contraction in prone. The participant was prone, shoes off with feet hanging unsupported off edge of the couch, and knees resting in 0 degrees extension. The trunk and lower extremities were anchored to the table by a strap just above the popliteal crease and across the pelvis at the level of the greater trochanters. The ankle position was maintained at 0 degrees neutral.

Then, a steel cable was connected to the carabiner and anchored to a fixed platform on the floor to the opposite side of the couch where the patient's head rested. A load cell connected between the steel cable and the platform measured the force produced by the subject during the isometric gastrocnemius contraction. In order to obtain an isometric contraction, before each trial, the cable was pre-loaded with 1 Kg tension. Each subject performed three familiarization trials and three maximal trials for each foot, with a 3-min recovery in between. At the end of each trial (both familiarization and maximal), pain intensity scale was shown to the subjects and measured with a 5-point Likert scale (0 = no pain, 1 = low pain intensity, 2 = medium pain intensity, 3 = high pain intensity, and 4 = severe pain intensity) [24]. Both for the MVIC and the pain scale, the highest scores between the three maximal trials were considered for the analysis.

2.4. Biochemical Assessment

To support the clinical and functional evaluation of the HA treatment, we also analyzed specific pro-inflammatory mediators in the peritendinous effusion aspirated after HA treatment. Quantification of IL-1β and MMP-3 levels was performed using Enzyme-linked Immunosorbent assay (ELISA) test. Human IL-1 beta/IL-1F2 (HSLB00D) and Human Total MMP-3 (DMP300) Quantikine High Sensitivity ELISA Kits were used (R&D Systems, Milan, Italy). The results were detected at a wavelength of 450 nm using a spectrophotometer reader.

2.5. Statistical Analyses

Descriptive statistics of variables considered were performed reporting means and standard deviations at different time measurements. In order to verify changes during time in treated and untreated arms, two-way mixed designs (MANOVA for repeated measures) were performed. Time was within-subjects 4 levels factor (T0, T1, T2, T3). Unilateral tendon (treated-injured vs. untreated-healthy condition) was 2 levels between group's factors; age and BMI were covariates; pain level, MVIC, frequency, and stiffness were dependent variables. Contrasts are used to test for differences among the levels of a between-subjects factor; difference contrast compares the mean of each level (T1, T2, T3) to the previous level. IL-1β and MMP3 levels at T0 and T2 were compared using MANOVA for repeated measures. Overall and partial Eta squared was used as effect size estimation. When epsilon was >0.75, the Huynh–Feldt correction was applied and when epsilon was <0.75, the Greenhouse-Geisser correction was applied. All elaborations were conducted with alpha = 0.05. Elaborations and graphics were obtained using Excel 365 (Microsoft) and SPSS version 20.0 (SPSS Inc., Chicago, IL, USA).

3. Results

Clinical exams confirmed the diagnosis of AT, while MRI excluded severe lesions or tendon ruptures. The treatment proved to be safe and well tolerated, and no adverse effect was observed. Repeated measures MANOVA test was conducted to test injection effects on pain, MVIC, and viscoelastometric parameters. Mauchly's Sphericity test was not significant for pain, frequency, and stiffness, while MVIC was significant ($p = 0.006$); for the latter variables, Huynh-Feldt or Greenhouse-Geisser correction was applied. The results showed that during overall time (T0–T3), pain, MVIC, frequency, and stiffness were significantly different between injured and contralateral tendon ($p = 0.028$; $p = 0.023$; $p = 0.047$, respectively); this is mainly due to the difference in T0; in later times the differences become very small. The results showed that during time, pain, MVIC, frequency, and stiffness were significantly different between healthy and injured tendon ($p = 0.028$; $p = 0.023$; $p = 0.047$, respectively). Considering the age and BMI as covariates, only frequency was related to these parameters ($p = 0.002$ and $p = 0.001$, respectively), while pain, MVIC, and stiffness were independent of age (see Table 1).

Table 1. Functional and viscoelastometric measurements.

Variables	T0		T1		T2		T3	
	Injured	Healthy	Injured	Healthy	Injured	Healthy	Injured	Healthy
Pain (AU)	2.57 (0.48)	1.40 (0.24)	1.29 (0.18)	1.40 (0.25)	1.43 (0.43)	1.40 (0.40)	1.07 (0.07)	1.04 (0.04)
MVIC (kg)	38.6 (5.35)	41.6 (6.08)	40.5 (5.01)	41.7 (5.91)	44.8 (4.90)	43.9 (6.22)	46.1 (4.34)	44.5 (5.78)
Tone (Hz)	32.2 (0.77)	33.3 (0.75)	33.0 (0.65)	33.1 (0.68)	33.0 (0.71)	32.8 (0.89)	32.9 (0.73)	32.7 (0.91)
Stiffness (N/m)	872 (29.1)	935 (35.6)	886 (22.4)	909 (31.9)	895 (28.1)	907 (39.6)	895 (25.3)	916 (30.1)

Mean (standard deviation) of pain, maximal voluntary isometric contraction (MVIC), frequency, and stiffness measured on injure and healthy tendons at different times: T0 (baseline), T1 (15d), T2 (30d), and T3 (45d).

Contrast analysis of differences highlighted when injured tendons got better until a non-significant difference in respect to the contralateral one was reached. The pain was higher in the injured tendon at T0; ΔT1-T0 contrast was significant ($p = 0.042$; $\eta^2 = 0.39$, see Figure 3a); T1-T0 decrease of pain in injured tendon was high and reached the average value of normal tendon; consequently, ΔT2-T1 and ΔT3-T2 were not significant ($p > 0.05$; $\eta^2 = 0.13$). Frequency showed a similar pattern: ΔT1-T0 showed a rise of frequency in injured tendons ($p = 0.048$; $\eta^2 = 0.40$), while there were not significant variations in the following time points (see Figure 3c). A post-hoc analysis of power was performed for stiffness and tone variables; a difference between two dependent means (matched pairs, T0-T1 interval) was considered. Stiffness variable, in T0, was 872 ± 29.1; in T1 it was 935 ± 35.6 for an effect size (Cohen d) = 1.94. Considering alpha = 0.05 and a two tailed t test for paired data, with eight subjects, we reached a power (1-beta) = 0.99. Tone variable, in T0, was 32.2 ± 0.77; in T1 it was 33.3 ± 0.75 for an effect size (Cohen d) = 1.05. Considering alpha = 0.05 and a two tailed t test for paired data, with eight subjects, we reached a power (1-beta) = 0.78.

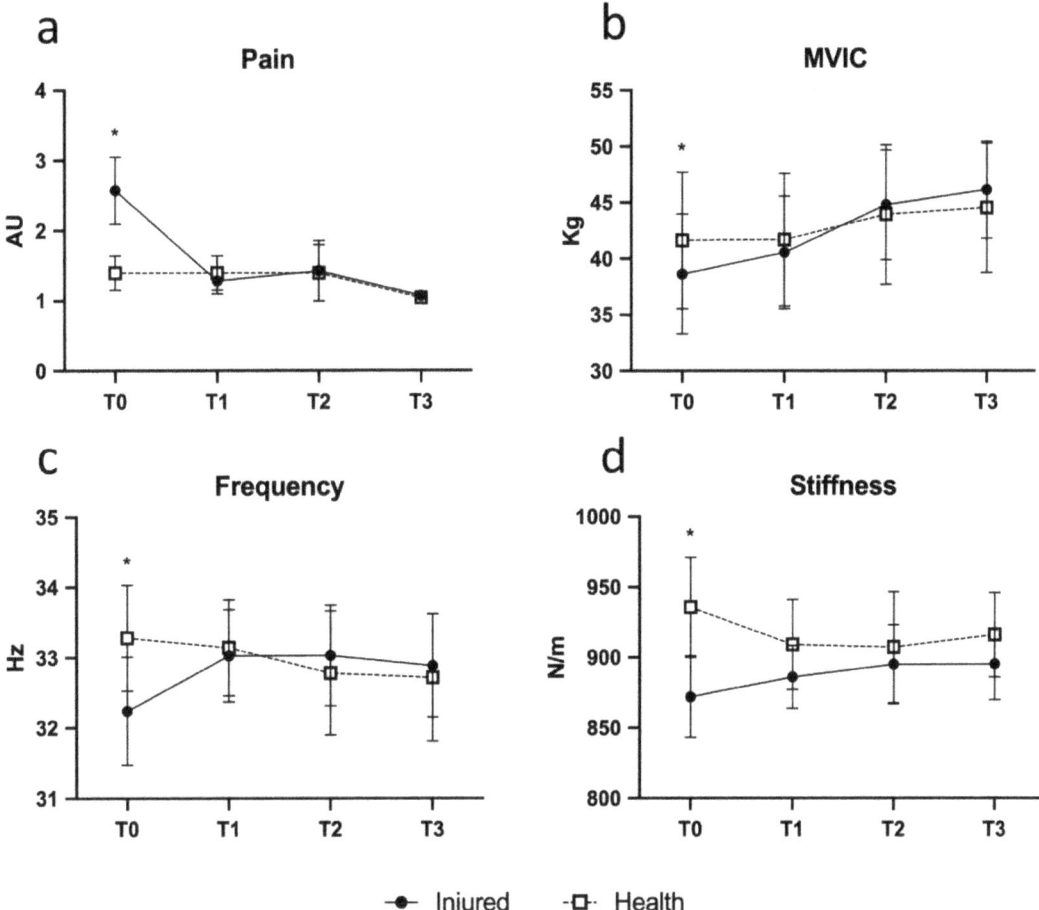

Figure 3. Time course variations of pain assessed with a 5-point Likert scale (**a**) (0 = no pain, 1 = low pain intensity, 2 = medium pain intensity, 3 = high pain intensity, and 4 = severe pain intensity), MVIC (**b**), frequency (**c**), and stiffness (**d**) in the Achilles tendinopathy (AT) (black dots) and contralateral healthy (white dots) tendon. Bars represent standard errors. * $p < 0.05$, intergroup comparison.

Similarly, MVIC ($p = 0.004$; $\eta^2 = 0.67$) and stiffness ($p = 0.035$; $\eta^2 = 0.44$) showed similar patterns (see Figure 3b,d). In brief, the first injection seems to account for the majority of the observed beneficial effects and the subsequent injections to maintain the improvements achieved. The volume of peritendinous effusion significantly dropped by about 57% at T2 (from 420.00 ± 40 uL to 238.75 ± 25 uL; $p = 0.018$; $\eta^2 = 0.63$) and was associated with a reduction of IL1-β and MMP-3 levels ($p = 0.027$; $\eta^2 = 0.58$) (Figure 4a,b).

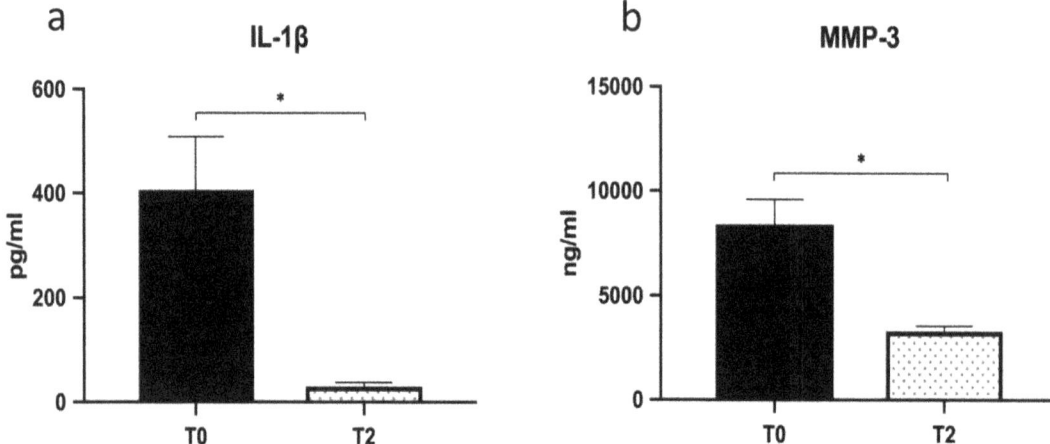

Figure 4. Peritendinous effusion levels of inflammation markers. IL-1β (**a**) and MMP-3 (**b**) levels were determined in peritendinous effusion at baseline (T0) and at one month (T2). Values are means ± SE. *, significantly different as compared to baseline ($p < 0.05$).

4. Discussion

This pilot study describes for the first time the effect efficacy of a cycle of three HA peritendinous injections over a forty-five-day period on clinical, viscoelastometric, functional, and biochemical parameters, in middle-aged recreational runners affected by unilateral AT.

Our data indicate that this treatment promoted a significant and rapid amelioration of the AT-associated alterations of the above parameters in all the patients. Relief from clinical symptoms such as tenderness on palpation and pain was very rapid; accordingly, peritendinous effusion volume reduction was observed after the treatment; the biochemical markers of inflammation significantly ameliorated at the selected checkpoints.

In addition, this pilot study is the first to adopt an experimental design combining the above determinations with tendon's viscoelastic—namely, tone and stiffness—and functional assessments over the course of the HA infiltrative treatment. In this regard, tone and stiffness are two parameters expressing the viscoelastic state of living tissues (muscles and tendons), which have been shown to reflect their biomechanical/functional status and integrity [14,27]. The tone and stiffness values augment with the increase of the contraction levels, exhaustive activity, and ageing [28,29]. Recently Morgan et al. [30] and Finnamore et al. [16] reported that AT induces appreciable alterations in Achilles tendon viscoelasticity suggesting a correlation between tendon integrity and its viscoelastic properties.

Here we report that all the considered parameters significantly varied over the treatment period in injured AT, reaching values similar or even superimposable to those of the contralateral healthy one. AT also resulted in functional impairment, as indicated by the decrease of MVIC in the homolateral limb. Interestingly, fifteen days after the first injection, all these parameters changed. It is worth considering that this implies that the functional and viscoelastometric asymmetries between the two limbs characterizing the pre-treatment stage tended to decrease and then disappear. In particular, the MVIC and the tone assessed in the AT tendon increased until they reached values similar and not statistically different from the healthy one. As to the stiffness values, fifteen days after the first injection, they equilibrated as well; however, in this case, it is worth noting that this achievement depended not only on the increase in AT tendon stiffness, but also on the concomitant slight reduction occurring in the healthy tendon. Concerning this, a likely hypothesis to explain this result may be that, in the absence of treatments, the healthy tendon stiffness increases in response to the altered/excessive distribution of loads obligatorily associated with the

AT which impacts on the contralateral limb biomechanical efficiency. The equilibrium in tone and stiffness between the healthy and inflamed tendon did not vary following the two injections at T2 and T3, while the MVIC increased constantly and symmetrically on both sides. In parallel with the balancing of the viscoelastic and functional parameters, the perceived pain drastically dropped after the first injection to the same values of the healthy tendon and did not vary up to the last clinical assessment.

Hence, these parameters may help, especially in runners, to accurately identify when the two limbs equilibrate each other and the athlete can return to normal activity, limiting the risk of underestimating the residual injury and of AT recurrence; however, further research is needed to generate basic data for specific population groups that monitor these variables over time.

In line with the clinical and functional amelioration due to the HA treatment, we also observed a significant reduction of specific pro-inflammatory mediators in the peritendinous effusion aspirated after HA treatment. Indeed, IL-1β, which is recognized as the initiator of tendinopathy since it induces inflammation, apoptosis, and ECM degradation by activating MMPs, drastically dropped out after HA treatment. In line with the fall of IL-1β and according to Del Buono et al. [31], we also found a significant reduction of MMP-3 levels, the endopeptidase that degrades the ECM and mediates the development of tendinopathy. Our data are in agreement with the finding of Wu et al. [24], who showed that high-molecular-weight HA attenuated tendinopathy by down regulating MMP-1 and -3 expression via CD44. Indeed, HA, beyond its physical and lubricating properties, is actively involved in regulating inflammatory responses mediated through the interactions with different substrates and receptors, among which CD44 represents a primary target [32] and has HA also effectively mitigated chondropathy and tendinopathy in clinical practice [33].

The HA utilized in this pilot study is a blend of different MW linear-HA similar in composition to that exhibiting a strong and prompt anti-inflammatory activity in a previous study on osteoarthrosis (OA) from a previous study of our group [33]. Although completely different from each other, a common trait linking the two pathologies is the need to reduce the inflammatory process and its consequences, an effect that both the blends of HA proved to afford. Indeed, in strict analogy with previous data on OA, here, we found that the AT-inflammatory hallmarks IL-1β and MMP-3 were rapidly and strongly reduced immediately after the first injection. Differently from OA, where very high MW HA is required—and usually included in injectable preparations—to afford viscosupplementation within the joint [33], in AT is unneeded. Rather, it is important that HA has some chance to diffuse around and through the paratenon sheath to reach the surrounding inflammation sites, a feature which is inversely related to MW; secondarily, some positive mechanical effect may derive from the lubrication of injured tendon, a property which is retained by the heavier HA fraction around 1.000 KDa.

Taken together these results confirm that the treatment with peritendinous HA injections allows a reduction of the main symptoms characterizing AT and allows the patient to resume the main basic functions. These data are in agreement with the recent clinical evidence [22–24]. Here, our pilot study shows that AT is accompanied by alterations of stiffness and tone of the tendon body, supporting the concept that tissue mechanical properties are a marker of disease. Since stiffness and tone can be precisely and reliably determined, their measurement provides the clinician with a simple, rapid, and non-invasive method to objectively quantitate the extent of tendon recovery.

5. Strengths and Weaknesses of the Study

The strength of the present study, as compared to previous ones on the same or similar topics [16,17,24] is that it is the first one adopting a multi-methodological approach in a longitudinal setting. Indeed, this approach—that could be extended to larger clinical studies—allows to gather an integrated, complex data set accurately and objectively reflecting the quali-quantitative state of the AT changes induced by HA treatment. Furthermore, we highlight the capacity of viscoelastometry to easily, rapidly, and non-invasively assess the state of AT with the additional advantage of providing quantitative parameters.

Conversely, the main limitations were the small number of the enrolled sample and the lack of a control group of AT runners treated according to the standard of care. Although this limitation is not uncommon in similar studies focusing on "real life" settings, it is of worth that the aim of this pilot study was to set the basis for future, larger clinical studies, rather than comparing the efficacy of HA with the standard of care. Moreover, another limitation is that the patients enrolled in this study—the recreational runners—while likely representative of sport practitioners and athletes suffering of AT, might not necessarily reflect the situation of other AT population subgroups, i.e., sedentary and/or elderly and/or overweight people. Again, future clinical studies should include these population subgroups as well as a standard of care group.

6. Conclusions

In conclusion, our results point out the therapeutic potential of low to medium MW HA in treating one of the most diffused tendon pathologies. In particular, we noticed a progressive improvement of all the tested parameters over the treatment with HA, leading to a significant reduction of functional and mechanical asymmetries between AT and Healthy limbs. Furthermore, this study proposes a new multi-methodological and integrated approach which might pave the way to larger clinical studies focusing on the pharmacological treatment of AT, a very common and subtle condition.

Author Contributions: Conceptualization, P.S., M.G., I.C. and E.B.; methodology, M.G., P.S., E.B. and G.A.; statistical analysis, M.B.L.R., D.S., S.A. and M.G.; investigation, M.G., P.S., E.B., V.C. and I.C.; resources, V.S., P.S. and E.B.; data curation, M.G., G.A. and G.V.; writing—original draft preparation, M.G., P.S. and E.B.; writing—review and editing, M.G., G.V., S.D.Z. and P.S. supervision, P.S. and V.S.; project administration, M.G., P.S. and E.B.; funding acquisition, P.S., E.B. and V.S. All authors have read and agreed to the published version of the manuscript.

Funding: This research received no external funding.

Institutional Review Board Statement: The protocol for the pilot study project has been approved by the Institutional Ethics Committee of the Stella Maris Hospital (San Benedetto del Tronto, Italy) on 26 November 2018, and it conforms to the provisions of the Declaration of Helsinki.

Informed Consent Statement: Informed consent was obtained from all subjects involved in the study.

Data Availability Statement: The data presented in this study are available on request from the corresponding author. The data are not publicly available for ethical and privacy reasons.

Acknowledgments: We thank Antonio Romani of the Clinic Stella Maris San Benedetto del Tronto, Italy, for technical assistance.

Conflicts of Interest: The authors declare no conflict of interest.

References

1. Lipman, K.; Wang, C.; Ting, K.; Soo, C.; Zheng, Z. Tendinopathy: Injury, repair, and current exploration. *Drug Des. Dev. Ther.* **2018**, *12*, 591–603. [CrossRef] [PubMed]
2. McLauchlan, G.J.; Handoll, H.H. Interventions for treating acute and chronic Achilles tendinitis. *Cochrane Database Syst. Rev.* **2001**, CD000232. [CrossRef]
3. Malvankar, S.; Khan, W.S. Evolution of the Achilles tendon: The athlete's Achilles heel? *Foot* **2011**, *21*, 193–197. [CrossRef] [PubMed]
4. Schepsis, A.A.; Jones, H.; Haas, A.L. Achilles tendon disorders in athletes. *Am. J. Sports Med.* **2002**, *30*, 287–305. [CrossRef]
5. Clancy, W.G., Jr. Specific rehabilitation for the injured recreational runner. *Instr. Course Lect.* **1989**, *38*, 483–486.
6. Longo, U.G.; Ronga, M.; Maffulli, N. Achilles tendinopathy. *Sports Med. Arthrosc. Rev.* **2009**, *17*, 112–126. [CrossRef] [PubMed]
7. Mobasheri, A.; Shakibaei, M. Is tendinitis an inflammatory disease initiated and driven by pro-inflammatory cytokines such as interleukin 1beta? *Histol. Histopathol.* **2013**, *28*, 955–964. [CrossRef]
8. Ahmad, J.; Repka, M.; Raikin, S.M. Treatment of myotendinous Achilles ruptures. *Foot Ankle Int.* **2013**, *34*, 1074–1078. [CrossRef] [PubMed]

9. Maffulli, N.; Kenward, M.G.; Testa, V.; Capasso, G.; Regine, R.; King, J.B. Clinical diagnosis of Achilles tendinopathy with tendinosis. *Clin. J. Sport Med. Off. J. Can. Acad. Sport Med.* **2003**, *13*, 11–15. [CrossRef]
10. Cook, J.L.; Purdam, C.R. Is tendon pathology a continuum? A pathology model to explain the clinical presentation of load-induced tendinopathy. *Br. J. Sports Med.* **2009**, *43*, 409–416. [CrossRef]
11. Romero-Morales, C.; Martin-Llantino, P.J.; Calvo-Lobo, C.; Almazan-Polo, J.; Lopez-Lopez, D.; de la Cruz-Torres, B.; Palomo-Lopez, P.; Rodriguez-Sanz, D. Intrinsic foot muscles morphological modifications in patients with Achilles tendinopathy: A novel case-control research study. *Phys. Ther. Sport Off. J. Assoc. Chart. Physiother. Sports Med.* **2019**, *40*, 208–212. [CrossRef]
12. Romero-Morales, C.; Martin-Llantino, P.J.; Calvo-Lobo, C.; Lopez-Lopez, D.; Sanchez-Gomez, R.; De-La-Cruz-Torres, B.; Rodriguez-Sanz, D. Ultrasonography Features of the Plantar Fascia Complex in Patients with Chronic Non-Insertional Achilles Tendinopathy: A Case-Control Study. *Sensors* **2019**, *19*, 2052. [CrossRef] [PubMed]
13. Romero-Morales, C.; Martin-Llantino, P.J.; Calvo-Lobo, C.; Sanchez-Gomez, R.; Lopez-Lopez, D.; Pareja-Galeano, H.; Rodriguez-Sanz, D. Ultrasound evaluation of extrinsic foot muscles in patients with chronic non-insertional Achilles tendinopathy: A case-control study. *Phys. Ther. Sport Off. J. Assoc. Chart. Physiother. Sports Med.* **2019**, *37*, 44–48. [CrossRef]
14. Schneebeli, A.; Falla, D.; Clijsen, R.; Barbero, M. Myotonometry for the evaluation of Achilles tendon mechanical properties: A reliability and construct validity study. *BMJ Open Sport Exerc. Med.* **2020**, *6*, e000726. [CrossRef] [PubMed]
15. Coombes, B.K.; Tucker, K.; Vicenzino, B.; Vuvan, V.; Mellor, R.; Heales, L.; Nordez, A.; Hug, F. Achilles and patellar tendinopathy display opposite changes in elastic properties: A shear wave elastography study. *Scand. J. Med. Sci. Sports* **2018**, *28*, 1201–1208. [CrossRef] [PubMed]
16. Finnamore, E.; Waugh, C.; Solomons, L.; Ryan, M.; West, C.; Scott, A. Transverse tendon stiffness is reduced in people with Achilles tendinopathy: A cross-sectional study. *PLoS ONE* **2019**, *14*, e211863. [CrossRef]
17. McAuliffe, S.; Tabuena, A.; McCreesh, K.; O'Keeffe, M.; Hurley, J.; Comyns, T.; Purtill, H.; O'Neill, S.; O'Sullivan, K. Altered Strength Profile in Achilles Tendinopathy: A Systematic Review and Meta-Analysis. *J. Athl. Train.* **2019**, *54*, 889–900. [CrossRef]
18. Li, H.Y.; Hua, Y.H. Achilles Tendinopathy: Current Concepts about the Basic Science and Clinical Treatments. *Biomed. Res. Int.* **2016**, *2016*, 6492597. [CrossRef]
19. Wilson, A. Use of combined inhalers for stable chronic obstructive pulmonary disease. *Nurs. Stand.* **2018**, *32*, 47–48. [CrossRef]
20. Noble, P.W. Hyaluronan and its catabolic products in tissue injury and repair. *Matrix Biol. J. Int. Soc. Matrix Biol.* **2002**, *21*, 25–29. [CrossRef]
21. Necas, J.; Bartosikova, L.; Brauner, P.; Kolar, J. Hyaluronic acid (hyaluronan): A review. *Vet. Med. Czech* **2008**, *53*, 397–411. [CrossRef]
22. Fogli, M.; Giordan, N.; Mazzoni, G. Efficacy and safety of hyaluronic acid (500-730kDa) Ultrasound-guided injections on painful tendinopathies: A prospective, open label, clinical study. *MusclesLigaments Tendons J.* **2017**, *7*, 388–395. [CrossRef]
23. Frizziero, A.; Oliva, F.; Vittadini, F.; Vetrano, M.; Bernetti, A.; Giordan, N.; Vulpiani, M.C.; Santilli, V.; Masiero, S.; Maffulli, N. Efficacy of ultrasound-guided hyaluronic acid injections in achilles and patellar tendinopathies: A prospective multicentric clinical trial. *MusclesLigaments Tendons J.* **2019**, *9*, 305–313. [CrossRef]
24. Wu, P.T.; Kuo, L.C.; Su, F.C.; Chen, S.Y.; Hsu, T.I.; Li, C.Y.; Tsai, K.J.; Jou, I.M. High-molecular-weight hyaluronic acid attenuated matrix metalloproteinase-1 and -3 expression via CD44 in tendinopathy. *Sci. Rep.* **2017**, *7*, 40840. [CrossRef]
25. Chiodo, C.P.; Logan, C.; Blauwet, C.A. Aspiration and Injection Techniques of the Lower Extremity. *J. Am. Acad. Orthop. Surg.* **2018**, *26*, e313–e320. [CrossRef]
26. Peters, S.E.; Laxer, R.M.; Connolly, B.L.; Parra, D.A. Ultrasound-guided steroid tendon sheath injections in juvenile idiopathic arthritis: A 10-year single-center retrospective study. *Pediatric Rheumatol. Online J.* **2017**, *15*, 22. [CrossRef]
27. Sohirad, S.; Wilson, D.; Waugh, C.; Finnamore, E.; Scott, A. Feasibility of using a hand-held device to characterize tendon tissue biomechanics. *PLoS ONE* **2017**, *12*, e0184463. [CrossRef] [PubMed]
28. Gervasi, M.; Sisti, D.; Amatori, S.; Andreazza, M.; Benelli, P.; Sestili, P.; Rocchi, M.B.L.; Calavalle, A.R. Muscular viscoelastic characteristics of athletes participating in the European Master Indoor Athletics Championship. *Eur. J. Appl. Physiol.* **2017**, *117*, 1739–1746. [CrossRef]
29. Gervasi, M.; Sisti, D.; Benelli, P.; Fernandez-Pena, E.; Calcabrini, C.; Rocchi, M.B.L.; Lanata, L.; Bagnasco, M.; Tonti, A.; Vilberto, S.; et al. The effect of topical thiocolchicoside in preventing and reducing the increase of muscle tone, stiffness, and soreness: A real-life study on top-level road cyclists during stage competition. *Medicine* **2017**, *96*, e7659. [CrossRef]
30. Morgan, G.E.; Martin, R.; Williams, L.; Pearce, O.; Morris, K. Objective assessment of stiffness in Achilles tendinopathy: A novel approach using the MyotonPRO. *BMJ Open Sport Exerc. Med.* **2018**, *4*, e000446. [CrossRef]
31. Del Buono, A.; Oliva, F.; Longo, U.G.; Rodeo, S.A.; Orchard, J.; Denaro, V.; Maffulli, N. Metalloproteases and rotator cuff disease. *J. Shoulder Elb. Surg.* **2012**, *21*, 200–208. [CrossRef] [PubMed]
32. Vasvani, S.; Kulkarni, P.; Rawtani, D. Hyaluronic acid: A review on its biology, aspects of drug delivery, route of administrations and a special emphasis on its approved marketed products and recent clinical studies. *Int. J. Biol. Macromol.* **2019**. [CrossRef] [PubMed]
33. Barbieri, E.; Capparucci, I.; Mannello, F.; Annibalini, G.; Contarelli, S.; Vallorani, L.; Gioacchini, A.M.; Ligi, D.; Maniscalco, R.; Gervasi, M.; et al. Efficacy of a Treatment for Gonarthrosis Based on the Sequential Intra-Articular Injection of Linear and Cross-Linked Hyaluronic Acids. *MuscleLigaments Tendons J.* **2019**, *9*, 606–614. [CrossRef]

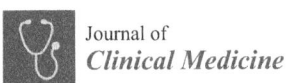

Review

Cardiac Rehabilitation in Patients with Peripheral Artery Disease—A Literature Review in COVID-19 Era

Razvan Anghel [1,†], Cristina Andreea Adam [1,†], Dragos Traian Marius Marcu [2], Ovidiu Mitu [2,3,*] and Florin Mitu [1,2]

1. Clinical Rehabilitation Hospital, Cardiovascular Rehabilitation Clinic, Pantelimon Halipa Street nr 14, 700661 Iasi, Romania; razvan0312@gmail.com (R.A.); adam.cristina93@gmail.com (C.A.A.); mitu.florin@yahoo.com (F.M.)
2. Department of Internal Medicine, University of Medicine and Pharmacy "Grigore T. Popa", University Street nr 16, 700115 Iasi, Romania; dragos.marcu11@yahoo.com
3. "Sf. Spiridon" Clinical Emergency Hospital, Independence Boulevard nr 1, 700111 Iasi, Romania
* Correspondence: mituovidiu@yahoo.co.uk
† These authors contributed equally to this work.

Abstract: Cardiac rehabilitation (CR) is an integral part of the management of various cardiovascular disease such as coronary artery disease (CAD), peripheral artery disease (PAD), or chronic heart failure (CHF), with proven morbidity and mortality benefits. This article aims to review and summarize the scientific literature related to cardiac rehabilitation programs for patients with PAD and how they were adapted during the COVID-19 pandemic. The implementation of CR programs has been problematic since the COVID-19 pandemic due to social distancing and work-related restrictions. One of the main challenges for physicians and health systems alike has been the management of PAD patients. COVID-19 predisposes to coagulation disorders that can lead to severe thrombotic events. Home-based walking exercises are more accessible and easier to accept than supervised exercise programs. Cycling or other forms of exercise are more entertaining or challenging alternatives to exercise therapy. Besides treadmill exercises, upper- and lower-extremity ergometry also has great functional benefits, especially regarding walking endurance. Supervised exercise therapy has a positive impact on both functional capacity and also on the quality of life of such patients. The most effective manner to acquire this seems to be by combining revascularization therapy and supervised exercise. Rehabilitation programs proved to be a mandatory part of the integrative approach in these cases, increasing quality of life, and decreasing stress levels, depression, and anxiety.

Keywords: cardiac rehabilitation; peripheral artery disease; COVID-19; intermittent claudication; quality of life; review

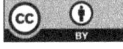

1. Introduction

Cardiovascular diseases (CVD) are still the main cause of mortality and morbidity despite a downwards trend due to earlier diagnostic facilities and advanced interventional techniques. Cardiac rehabilitation (CR) (alongside risk-factor management) is an integral part of the management of various CVD such as coronary artery disease (CAD), peripheral artery disease (PAD), chronic heart failure (CHF) or valvular heart disease (VHD), with proven morbidity and mortality benefits [1]. Physical exercise is an important element of rehabilitation, but in order to obtain a secondary prevention through CR we need to focus also on other aspects such as dietary advice, psychotherapy, smoking cessation programs, weight management or drug therapy. Improving functional capacity, psychological adaptation to chronic illness, applying lifestyle changes or maintaining the independence of daily activities are central objectives in CR to favorably influence the long-term prognosis (Figure 1) [2–4]. This article aims to review and summarize the scientific literature related to current cardiac rehabilitation programs for patients with PAD and how they were adapted during the COVID-19 pandemic through telemedicine. Besides that, in the light of the information available to date, we have assessed the effectiveness of home-based CR programs for patients with PAD who face multiple challenges in the context of the COVID-19 pandemic. Different databases were exploited and brief descriptions of the different types of exercise are presented in this article. From pathophysiology to comparisons between traditional and novel exercise types, benefits of CR programs and challenges due to the COVID-19 pandemic, all of these issues are discussed in terms of efficacy and prognostic value.

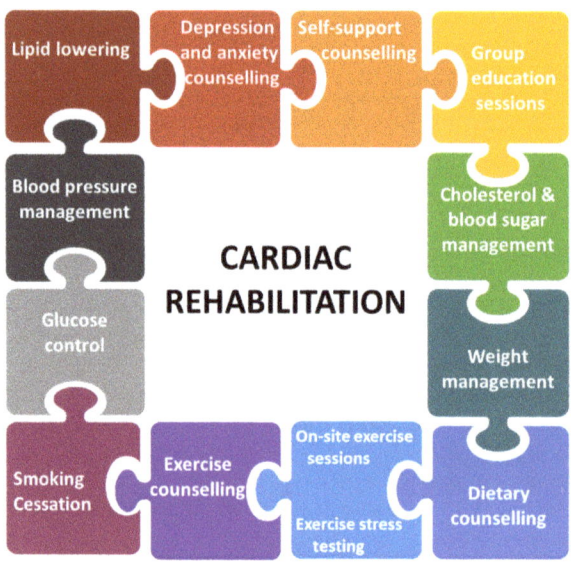

Figure 1. Components of cardiac rehabilitation.

2. Literature Research

We conducted a search using the PubMed and SCIENCE DIRECT in November 2021 using the terms and phrases, "Coronavirus", "COVID-19", "cardiac rehabilitation", "peripheral artery disease" and "exercise training" under different word associations. We focused on studies related to the impact of COVID-19 on cardiovascular rehabilitation programs. For inclusion, we selected observational cohort studies of patients with PAD previously confirmed by an ABI less than 0.9 or using imaging methods (duplex ultrasound, angiography) or with a history of lower-limb endovascular or open-surgical revascularization. Interventional studies, case reports, editorials and letters were excluded.

3. Cardiac Rehabilitation during the COVID-19 Pandemic

The implementation of CR programs has been problematic since the COVID-19 pandemic due to social distancing and work-related restrictions ("smart working"). Worldwide CR programs have been interrupted or have been reduced as they are considered non-essential in the pandemic emergency [5].

The suspension of CR based centers has significant consequences for both shorter- and longer-term prognoses as well as increased rates of acute coronary events and hence exposure to infection [6]. The appearance of mental health problems, increasing sedentary lifestyle, inadequate nutrition and giving up or decreasing regular physical activities are factors associated with negative long-term consequences [5,7]. The occurrence of PAD before the age of 50 years is currently defined as premature PAD and unfortunately remains undertreated despite the continued increase in prevalence [8,9]. Both the medical and economic impact of COVID-19 infection increases with age and the number of associated comorbidities. Wu and McGoogan pointed out that the mortality rate increased from 8.0%

in 70–79 years old patients to 14.8% in patients over 80 years old [10]. Given the prevalence of CVD in patients over 65 years old, with great impact on both morbidity and mortality, the improvement in health status secondary to CR programs is essential.

Virtual CR (VCR) is an alternative for center-based CR programs, with the same patient outcomes and safety profiles for cardiac patients with low to moderate cardiovascular risk. Tele-medicine alternatives-telephone, video conferencing and other resources are some of the methods used in VCR [11].

There are some disadvantages such as resource limitations, communication difficulties, as well as risk stratification and supervision associated issues especially in elderly and frail cardiovascular patients with several associated comorbidities. Risk stratification is important in both traditional CR programs and VCR, especially when patients associates residual ischemia, reduced left ventricular ejection fraction (less than 40%), arrhythmias, or variable hemodynamic responses induced by exercise [12,13].

Italy has been one of the most affected countries by the COVID-19 pandemic. There, the Italian Association of Preventive and Rehabilitative Clinical Cardiology (AICPR) conducted a national survey on the activity of CR centers during the COVID-19 pandemic. They collected information from 75 centers (one-third of the national network) and showed that 14% of CR units continued their activities without any reorganization, 61% reduced or reshaped their programs and 25% completely stopped all of their activities. Half of CR units have implemented programs dedicated to COVID-19 patients and were managed by a multidisciplinary team that involved various health specialties (especially physiatrists and pulmonologists) [14].

Besides Italy, Canada is another country which has experienced negative impacts of the COVID pandemic on their health system. The Canadian Cardiac Rehabilitation Association implemented special home-based CR programs for PAD patients with low and moderate risk. With limited hospital visits and counselling via telemedicine, the patients completed their exercise programs in a safe and familiar environment [15–18]. At the beginning of the COVID-19 pandemic, 41.2% of the CR centers closed due to restrictions and staff redeployment and therefore a large proportion of PAD patients discontinued their CR programs. The inclusion criteria have also been modified, with patients with less complex pathologies, less motor disorders and without severe cognitive disorders being enrolled [19].

The need for alternative delivery models such as tele-cardiology, home CR programs or the use of digital health tools that allow for increased access and participation has never been more urgent. Patients with pre-existing cardiovascular diseases who have contracted COVID-19 must be considered a priority for CR centers, especially due to the long-term impact of the virus on cardiovascular and pulmonary function. As the CR programs have been reduced or interrupted worldwide due to the pandemic, we should very carefully balance the decision of excluding the high-risk patients from VCR, as studies have shown benefit of appropriately prescribed physical activity in these patients [20]. Patient education and independence are key elements of self-manage for PAD patients. The role of telerehabilitation has become increasingly important in the context of COVID-19 through the rapid development of online education programs designed to replace traditional exercise programs.

Anderson et al. demonstrated in a Cochrane Database Systematic Review that home-based exercise programs and center groups CR programs have the same results in terms of mortality, occurrence of acute cardiac events, improvement of physical parameters and correction of risk factors, with greater adherence for the first category [20]. The concept of telehealth improved during the COVID-19 pandemic and nowadays has become a relevant alternative to traditional CR programs. Through telephone, internet or videoconferencing, telerehabilitation is a cost-effective method, impacting the quality of life and mortality rate of PAD patients [21–23]. Telerehabilitation has both advantages and limitations. Greater independence, lower costs and privacy are factors that increase patient adherence to CR programs, while the lack of social contact, the need for at least a minimal knowledge of technology in the digital era and data security and confidentiality can be perceived as barriers [24–26].

The target of the VCR programs should be reaching the expected functional benefit with the least level of physical activity and with exercise intensity lower than moderate. Two important aspects of VCR are the patient's education regarding symptom and intensity assessment which can be achieved through heart rate check-up by palpation or by using wearable heart rate monitors as well as communication with the specialists from the CR center who coordinates the exercise [17,20].

O'Doherty et al., in association with the British Association for Cardiovascular Prevention and Rehabilitation, conducted an international study based on a mixed methods survey, which aim was to investigate whether CR centers for PAD patients continued their exercise programs during the COVID-19 pandemic. Approximately half of the centers noted that CR programs were stopped due to COVID-19. The telephone was most used in VCR, as well as teleconferencing in centers where both physicians and patients had access to this type of advanced technology. The study also identified some limitations regarding the impact of technology in exercise-based CR programs such as lack of patient confidence, technical difficulties (patients without access to computers/tablets/smartphones or internet connection), concerns about patient safety (from both professionals and patients) or internet security and patient confidentiality concerns [17,27–30]. Both physical and psychological benefits of exercise training depend on the weekly exercise time and long-term adherence to the program [31].

Patients with PAD infected with COVID-19 require rigorous supervision due to the persistent systemic inflammatory state, defined as, "long COVID" [32]. Cardiac rehabilitation through physical exercises adapted to each patient and carefully supervised are essential after COVID-19 in order to decrease endothelial inflammation [33]. The 6 Minute Walking Test (6MWT) is easy and simple to use during recovery from COVID-19 in order to evaluate the physical function and to identify any potential deficiencies in daily life activities. During exercise, saturation, blood pressure, heart rate and worsening of symptoms need to be permanently evaluate (Table 1) [34–38].

Table 1. Parameters evaluated during the 6 Minute Walking Test after COVID-19 (adapted after [34]).

Parameters	Value
Saturation	>92–93%
Heart rate	An increase up to 20 beats per minute from the baseline
Systolic blood pressure	$\geq$90 mmHg and $\leq$180 mmHg
Symptoms	The Borg Scale–dyspnea with a score < 4 Rate of perceived exertion–fatigue with a score < 11–12

COVID-19 has multiple implications on the morbidity and mortality of patients with PAD. SARS-CoV2 infection causes the appearance of a pro-inflammatory status accompanied by cytokine storms that cause secondary vascular inflammation and endothelial dysfunction. SARS-CoV2 infection can cause arterial and venous thromboembolic complications in patients with previous CVD [39–41]. Patients with PAD and COVID-19 may develop acute limb ischemia secondary to thrombosis of the aorta or peripheral arteries secondary to endothelial dysfunction [41,42]. Both PAD and COVID-19 causes hypercoagulability, but it is currently not well defined whether PAD patients associate worse outcomes when infected with SARS-CoV2. Smolderen et al. demonstrated that PAD patients have an increased risk of 40% when it comes major averse cardiovascular events in case of co-existence of infection with COVID-19 [43].

Enrolling these patients in cardiac rehabilitation programs after the acute phase has beneficial cardiovascular effects such as decrease in arterial stiffness, increased bioavailability of nitric oxide and endothelial function improvement through vasodilatation. Aerobic endurance training, interval training, high intensity interval training and resistance training are the types of exercise training most commonly used [44–46].

Studies have shown that in post-COVID-19 patients with moderate illness interval training is preferable and better tolerated as a first approach at an intensity of 2–3 METs with a frequency of 3 to 5 times a week [45,47,48]. High intensity interval training based on series of high intensity exercises interspersed with recovery periods lead to the improvement of endothelial dysfunction through the intensity variation within the same exercise. High intensity exercise programs such as these require a thorough initial evaluation and can be recommended in patients with a high level of fatigue and respiratory distress 2–3 times a week [34,49,50].

Resistance training involves different muscle groups, and it is based on anaerobic exercises of moderate intensity in which resistance is offered by an external load or body weight. Both high intensity interval training and resistance training programs should be adjusted according to the clinical particularities and vitals of the patients [34]. Circuit training programs consist of anaerobic exercises in which all of the muscle groups are included which secondly leads to a more hypotensive response. Compared to endurance training, resistance training is associated with diminished endothelial function improvements and vasodilatation [51,52].

In addition to the benefits mentioned above, there are a number of risks and adverse events during cardiac rehabilitation in post-COVID patients which require further evaluation in order to evaluate the need to participate exercise training programs such as body temperature, heart rate and blood pressure fluctuations or worsening of respiratory symptoms during exercise with no improvement after its discontinuation (Table 2) [36,53].

Table 2. Adverse hemodynamic events during cardiac rehabilitation, especially after COVID-19 (adapted after [34]).

Parameters	Value
Saturation	<88–93%
Heart rate	<40 beats per minute or >120 beats per minute
Systolic blood pressure	<90 mmHg and >180 mmHg
Body temperature fluctuations	>37.2 °C
Symptoms	Worsening of respiratory symptoms during exercise Chest tightness or pain Difficulty in breathing Palpitations Sweating
	Unclear vision

Respiratory rehabilitation is as important as cardiovascular rehabilitation in patients with CVD and COVID-19. The majority of patients enrolled in exercise training programs associate respiratory problems [36]. Improving ventilation of the deep lung by chest expansion exercises [54,55] and airway clearance by methods based on exploit positive expiratory pressure are the main goals of respiratory rehabilitation which ameliorate dyspnea, reduce morbidity and improves quality of life in patients with COVID-19 and CVD such as PAD [56].

Recovery after COVID-19 can be long, especially for patients with associated comorbidities such as PAD. There are so far unknown long-term effects that influence the quality of life and functional status. These patients may present several limitations in terms of pulmonary dysfunction that do not allow them to undertake a physical effort in the same way as a patient who was never infected.

In the implementation of telerehabilitation, monitoring devices play an essential role through real-time monitoring [57]. Smartwatches, smartphones, pedometers, or sensor devices allow assessment of multiple parameters, both clinical and physical. The impact on quality of life can also be estimated via depression scales, sleep quality monitoring or cognitive tests [5]. Rosen et al. consider telemedicine as an electronic personal protective equipment by reducing both the risks of exposure and contamination between rehabilitation therapists and patients [58]. Group sessions, easy to apply exercise programs and facilitating the access to telerehabilitation for vulnerable patients are practical tips which are easy to apply. Lending devices such as smartphones or smart tables to patients in order to participate in individual session increases adherence among PAD patients enrolled in CR programs [5,59]. As an alternative to traditional exercise programs, during the COVID-19 pandemic patients were encouraged to perform gymnastic movements of muscular strengthening, stretching training and online relaxation sessions previously explained via videos [7,59]. The devices used are often equipped with a series of sensors designed to monitor vital parameters in order to prevent complications and store them in servers easily accessible by healthcare professionals [13,60].

4. Physical Training—Mechanisms & Benefits

Loss of exercise tolerance leads to weight gain and influences the lipid metabolism and serum glucose levels, all of which may contribute to the development of atherosclerosis and to an increase in the degree of disability [3].

Increasing exercise capacity is the main goal of physical training in cardiac rehabilitation. The increase in the maximum volume of oxygen (VO2 max) is variable (10–30% usually) and depends on the degree of physical deconditioning of the patient and the intensity of training. Effort adaptation is achieved through central mechanisms such as increases in cardiac contractility or heart rate as well as through peripheral mechanisms such as vasodilation of skeletal muscle arterioles during exercise, an increased oxygen extraction fraction or arterial and venous constriction in the rest of the territories [2,3]. The more trained the patient is, the later the central mechanisms will be involved during the physical training. This reduced vascularization causes a lack in oxygen supply leading to reduced aerobic generation of adenosine triphosphate (ATP) and thus a dependency on anaerobic metabolism. This increases creatine phosphate and lactate levels, which subsequently leads to muscular pain.

Physical training induces morphological, hemodynamic, and metabolic changes. The hemodynamic effects are the most obvious after training. The main hemodynamic changes are reduced blood pressure, increased blood volume or increases in maximal oxygen uptake (Figure 2) [61].

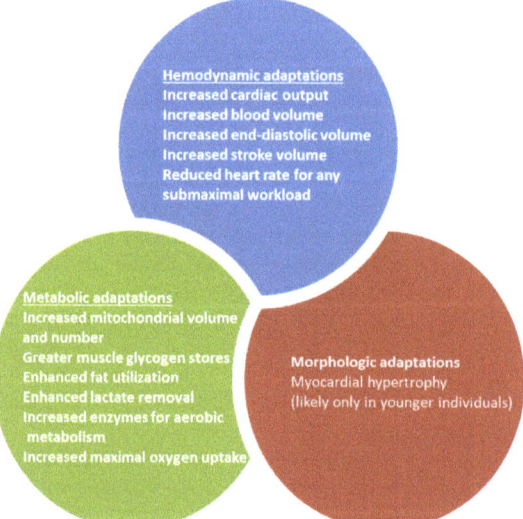

Figure 2. Physiologic adaptations to physical training in humans. Physical training involves hemodynamic, metabolic, and morphologic adaptations.

Exercise therapy leads to an increase in blood flow through various mechanisms which include but are not limited to arterial collateralization, increased vascular endothelial growth factor levels, increased release of nitric oxide, increased mitochondrial function leading to enhanced oxygen extraction ratios, or decreased endothelial inflammation [62,63].

5. Initial Evaluation

Before entering a home-based exercise program, PAD patients willing to be enrolled in a CR program should perform a baseline treadmill cardiac stress test at a specialized center to identify silent or residual ischemia which may lead to an acute event during CR programs. If the stress test indicates coronary ischemia, patients should be further evaluated before being enrolled in a CR program [61]. For PAD patients, a walking assessment is used to establish claudication thresholds and walking time which serve as parameters for determining exercise intensity and subsequently as prognostic indicators.

6. Cardiac Rehabilitation—Where Do We Stand

The main objectives of medical and endovascular treatment in PAD patients are to prevent any acute cardiovascular events as well as to improve quality of life appreciated indirectly through physical capacity, stress levels, depression, and social functioning [62].

The addressability or accessibility of PAD patients to CR programs is low and there are several possible explanations for this including the physician, the patient, and health care system levels. Current studies have repeatedly shown that for PAD patients, going to an exercise center for at least 3 times a week for supervised exercise is fairly difficult [3,4,62].

The beneficial role of CR (both functional and social) has been demonstrated in trials based on various exercise programs. Supervised exercise therapy improves cardiorespiratory fitness as well as over-ground and treadmill walking performance in PAD patients, along with a decrease in the mortality rate [63]. An increased exercise capacity is associated with a higher degree of cardiorespiratory fitness and therefore with a superior benefit on morbidity and mortality for PAD patients. CR programs with a low impact on symptomatology should be considered in patients with severe IC or walking disability who cannot participate in supervised programs or have no benefit from it. Women, patients with osteoarticular disease or end-stage renal disease have a higher risk of sedentary behavior [63–69].

Another issue is that some patients with PAD are reluctant about the efficacy of exercise, especially when it is uncomfortable or painful. The main inconvenience for patients with PAD is pain, followed by low walking capacity with few exercise facilities, and rest places. Alternative modes of exercise combined with low pain exercises increase adherence and participation in CR programs. Claudication increases during walking such that PAD patients need to rest during exercise [62,63,70–74].

Patients with intermittent claudication (IC) usually walk at a moderate speed up to the point of submaximal pain, resuming exercise after the pain has passed. With a total session duration of 30 min (more than 3 times per week), the main objective should be to determine the appearance of IC within 5 min and severe pain within 10 min following rests and repeats. Significant functional improvements are not achieved by walking to near-maximal pain as claudication pain leads to catabolic status with negative impact on skeletal muscles [75,76]. Exercise therapy plays an essential role in the therapeutic management of all patients with PAD except of those with acute arterial occlusion or critical limb ischemia with infection [77].

7. Cardiac Rehabilitation Programs

7.1. Treadmill Exercise

CR programs based on either supervised treadmill exercise or home-based walking exercise improve walking ability in PAD patients. A total of 3 randomized trials in which a number of 493 patients diagnosed with PAD were included, demonstrated that home-based walking exercise programs combined with behavioral change techniques improves the 6-min walk test performance more than supervised treadmill exercise interventions (45–54 m vs. 33–35 m) as well as walking ability [62,76].

In 1995, Gardner et al. performed a meta-analysis of 21 studies on PAD patients and concluded that supervised treadmill walking improved maximum treadmill walking distance from 125.9 ± 57.3 m to 351.2 ± 188.7 m ($p < 0.001$, increase by 179%) and pain-free treadmill walking distance from 325.8 ± 148.1 m to 723.3 ± 591.5 m ($p < 0.001$, increase by 122%) [78]. They also identified that increases in the distances to onset and to maximal claudication pain during treadmill exercise are independently related to three essential parts of a CR program which can be considered predictors of the changes in claudication pain distances: claudication pain end point used during the exercise training program, the length of the program and the type of exercise. Based on the results from the meta-regression analysis, Gardner et al. concluded that the most effective exercise programs for patients with PAD include 3 sessions per week, 30 min each, at intensity close to the point of maximum or near-maximum pain onset during exercise for at least 6 months [76,79].

Later, in 2012, Fakhry et al. summarized in a meta-analysis the results of 25 randomized clinical trials of supervised walking CR programs in which 1054 symptomatic PAD patients were included. Improvements in both maximal walking distance and pain-free walking distance were achieved in supervised walking exercise group (increase of 180 m, 95% CI, 130–230 m and 128 m, 95% CI, 92–165 m), compared to the control group without exercise. A total of 60% of the trials had a total duration between 12 and 26 weeks. In a subgroup analysis based on the length of the programs (<12 weeks, 12–26 weeks and >26 weeks), using multivariate meta-regression, Fakhry et al. observed the tendency to greater mean improvement in maximum walking distance and pain free walking distance in programs with a duration of 12–26 weeks, that those shorter or longer duration, suggesting a maximum benefit for PAD patients enrolled in CR programs with a duration between 12 and 26 weeks, with 3 sessions per week and 30 min of walking in each session [78,80]. The meta-analysis demonstrated significant functional benefits in treadmill walking performance in patients with PAD after finalizing the supervised CR program, with the reported results suggesting a lower final effect than the one obtained in the meta-analysis reported by Gardner et al. since it included only randomized trials [75,76].

7.1.1. Intensity

It is unclear if walking up to the maximal ischemic pain or rather just up to pain's onset is more beneficial for the PAD patients, moreover since available trials did not show any difference between these strategies [70].

7.1.2. Program Length

Fakhry et al. reported significant increases in both pain-free treadmill walking time and maximum treadmill walking time regardless of CR program length (short: 4–11 weeks, medium: 12–26 weeks and long: more than 26 weeks). After 4 weeks of exercise the initial benefit is observed while the maximum benefit of the treadmill walking is achieved after 8–12 weeks of CR. The parameters associated with the 6-min walk test gradually improve due to the fact that the treadmill exercise trains the patient to measure the treadmill walking result (Figure 3) [76].

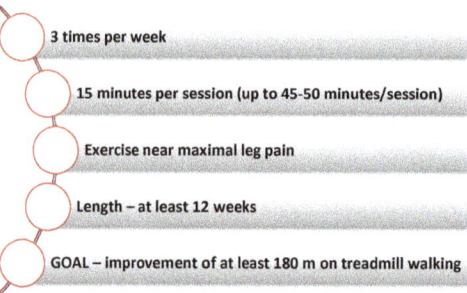

Figure 3. Key elements of an exercise training program.

7.2. Home-Based Walking Exercise

Home-based exercise, including behavioral changes, represents an acceptable and affordable alternative to supervised weekly exercise, as it saves time and effort associated to traveling to a dedicated medical center. Home-based walking exercises are more accessible and easier to accept for PAD patients. Regardless of the presence or absence of symptoms, they improve both treadmill walking performance and walk distance in the 6MWT [76,79,81,82]. Furthermore, the benefits of home-based walking sessions in improving both walking capacity and the 6MWT parameters, compared to supervised treadmill exercise programs, have been proved since 2011 through several randomized trials.

Gardner et al. enrolled 119 men and women with symptomatic PAD to 1 of 3 groups (supervised treadmill exercise, home-based walking exercise, or a control group) for a total duration of 12 weeks. Patients randomly assigned to the home exercise group were instructed to perform exercise or walking sessions of at least 45 min, 3 times a week, at their own pace. At the 12-week follow-up, both patients from the home exercise group and the supervised exercise group showed a remarkable improvement in walking distance without the occurrence of IC and an increasing of the maximum exercise duration compared to the control group. Adherence to exercise programs was similar in the 2 groups ($p > 0.05$). PAD patients from the first group walked longer in each session ($p < 0.001$), but with a slower cadence than those in the second group ($p < 0.05$), resulting in a similar total exercise volume, expressed as MET-minutes ($p > 0.05$). No statistically significant differences were identified between the two groups in terms of treadmill walking ability or perimeter walking without IC. It is noteworthy that the study had an overall dropout rate of 23% in the home exercise group and 28% in the supervised treadmill exercise group, pointing difficulties in terms of adherence for PAD patients especially during COVID-19 pandemic [76,79,81–84].

In the second randomized trial, Gardner et al. randomized 180 PAD patients with IC to 3 groups: supervised treadmill exercise, home-based walking exercise and a light resistance training group. At the 12-week follow-up, patients from the first group had significantly greater improvement in treadmill walking compared to home-based exercise (192 ± 190 s vs. 110 ± 193 s vs. 22 ± 159 s) and in the time to onset of claudication pain on the treadmill (+170 s vs. +104 s vs. +17 s). Beneficial effects were also observed in the 6-minute walking distance which improved by 45 m in the home-based walking group compared to 15 m in the supervised treadmill group and 4 m in the control one [80,83].

The Group Oriented Arterial Leg Study (GOALS) is the only randomized clinical trial of home-based exercise for PAD patients both with and without IC. A total of 192 participants were randomized to a Group Mediated Cognitive Behavioral (GMCB) intervention group or to a control group. The GMCB intervention methods included social cognitive behavioral change theory and group support in order to increase adherence to home-based walking exercise programs and therefore increasing the walking performance. The intervention group had weekly meetings at the medical center with other PAD patients and a facilitator. At the 6 months follow-up, the intervention group had a significantly improved 6-minute walk performance compared to the control group (+42.4 m vs. 11.1 m). Improvements were also observed in the case of pain-free treadmill walking time (+1.01 min compared to the control group) and in maximum treadmill walking time. Support sessions were discontinued after the first 6 months, but the benefits on functional status persisted at the 12-month follow-up [82,85,86].

CR programs for PAD patients should be permanently adapted to the associated comorbidities and needs in order to achieve the desired results. The aim is to achieve a total exercise session duration of up to 50 min, with a gradual increase of 5 min each week, starting from a minimum duration of 30 min per session. The PAD patient should walk until close to reaching maximum leg pain. Even so, trials demonstrated that walking until the onset of intermittent claudication is also beneficial. Rest breaks are acceptable for PAD patients, with the recommendation to resume walking exercise as soon as leg pain has subsided (Table 3) [76,79,81–84].

Table 3. Change in Walking Distance after cardiac rehabilitation programs in patients with PAD. For PAD patients enrolled in different cardiac rehabilitation programs, there is a direct proportionality between duration and claudication onset distance or change in peak walking distance.

Supervised Program (Studies until 2021)	Claudication Onset Distance (Mean ± SD, %)	Peak Walking Distance (Mean ± SD, %)
12 weeks (8 studies)	156.60 ± 46.97 m (103%)	283.10 ± 69.32 m (79%)
24–52 weeks (7 studies)	251.23 ± 75.72 m (167%)	334.06 ± 78.14 m (92%)
Overall (15 studies)	203.93 ± 77.93 m (128%)	307.45 ± 75.58 m (82%)

Collins et al. also investigated the role of behavioral intervention methods on the adherence of PAD patients to home-based exercise programs. A total of 145 patients with PAD and diabetes were enrolled for 6 months and randomized into 2 groups: a behavioral intervention group vs. an attention control group. The patients from the first group had an individualized counseling session at enrollment, followed by a walking session weekly with an instructor and other patients with PAD at an exercise center and 3 days of walking at home (with a total of 50 min of exercise per session). All patients received bi-weekly phone calls, to evaluate progress in the first group. Compared to the previous study, at the six-month follow-up the investigators found no statistically significant differences in treadmill walking parameters between the two groups [34,82,87].

The impact of COVID-19 pandemic on home-based CR programmes has been assessed by Lamberti et al. in a study in which 83 patients with PAD were enrolled within 9-month before the lockdown. The physical activity consisted of twice a day 8 min sessions of slow and intermittent in-home walking. During lockdown, the patients received regular telehone questionnaires regarding general health, adherence to exercise program and evolution of symptoms. Only 80% of the PAD patients showed up for the follow-up after lockdown. The pain-free walking distance improved improved directly proportional to the time since enlistment before the lockdown ($p < 0.001$) regardless of gender and comorbidities. Improvements were also observed regarding body weight, blood pressure and ankle-brachial index [88].

7.3. Alternative Forms of Exercise–Ergometry, Cycling and Strength Training

7.3.1. Ergometry

Classic CR programs such as home-based walking exercise or supervised treadmill exercise have more entertaining or challenging alternatives such as cycling, strength training, and upper arm ergometry. Upper-limb exercise determine greater heart rate, intra-arterial blood pressure, and pulmonary ventilation than lower-limb exercise for a specific level of submaximal work [89–91]. Multiple randomized trials concluded that both upper- and lower-extremity ergometry have significantly functional benefits especially improving walking endurance in PAD [92].

Zwierska et al. randomized 104 PAD patients into 3 major groups: upper-limb aerobic ergometry, lower-limb aerobic ergometry and a non-exercise control group for a total duration of CR program of 6 months. Each patient performed 2 weekly exercise sessions consisting of 10 cycles of 2 min each of arm (or leg) ergometer cycling, followed by 2 min of rest, with a total duration of 20 min of exercise each session. At the 6-month follow-up, maximum walking distance increased in both upper-limb and lower-limb ergometry groups (29% in the first group and 31% the second group). A beneficial effect was also identified in the peak oxygen uptake, suggesting a link between walking endurance and cardiovascular fitness [84].

Another alternative exercise modality for patients with PAD and IC is arm cranking. Tew et al. randomized a total of 57 patients with IC to an arm-crank exercise group and a non-exercise control group. Patients were evaluated at baseline and at the 12 weeks follow-up. The results showed an incremental improvement to maximum exercise tolerance on both an arm-crank ergometer and a treadmill. In the study group, increases in walking distance (from 496 ± 250 to 661 ± 324 m) and VO2 maximal values (from 17.2 ± 2.7 to 18.2 ± 3.4 mL·kg^{-1} body mass·min^{-1}) were recorded in the treadmill walking test ($p < 0.05$). After training, an increase in time to reach minimum tissue O2 saturation (from 268 ± 305 s to 410 ± 366 s), as well as an increase in VO2 kinetics (from 44.7 ± 10.4 to 41.3 ± 14.4 s) and an increase in submaximal StO2 were observed during the treadmill walking test ($p < 0.05$). The increase in walking distance without the occurrence of IC as well as in maximum walking perimeter after arm crank exercise in patients with PAD is partly attributed to improved lower-limb oxygen delivery [93–95].

Walker et al. enrolled 67 patients with moderate and severe IC and randomized them in an upper-limb training group (26 patients), a lower-limb training group (26 patients) and a control group (15 patients). The patients from the training group had twice a week 40-min exercise sessions (2 min of exercise followed by 2 min of rest), for 6 weeks. At the follow-up, the pain free walking distance increased by 122% in the first group and by 93% in the second one ($p < 0.001$). Improvements have also been observed in the maximum walking distance which increased by 47% in the upper-limb group ($p < 0.05$) and by 50% in the lower-limb group ($p < 0.001$) [92,96].

7.3.2. Cycling

Lauret et al. included 135 patients from 5 studies that compared different training modalities, including supervised walking exercises. From the results, there was no statistically significant difference regarding reaching the maximum walking distance between supervised walking group and alternative training modalities (8.15 metabolic equivalent <METs>, 95% CI −2.63 to 18.94, $p > 0.05$, equivalent to an increase of 173 m, 95% CI −56 m to 401 m), on the treadmill without incline, for an average speed comparable to everyday life walking (3.2 km/h). At the same time, no statistically significant differences were observed for reaching the maximum walking perimeter without the occurrence of intermittent claudication (6.42 METs, 95% CI −1.52 to 14.36, $p > 0.05$, equivalent to an increase of 136 m, 95% CI −32 m to 304 m), with parameters associated with quality-of-life showing important improvements in both groups [95,97].

Sanderson et al. randomized 42 patients with PAD and IC in 3 different groups: a treadmill exercise group, a cycling one and a control group. The first 2 groups trained 3 times a week for 6 weeks. The exercise consisted of 10 rounds of 2 min each of exercise, interspersed with 2-min breaks, for a total of 20 min of exercise in each session. Cycle training improved cycle performance, but not walking performance. Treadmill training improved maximal and pain-free exercise time by 25%, but not maximal cycle time. While IC in the calf was the most common symptom in the first group, patients from the second group noted the presence of IC in the quadriceps. The difference between the location of IC in the two modes of exercise raise the observation that cycling would not have functional benefit for PAD patients who frequently experience IC in the calf. Sanderson et al. observed in PAD patients with limiting symptoms during cycling and walking a cross-transfer effect between the training modes, suggesting cycling as an exercise alternative for these patients [92,98].

7.3.3. Resistance Exercise Training

Strength training has been used in randomized trials to demonstrate the potential role in improving walking performance for PAD patients. Studies have shown that lower extremity strength training improves maximal treadmill walking time compared to a non-exercise control group. Following resistance training there is an increase in lower extremity skeletal muscle capillary growth. McDermott et al. reported no change in the primary outcome of 6-min walk distance in the strength training group, while supervised treadmill exercise significantly improved 6-min walk distance, leading to the conclusion that walking exercise is more effective than strength training in PAD patients [76,92].

Gomes et al. conducted a randomized controlled trial to evaluate resistance training effects on cardiovascular function. In total, 30 patients with PAD were enrolled and randomly allocated to a control group (15 patients, stretching and relaxation exercises) or resistance training group (15 patients, 3 sets of 10 repetitions of eight whole body exercises, with a pause of 2 minutes between sets). Resting and 24-h blood pressure (BP), cardiac output, systemic vascular resistance, and autonomic variables were obtained before and after 12 weeks of intervention. There was a time effect reduction in heart rate as well as statistically significant changes in cardiac autonomic modulation ($p < 0.05$). In the resistance training group, the blood pressure variability decreased in systolic, diastolic, and mean values ($p < 0.05$). At the 12-week follow-up the resting and 24-h BP, or their hemodynamic and autonomic determinants did not change in the PAD patients enrolled in the training group. However, there were decreases in BP variability, indicating that it could be considered as an alternative to reduce cardiovascular risk (Table 4) [64,76,92,99–101].

Table 4. Comparison of resistance exercise training programs in patients with PAD. High-intensity resistance training is superior to treadmill exercise training in improving walking distance in PAD patients.

	Group	Increase Peak Walking Distance (Mean)	Increase Claudication Onset Distance (Mean)	Increase the 6 Minute Walking Test Distance (Mean)
Hiatt et al. [99]	Resistance Training Group	+107 m	+1.6 m	NA
	Treadmill Walking Group	+273 m	+182	NA
McDermott et al. [76]	Resistance Training Group	+129 m	+102	−3 m
	Treadmill Walking Group	+212 m	+156 m	+20.9 m
Ritti-Dias et al. [100]	Resistance Training Group	+157 m *	+146	-
	Treadmill Walking Group	+149 m *	+127 m	-
Parmenter et al. [101]	Resistance Training Group	-	-	+60 m
	Treadmill Walking Group	-	-	−9 m

* Change with high-intensity resistance training.

8. Revascularization and Supervised Exercise

Supervised exercise therapy has a positive impact on both functional capacity and quality of life in patients with IC. The combined effect seems to be superior, regardless of order (in a parallel or sequential manner). Studies have shown that supervised exercise has an additional functional benefit in PAD patients. In the randomized ERASE trial, patients were divided into 2 groups: those who received endovascular therapy and additional participated in supervised exercise programs (106 patients) and those who were enrolled in CR programs based on supervised exercise alone (106 patients). At the one-year follow-up, in both groups functional and quality-of-life related parameters were achieved, both groups showing improvements in maximal walking distance, pain-free walking distance, and quality of life.

Fakhry et al. demonstrated in a randomized clinical trial of 212 patients (allocated to either endovascular revascularization and supervised exercise or supervised exercise only) that among patients with IC, at the 1-year follow-up, endovascular revascularization followed by supervised exercise had better results in walking distances and quality-of-life scores than supervised exercise only [76,83,102]. Combined therapy was associated with a significantly greater improvement in maximum walking distance and pain-free walking distance. Regarding the maximum walking distance, the mean difference between groups was of 282 m (improvement of 1237 m vs. 955 m) (99% CI, 60–505 m). The mean difference was bigger for the pain-free walking distance (408 m) with an improvement of 1120 m, respectively 712 m for the combined therapy group or supervised exercise only (99% CI, 195–622 m). A significantly greater improvement was also obtained in the disease-specific VascuQol score in both groups (1.34 in the combination therapy group vs. 0.73 in the exercise group; mean difference, 0.62 [99% CI, 0.20–1.03]) as well as in the score for the SF-36 physical functioning questionnaire (22.4 vs. 12.6 respectively; mean difference, 9.8 [99% CI, 1.4–18.2]). There were no differences in the SF-36 domains of physical role functioning, bodily pain and general health perceptions between the 2 groups [65,102].

9. Effects on Biomarkers after Cardiac Rehabilitation

Home-based exercise programs which can be overseen have multiple vascular benefits in patients with PAD with IC by ameliorating various biological markers such as blood glucose, circulating markers of endogenous antioxidant capacity, as well as inflammatory related to the inflammation of the endothelium. E-selectin, intercellular adhesion molecule (ICAM-1), and interleukin-6 (IL-6) are some of the vascular and inflammatory biomarkers reduced after participating in supervised CR programs [102]. Previous studies suggested that this effect is inconsistent on high-sensitivity C-reactive protein (hsCRP) [103,104]. Gardner et al. randomized 114 patients into 3 groups different by the intensity of exercise programs and supervision level: home-based programs, supervised programs of low intensity resistance training and walking to mild-to-moderate claudication pain for 12 weeks as well as a control group with unsupervised training. Upon enrolment and after finishing the 12-week exercise program, treadmill performance was evaluated, as well as circulating inflammatory biomarkers known the endothelial effects of circulating factors, using a cell culture-based bioassay on primary human arterial endothelial cells [83,104]. The statistical analysis showed that treadmill peak walking time improved in all groups except the control group ($p < 0.05$). Cultured endothelial cell apoptosis diminished in the first group (exercises performed at home, $p < 0.05$). The antioxidant capacity of the hydroxyl radical (HORAC) ($p < 0.05$) increased as well as the vascular endothelial growth factor A levels (VEGF-A) ($p < 0.05$). In particular, it was observed in patients from the first group that E-selectin ($p < 0.05$) and blood glucose levels decreased (decreases insulin resistance) ($p < 0.05$) [105–108].

In patients with IC or other PAD symptoms, the daily activity level was positively correlated with HORAC, suggesting that ischemic preconditioning is ameliorated after daily exercises due to circulating antioxidant capacity. At the eight weeks follow-up E-selectin levels decreased after supervised exercise training, but studies suggest that this result is inconsistent. Gardner et al. demonstrated that VEGF-A serum levels increased after home-based exercise. A non-randomized exercise trial found that VEGF-A serum levels were not modified after following non-supervised exercise programs but increased initially with a program of supervised exercise. Previous studies demonstrated that skeletal muscle VEGF-A was decreased following 12 weeks of supervised exercise and remained unchanged after a home-based exercise program [83].

Blood glucose level decreases after a home-based exercise program and does not change following supervised treadmill exercise. Its clinical significance is based on elevated fasting glucose in patients with symptomatic PAD being associated with peripheral circulation, patient-perceived walking ability, health-related quality of life, and sedentary behavior. Diabetes impairs microcirculation and metabolic syndrome impairs ABI and claudication distances in patients with PAD [106–111].

10. Physical Exercise Protocols

Exercise is an essential part of CR programs for PAD patients, with most functional benefits being observed in the first 2–3 months of supervised training. Current studies demonstrated that PAD patients should exercise at least 3 times every week, for about 30–60 min, with a total training volume of 1500–2000 min. Wang et al. demonstrated that exercise using an individual leg plantar flexion ergometer improves peak oxygen consumption (VO2), at that level 78% of the patients enrolled being symptom free [111,112].

Lower-limb resistance training based on knee extension and leg press/curl exercises is an alternative to treadmill workout, studies suggesting that 1 repetition maximum improves the 6-minute walk test distance by 12.4 m comparing to a control group. PAD patients who associate important comorbidities such as heart failure and have difficulties in walking on a treadmill can use lower-limb resistance training as an alternative to treadmill exercises with a diminished total effect on symptoms, especially IC [111–113].

Upper-limb cycle ergometry ameliorates the walking distance and can be used as an alternative training method in PAD patients with functional impairment due to symptoms associated with IC. Its positive effect on symptoms suggests the presence of a cross-training effect on the lower-limb through several adaptive mechanisms. Further studies are much needed to determine the physiological mechanism [114–116].

Pole striding involves both upper- and lower-limb exercises. Its functional benefit was illustrated in a randomized controlled trial by improving both peak VO2 and pain-free walking distance in comparison to placebo or vitamin E groups. Taking into consideration the fact that it involves both upper- and lower-limb muscles, this alternative method of training may have additional benefits which require further research. Which types of exercises have the maximum functional effect, in which combination or duration, are some of the main questions needed to be answered in the near future in order to determine the best strategy regarding CR programs with maximum benefit in reducing IC symptoms and improving the long-term prognosis [116–121].

11. Psychological and Social Outcome

CR programs have multiple functional benefits and a great impact on the psychosocial status, increasing quality of life, decreasing depression and anxiety as well as reducing the stress levels [26]. After being part of a CR program, PAD patients testified that their energy levels increased. Unfortunately, up until now, studies regarding PAD patients enrolled in different types of CR programs have offered little information about psychosocial outcomes and although exercise programs have positive impact on the quality of life, further research on this topic are needed [63,92].

Stauber et al. coordinated a study in which 529 patients were included in a comprehensive 12-week outpatient CR program. All of the patients fulfilled psychosocial questionnaires upon inclusion in the study and at the 12-week follow-up. Hospital Anxiety and Depression Scale questionnaire (HADS) was used for analyzing the depression and anxiety levels of PAD patients, while the positive and negative impact of the cardiovascular disease was monitored with the Global Mood Scale. Different health-related aspects with impact on the quality of life were measured with the SF-36 Health Survey. The 12-week follow-up proved that exercise training programs had multiple benefits on anxiety ($p < 0.001$) and negative affect ($p < 0.001$), as well as in bodily pain as a health-related quality of life marker ($p < 0.001$) [3,4,120,121]. The 6MWT distance is independently and statistically associated with better physical and social aspects of psycho-emotional status in people with IC [122]. In terms of mental health and quality of life, COVID-19 has a negative impact. PAD typically limits social activities and interpersonal relations.

De Donato et al. enrolled 102 patients with PAD and, through a questionnaire, evaluated the quality of life between the "No-COVID-19 period" (July–December 2019) and the pandemic time period (January–June 2020). An increase in pain intensity has been highlighted during SARS-CoV2 pandemic (from a mean score of 4.7 ± 2.9 to 6.3 ± 2.9, $p < 0.0001$) but without an increase in the consumption of analgesic drugs ($p = 0.15$). The overall lower-limb health status worsened ($p = 0.0001$) due to the restrictions which limited the possibility of walking outside combined with the fear of infection in public places. All of these aspect influence mental health and have caused among patients enrolled in the study an increasing of the feeling of fear associated with disease worsening ($p < 0.0001$) [123].

12. Conclusions

Physical exercise remains an important element of rehabilitation in patients with CVD. The management of PAD during the COVID-19 pandemic has been a major challenge for both patients and medical personnel. Supervised exercise therapy has a positive impact on both functional capacity and quality of life in PAD, although the combination with revascularization therapy seems to be even more effective. Improving functional capacity, increasing quality of life, and preventing depression are some of the benefits seen in patients with PAD included in CR programs.

Author Contributions: R.A., C.A.A. and O.M. contributed equally to this work; R.A. and O.M. wrote the paper; D.T.M.M. helped revise the language and review editing; F.M. selected the figures and revised the final script. All authors have equally contributed. All authors have read and agreed to the published version of the manuscript.

Funding: This research received no external funding.

Conflicts of Interest: The authors declare no conflict of interest.

References

1. Sandercock, G.R.H.; Cardoso, F.; Almodhy, M.; Pepera, G. Cardiorespiratory Fitness Changes in Patients Receiving Comprehensive Outpatient Cardiac Rehabilitation in the UK: A Multicentre Study. *Heart* **2013**, *99*, 785–790. [CrossRef]
2. Cowie, A.; Buckley, J.; Doherty, P.; Furze, G.; Hayward, J.; Hinton, S.; Jones, J.; Speck, L.; Dalal, H.; Mills, J. Standards and Core Components for Cardiovascular Disease Prevention and Rehabilitation. *Heart* **2019**, *105*, 510–515. [CrossRef]
3. Gerhard-Herman, M.D.; Gornik, H.L.; Barrett, C.; Barshes, N.R.; Corriere, M.A.; Drachman, D.E.; Fleisher, L.A.; Fowkes, F.G.R.; Hamburg, N.M.; Kinlay, S.; et al. 2016 AHA/ACC Guideline on the Management of Patients With Lower Extremity Peripheral Artery Disease: A Report of the American College of Cardiology/American Heart Association Task Force on Clinical Practice Guidelines. *Circulation* **2017**, *135*, e726–e779. [CrossRef]
4. Writing Committee Members; Gerhard-Herman, M.D.; Gornik, H.L.; Barrett, C.; Barshes, N.R.; Corriere, M.A.; Drachman, D.E.; Fleisher, L.A.; Fowkes, F.G.R.; Hamburg, N.M.; et al. 2016 AHA/ACC Guideline on the Management of Patients with Lower Extremity Peripheral Artery Disease: Executive Summary. *Vasc. Med.* **2017**, *22*, NP1–NP43. [CrossRef] [PubMed]
5. Moulson, N.; Bewick, D.; Selway, T.; Harris, J.; Suskin, N.; Oh, P.; Coutinho, T.; Singh, G.; Chow, C.-M.; Clarke, B.; et al. Cardiac Rehabilitation During the COVID-19 Era: Guidance on Implementing Virtual Care. *Can. J. Cardiol.* **2020**, *36*, 1317–1321. [CrossRef]
6. Ji, H.; Fang, L.; Yuan, L.; Zhang, Q. Effects of Exercise-Based Cardiac Rehabilitation in Patients with Acute Coronary Syndrome: A Meta-Analysis. *Med. Sci. Monit.* **2019**, *25*, 5015–5027. [CrossRef]
7. Besnier, F.; Gayda, M.; Nigam, A.; Juneau, M.; Bherer, L. Cardiac Rehabilitation During Quarantine in COVID-19 Pandemic: Challenges for Center-Based Programs. *Arch. Phys. Med. Rehabil.* **2020**, *101*, 1835–1838. [CrossRef]
8. Barretto, S.; Ballman, K.V.; Rooke, T.W.; Kullo, I.J. Early-Onset Peripheral Arterial Occlusive Disease: Clinical Features and Determinants of Disease Severity and Location. *Vasc. Med.* **2003**, *8*, 95–100. [CrossRef] [PubMed]
9. Mehta, A.; Dhindsa, D.S.; Hooda, A.; Nayak, A.; Massad, C.S.; Rao, B.; Makue, L.F.; Rajani, R.R.; Alabi, O.; Quyyumi, A.A.; et al. Premature Atherosclerotic Peripheral Artery Disease: An Underrecognized and Undertreated Disorder with a Rising Global Prevalence. *Trends Cardiovasc. Med.* **2021**, *31*, 351–358. [CrossRef]
10. Wu, Z.; McGoogan, J.M. Characteristics of and Important Lessons From the Coronavirus Disease 2019 (COVID-19) Outbreak in China: Summary of a Report of 72 314 Cases From the Chinese Center for Disease Control and Prevention. *JAMA* **2020**, *323*, 1239–1242. [CrossRef]
11. Frederix, I.; Vanhees, L.; Dendale, P.; Goetschalckx, K. A Review of Telerehabilitation for Cardiac Patients. *J. Telemed. Telecare* **2015**, *21*, 45–53. [CrossRef] [PubMed]
12. Thomas, R.J.; Beatty, A.L.; Beckie, T.M.; Brewer, L.C.; Brown, T.M.; Forman, D.E.; Franklin, B.A.; Keteyian, S.J.; Kitzman, D.W.; Regensteiner, J.G.; et al. Home-Based Cardiac Rehabilitation. *J. Am. Coll. Cardiol.* **2019**, *74*, 133–153. [CrossRef] [PubMed]
13. Babu, A.S.; Arena, R.; Ozemek, C.; Lavie, C.J. COVID-19: A Time for Alternate Models in Cardiac Rehabilitation to Take Centre Stage. *Can. J. Cardiol.* **2020**, *36*, 792–794. [CrossRef] [PubMed]
14. Gian Francesco, M.; Francesco, G.; Elio, V.; Francesco, F.; Marco, A. Cardiologia riabilitativa e prevenzione secondaria durante la pandemia COVID-19: Stato dell'arte e prospettive. *G. Ital. Cardiol.* **2020**, *20*, 527–528. [CrossRef]
15. Sandesara, P.B.; Dhindsa, D.; Khambhati, J.; Lee, S.K.; Varghese, T.; O'Neal, W.T.; Harzand, A.; Gaita, D.; Kotseva, K.; Connolly, S.B.; et al. Reconfiguring Cardiac Rehabilitation to Achieve Panvascular Prevention: New Care Models for a New World. *Can. J. Cardiol.* **2018**, *34*, S231–S239. [CrossRef] [PubMed]
16. Canadian Association of Cardiac Rehabilitation. *Canadian Guidelines for Cardiac Rehabilitation and Cardiovascular Disease Prevention: Translating Knowledge into Action*; Canadian Association of Cardiac Rehabilitation: Winnipeg, MB, Canada, 2009; ISBN 978-0-9685851-3-9.
17. Grace, S.L.; Turk-Adawi, K.; Santiago de Araújo Pio, C.; Alter, D.A. Ensuring Cardiac Rehabilitation Access for the Majority of Those in Need: A Call to Action for Canada. *Can. J. Cardiol.* **2016**, *32*, S358–S364. [CrossRef]
18. Pfaeffli Dale, L.; Whittaker, R.; Dixon, R.; Stewart, R.; Jiang, Y.; Carter, K.; Maddison, R. Acceptability of a Mobile Health Exercise-Based Cardiac Rehabilitation Intervention: A Randomized Trial. *J. Cardiopulm. Rehabil. Prev.* **2015**, *35*, 312–319. [CrossRef] [PubMed]
19. Marzolini, S.; Ghisi, G.L.d.M.; Hébert, A.-A.; Ahden, S.; Oh, P. Cardiac Rehabilitation in Canada During COVID-19. *CJC Open* **2021**, *3*, 152–158. [CrossRef] [PubMed]
20. Anderson, L.J.; Taylor, R.S. Cardiac Rehabilitation for People with Heart Disease: An Overview of Cochrane Systematic Reviews. *Int. J. Cardiol.* **2014**, *177*, 348–361. [CrossRef]
21. Anderson, L.; Oldridge, N.; Thompson, D.R.; Zwisler, A.-D.; Rees, K.; Martin, N.; Taylor, R.S. Exercise-Based Cardiac Rehabilitation for Coronary Heart Disease. *J. Am. Coll. Cardiol.* **2016**, *67*, 1–12. [CrossRef] [PubMed]

22. Wong, W.P.; Feng, J.; Pwee, K.H.; Lim, J. A Systematic Review of Economic Evaluations of Cardiac Rehabilitation. *BMC Health Serv. Res.* **2012**, *12*, 243. [CrossRef] [PubMed]
23. Jin, K.; Khonsari, S.; Gallagher, R.; Gallagher, P.; Clark, A.M.; Freedman, B.; Briffa, T.; Bauman, A.; Redfern, J.; Neubeck, L. Telehealth Interventions for the Secondary Prevention of Coronary Heart Disease: A Systematic Review and Meta-Analysis. *Eur. J. Cardiovasc. Nurs.* **2019**, *18*, 260–271. [CrossRef] [PubMed]
24. Batalik, L.; Filakova, K.; Batalikova, K.; Dosbaba, F. Remotely Monitored Telerehabilitation for Cardiac Patients: A Review of the Current Situation. *World J. Clin. Cases* **2020**, *8*, 1818–1831. [CrossRef] [PubMed]
25. Batalik, L.; Dosbaba, F.; Hartman, M.; Batalikova, K.; Spinar, J. Benefits and Effectiveness of Using a Wrist Heart Rate Monitor as a Telerehabilitation Device in Cardiac Patients: A Randomized Controlled Trial. *Medicine* **2020**, *99*, e19556. [CrossRef]
26. Stefanakis, M.; Batalik, L.; Papathanasiou, J.; Dipla, L.; Antoniou, V.; Pepera, G. Exercise-Based Cardiac Rehabilitation Programs in the Era of COVID-19: A Critical Review. *Rev. Cardiovasc. Med.* **2021**, *22*, 1143–1155. [CrossRef]
27. O'Doherty, A.F.; Humphreys, H.; Dawkes, S.; Cowie, A.; Hinton, S.; Brubaker, P.H.; Butler, T.; Nichols, S. How Has Technology Been Used to Deliver Cardiac Rehabilitation during the COVID-19 Pandemic? An International Cross-Sectional Survey of Healthcare Professionals Conducted by the BACPR. *BMJ Open.* **2021**, *11*, e046051. [CrossRef] [PubMed]
28. Abell, B.; Glasziou, P.; Hoffmann, T. The Contribution of Individual Exercise Training Components to Clinical Outcomes in Randomised Controlled Trials of Cardiac Rehabilitation: A Systematic Review and Meta-Regression. *Sports Med. Open* **2017**, *3*, 19. [CrossRef] [PubMed]
29. Mann, D.M.; Chen, J.; Chunara, R.; Testa, P.A.; Nov, O. COVID-19 Transforms Health Care through Telemedicine: Evidence from the Field. *J. Am. Med. Inform. Assoc.* **2020**, *27*, 1132–1135. [CrossRef]
30. Strain, T.; Wijndaele, K.; Brage, S. Physical Activity Surveillance Through Smartphone Apps and Wearable Trackers: Examining the UK Potential for Nationally Representative Sampling. *JMIR MHealth UHealth* **2019**, *7*, e11898. [CrossRef]
31. Hammill, B.G.; Curtis, L.H.; Schulman, K.A.; Whellan, D.J. Relationship Between Cardiac Rehabilitation and Long-Term Risks of Death and Myocardial Infarction Among Elderly Medicare Beneficiaries. *Circulation* **2010**, *121*, 63–70. [CrossRef] [PubMed]
32. Manson, J.J.; Crooks, C.; Naja, M.; Ledlie, A.; Goulden, B.; Liddle, T.; Khan, E.; Mehta, P.; Martin-Gutierrez, L.; Waddington, K.E.; et al. COVID-19-Associated Hyperinflammation and Escalation of Patient Care: A Retrospective Longitudinal Cohort Study. *Lancet Rheumatol.* **2020**, *2*, e594–e602. [CrossRef]
33. Bektas, A.; Schurman, S.H.; Franceschi, C.; Ferrucci, L. A Public Health Perspective of Aging: Do Hyper-Inflammatory Syndromes Such as COVID-19, SARS, ARDS, Cytokine Storm Syndrome, and Post-ICU Syndrome Accelerate Short- and Long-Term Inflammaging? *Immun. Ageing* **2020**, *17*, 23. [CrossRef] [PubMed]
34. Calabrese, M.; Garofano, M.; Palumbo, R.; Di Pietro, P.; Izzo, C.; Damato, A.; Venturini, E.; Iesu, S.; Virtuoso, N.; Strianese, A.; et al. Exercise Training and Cardiac Rehabilitation in COVID-19 Patients with Cardiovascular Complications: State of Art. *Life* **2021**, *11*, 259. [CrossRef] [PubMed]
35. Celis-Morales, C.A.; Welsh, P.; Lyall, D.M.; Steell, L.; Petermann, F.; Anderson, J.; Iliodromiti, S.; Sillars, A.; Graham, N.; Mackay, D.F.; et al. Associations of Grip Strength with Cardiovascular, Respiratory, and Cancer Outcomes and All Cause Mortality: Prospective Cohort Study of Half a Million UK Biobank Participants. *BMJ* **2018**, *361*, k1651. [CrossRef]
36. Zhao, H.-M.; Xie, Y.-X.; Wang, C. Recommendations for Respiratory Rehabilitation in Adults with Coronavirus Disease 2019. *Chin. Med. J.* **2020**, *133*, 1595–1602. [CrossRef]
37. Kamiya, K.; Hamazaki, N.; Matsue, Y.; Mezzani, A.; Corrà, U.; Matsuzawa, R.; Nozaki, K.; Tanaka, S.; Maekawa, E.; Noda, C.; et al. Gait Speed Has Comparable Prognostic Capability to Six-Minute Walk Distance in Older Patients with Cardiovascular Disease. *Eur. J. Prev. Cardiol.* **2018**, *25*, 212–219. [CrossRef] [PubMed]
38. Chinese Association of Rehabilitation Medicine; Respiratory Rehabilitation Committee of Chinese Association of Rehabilitation Medicine; Cardiopulmonary Rehabilitation Group of Chinese Society of Physical Medicine and Rehabilitation. Recommendations for respiratory rehabilitation of coronavirus disease 2019 in adult. *Zhonghua Jie He He Hu Xi Za Zhi Zhonghua Jiehe He Huxi Zazhi Chin. J. Tuberc. Respir. Dis.* **2020**, *43*, 308–314. [CrossRef]
39. Tang, N.; Bai, H.; Chen, X.; Gong, J.; Li, D.; Sun, Z. Anticoagulant Treatment Is Associated with Decreased Mortality in Severe Coronavirus Disease 2019 Patients with Coagulopathy. *J. Thromb. Haemost.* **2020**, *18*, 1094–1099. [CrossRef]
40. Madjid, M.; Safavi-Naeini, P.; Solomon, S.D.; Vardeny, O. Potential Effects of Coronaviruses on the Cardiovascular System: A Review. *JAMA Cardiol.* **2020**, *5*, 831–840. [CrossRef]
41. Panzavolta, C.; Zalunardo, B.; Irsara, S.; Ferretto, L.; Visonà, A. Peripheral Artery Disease, the 'Lost Syndrome' during Lockdown for COVID-19: A Report of Three Cases. *Med. Int.* **2021**, *1*, 15. [CrossRef]
42. Gonzalez Cañas, E.; Gimenez Gaibar, A.; Rodriguez Lorenzo, L.; Castro Rios, J.G.; Martinez Toiran, A.; Bella Cueto, M.R.; Bella Burgos, P.; Espasa Soley, M. Acute Peripheral Arterial Thrombosis in COVID-19. Role of Endothelial Inflammation. *Br. J. Surg.* **2020**, *107*, e444–e445. [CrossRef]
43. Smolderen, K.G.; Lee, M.; Arora, T.; Simonov, M.; Mena-Hurtado, C. Peripheral Artery Disease and COVID-19 Outcomes: Insights from the Yale DOM-CovX Registry. *Curr Probl Cardiol.* **2021**, *7*, 101007. [CrossRef]
44. Qiu, S.; Cai, X.; Yin, H.; Sun, Z.; Zügel, M.; Steinacker, J.M.; Schumann, U. Exercise Training and Endothelial Function in Patients with Type 2 Diabetes: A Meta-Analysis. *Cardiovasc. Diabetol.* **2018**, *17*, 64. [CrossRef]
45. Ashor, A.W.; Lara, J.; Siervo, M.; Celis-Morales, C.; Mathers, J.C. Effects of Exercise Modalities on Arterial Stiffness and Wave Reflection: A Systematic Review and Meta-Analysis of Randomized Controlled Trials. *PLoS ONE* **2014**, *9*, e110034. [CrossRef]

46. Lavie, C.J.; Arena, R.; Swift, D.L.; Johannsen, N.M.; Sui, X.; Lee, D.; Earnest, C.P.; Church, T.S.; O'Keefe, J.H.; Milani, R.V.; et al. Exercise and the Cardiovascular System: Clinical Science and Cardiovascular Outcomes. *Circ. Res.* **2015**, *117*, 207–219. [CrossRef]
47. Arias-Fernández, P.; Romero-Martin, M.; Gómez-Salgado, J.; Fernández-García, D. Rehabilitation and Early Mobilization in the Critical Patient: Systematic Review. *J. Phys. Ther. Sci.* **2018**, *30*, 1193–1201. [CrossRef]
48. Jones, H.; Taylor, C.E.; Lewis, N.C.S.; George, K.; Atkinson, G. Post-Exercise Blood Pressure Reduction Is Greater Following Intermittent Than Continuous Exercise and Is Influenced Less by Diurnal Variation. *Chronobiol. Int.* **2009**, *26*, 293–306. [CrossRef] [PubMed]
49. Boff, W.; da Silva, A.M.; Farinha, J.B.; Rodrigues-Krause, J.; Reischak-Oliveira, A.; Tschiedel, B.; Puñales, M.; Bertoluci, M.C. Superior Effects of High-Intensity Interval vs. Moderate-Intensity Continuous Training on Endothelial Function and Cardiorespiratory Fitness in Patients With Type 1 Diabetes: A Randomized Controlled Trial. *Front. Physiol.* **2019**, *10*, 450. [CrossRef]
50. Molmen-Hansen, H.E.; Stolen, T.; Tjonna, A.E.; Aamot, I.L.; Ekeberg, I.S.; Tyldum, G.A.; Wisloff, U.; Ingul, C.B.; Stoylen, A. Aerobic Interval Training Reduces Blood Pressure and Improves Myocardial Function in Hypertensive Patients. *Eur. J. Prev. Cardiol.* **2012**, *19*, 151–160. [CrossRef] [PubMed]
51. Casonatto, J.; Goessler, K.F.; Cornelissen, V.A.; Cardoso, J.R.; Polito, M.D. The Blood Pressure-Lowering Effect of a Single Bout of Resistance Exercise: A Systematic Review and Meta-Analysis of Randomised Controlled Trials. *Eur. J. Prev. Cardiol.* **2016**, *23*, 1700–1714. [CrossRef]
52. Yamamoto, S.; Hotta, K.; Ota, E.; Mori, R.; Matsunaga, A. Effects of Resistance Training on Muscle Strength, Exercise Capacity, and Mobility in Middle-Aged and Elderly Patients with Coronary Artery Disease: A Meta-Analysis. *J. Cardiol.* **2016**, *68*, 125–134. [CrossRef]
53. Yang, L.-L.; Yang, T. Pulmonary Rehabilitation for Patients with Coronavirus Disease 2019 (COVID-19). *Chronic Dis. Transl. Med.* **2020**, *6*, 79–86. [CrossRef]
54. Lewis, L.K.; Williams, M.T.; Olds, T.S. The Active Cycle of Breathing Technique: A Systematic Review and Meta-Analysis. *Respir. Med.* **2012**, *106*, 155–172. [CrossRef]
55. Ozalp, O.; Inal-Ince, D.; Cakmak, A.; Calik-Kutukcu, E.; Saglam, M.; Savci, S.; Vardar-Yagli, N.; Arikan, H.; Karakaya, J.; Coplu, L. High-intensity Inspiratory Muscle Training in Bronchiectasis: A Randomized Controlled Trial. *Respirology* **2019**, *24*, 246–253. [CrossRef]
56. Vitacca, M.; Carone, M.; Clini, E.M.; Paneroni, M.; Lazzeri, M.; Lanza, A.; Privitera, E.; Pasqua, F.; Gigliotti, F.; Castellana, G.; et al. Joint Statement on the Role of Respiratory Rehabilitation in the COVID-19 Crisis: The Italian Position Paper. *Respiration* **2020**, *99*, 493–499. [CrossRef]
57. Rawstorn, J.C.; Gant, N.; Rolleston, A.; Whittaker, R.; Stewart, R.; Benatar, J.; Warren, I.; Meads, A.; Jiang, Y.; Maddison, R. End Users Want Alternative Intervention Delivery Models: Usability and Acceptability of the REMOTE-CR Exercise-Based Cardiac Telerehabilitation Program. *Arch. Phys. Med. Rehabil.* **2018**, *99*, 2373–2377. [CrossRef]
58. Rosen, K.; Patel, M.; Lawrence, C.; Mooney, B. Delivering Telerehabilitation to COVID-19 Inpatients: A Retrospective Chart Review Suggests It Is a Viable Option. *HSS J.* **2020**, *16*, 64–70. [CrossRef]
59. Sari, D.M.; Wijaya, L.C.G. Cardiac Rehabilitation via Telerehabilitation in COVID-19 Pandemic Situation. *Egypt. Heart J.* **2021**, *73*, 31. [CrossRef]
60. Ribeiro, F.; Santos, M. Exercise-Based Cardiac Rehabilitation in COVID-19 Times: One Small Step for Health Care Systems, One Giant Leap for Patients. *Rev. Esp. Cardiol. Engl. Ed.* **2020**, *73*, 969–970. [CrossRef]
61. Hamburg, N.M.; Balady, G.J. Exercise Rehabilitation in Peripheral Artery Disease: Functional Impact and Mechanisms of Benefits. *Circulation* **2011**, *123*, 87–97. [CrossRef]
62. Tran, B. Assessment and Management of Peripheral Arterial Disease: What Every Cardiologist Should Know. *Heart Br. Card. Soc.* **2021**, *107*, 1835–1843. [CrossRef]
63. Lamberti, N.; López-Soto, P.J.; Guerzoni, F.; Napoli, N.; Gasbarro, V.; Zamboni, P.; Tsolaki, E.; Taddia, M.C.; Rodríguez-Borrego, M.A.; Manfredini, R.; et al. Changes in Exercise Capacity and Risk of All-Cause Mortality in Patients with Peripheral Artery Disease: A 10-Year Retrospective Cohort Study. *Intern. Emerg. Med.* **2020**, *15*, 289–298. [CrossRef]
64. Gomes, A.P.F.; Correia, M.A.; Soares, A.H.G.; Cucato, G.G.; Lima, A.H.R.A.; Cavalcante, B.R.; Sobral-Filho, D.C.; Ritti-Dias, R.M. Effects of Resistance Training on Cardiovascular Function in Patients With Peripheral Artery Disease: A Randomized Controlled Trial. *J. Strength Cond. Res.* **2018**, *32*, 1072–1080. [CrossRef]
65. Akerman, A.P.; Thomas, K.N.; van Rij, A.M.; Body, E.D.; Alfadhel, M.; Cotter, J.D. Heat Therapy vs. Supervised Exercise Therapy for Peripheral Arterial Disease: A 12-Wk Randomized, Controlled Trial. *Am. J. Physiol.-Heart Circ. Physiol.* **2019**, *316*, H1495–H1506. [CrossRef]
66. Lamberti, N.; Straudi, S.; Lissia, E.; Cavazzini, L.; Buja, S.; Manfredini, R.; Basaglia, N.; Manfredini, F. Home-Based Exercise for Elderly Patients with Intermittent Claudication Limited by Osteoarticular Disorders—Feasibility and Effectiveness of a Low-Intensity Programme. *Vasa* **2018**, *47*, 227–234. [CrossRef]
67. Malagoni, A.M.; Catizone, L.; Mandini, S.; Soffritti, S.; Manfredini, R.; Boari, B.; Russo, G.; Basaglia, N.; Zamboni, P.; Manfredini, F. Acute and Long-Term Effects of an Exercise Program for Dialysis Patients Prescribed in Hospital and Performed at Home. *J. Nephrol.* **2008**, *21*, 871–878.

68. Manfredini, F.; Mallamaci, F.; D'Arrigo, G.; Baggetta, R.; Bolignano, D.; Torino, C.; Lamberti, N.; Bertoli, S.; Ciurlino, D.; Rocca-Rey, L.; et al. Exercise in Patients on Dialysis: A Multicenter, Randomized Clinical Trial. *J. Am. Soc. Nephrol.* **2017**, *28*, 1259–1268. [CrossRef]
69. Manfredini, R.; Lamberti, N.; Manfredini, F.; Straudi, S.; Fabbian, F.; Rodriguez Borrego, M.A.; Basaglia, N.; Carmona Torres, J.M.; Lopez Soto, P.J. Gender Differences in Outcomes Following a Pain-Free, Home-Based Exercise Program for Claudication. *J. Womens Health* **2019**, *28*, 1313–1321. [CrossRef]
70. Thomas, S.G.; Marzolini, S.; Lin, E.; Nguyen, C.H.; Oh, P. Peripheral Arterial Disease: Supervised Exercise Therapy Through Cardiac Rehabilitation. *Clin. Geriatr. Med.* **2019**, *35*, 527–537. [CrossRef]
71. McDermott, M.M. Exercise Rehabilitation for Peripheral Artery Disease: A REVIEW. *J. Cardiopulm. Rehabil. Prev.* **2018**, *38*, 63–69. [CrossRef]
72. Parmenter, B.J.; Dieberg, G.; Smart, N.A. Exercise Training for Management of Peripheral Arterial Disease: A Systematic Review and Meta-Analysis. *Sports Med.* **2015**, *45*, 231–244. [CrossRef] [PubMed]
73. Nguyen, C.H.; Marzolini, S.; Oh, P.; Thomas, S.G. Entering Cardiac Rehabilitation With Peripheral Artery Disease: A Retrospective Comparison to Coronary Artery Disease. *J. Cardiopulm. Rehabil. Prev.* **2020**, *40*, 255–262. [CrossRef]
74. McDermott, M.M.; Kibbe, M.R. Improving Lower Extremity Functioning in Peripheral Artery Disease: Exercise, Endovascular Revascularization, or Both? *JAMA* **2017**, *317*, 689–690. [CrossRef] [PubMed]
75. Fakhry, F.; van de Luijtgaarden, K.M.; Bax, L.; den Hoed, P.T.; Hunink, M.G.M.; Rouwet, E.V.; Spronk, S. Supervised Walking Therapy in Patients with Intermittent Claudication. *J. Vasc. Surg.* **2012**, *56*, 1132–1142. [CrossRef] [PubMed]
76. McDermott, M.M.; Ades, P.; Guralnik, J.M.; Dyer, A.; Ferrucci, L.; Liu, K.; Nelson, M.; Lloyd-Jones, D.; Van Horn, L.; Garside, D.; et al. Treadmill Exercise and Resistance Training in Patients with Peripheral Arterial Disease with and without Intermittent Claudication: A Randomized Controlled Trial. *JAMA* **2009**, *301*, 165–174. [CrossRef]
77. Yasu, T. Comprehensive Cardiac Rehabilitation Program for Peripheral Arterial Diseases. *J. Cardiol.* **2021**. [CrossRef]
78. Gardner, A.W.; Poehlman, E.T. Exercise Rehabilitation Programs for the Treatment of Claudication Pain. A Meta-Analysis. *JAMA* **1995**, *274*, 975–980. [CrossRef] [PubMed]
79. Sami, F.; Ranka, S.; Lippmann, M.; Weiford, B.; Hance, K.; Whitman, B.; Wright, L.; Donaldson, S.; Boyer, B.; Gupta, K. Cardiac Rehabilitation in Patients with Peripheral Arterial Disease after Revascularization. *Vascular* **2021**, *29*, 350–354. [CrossRef]
80. McDermott, M.M. Exercise Training for Intermittent Claudication. *J. Vasc. Surg.* **2017**, *66*, 1612–1620. [CrossRef] [PubMed]
81. Li, Y.; Li, Z.; Chang, G.; Wang, M.; Wu, R.; Wang, S.; Yao, C. Effect of Structured Home-Based Exercise on Walking Ability in Patients with Peripheral Arterial Disease: A Meta-Analysis. *Ann. Vasc. Surg.* **2015**, *29*, 597–606. [CrossRef] [PubMed]
82. McDermott, M.M.; Liu, K.; Guralnik, J.M.; Criqui, M.H.; Spring, B.; Tian, L.; Domanchuk, K.; Ferrucci, L.; Lloyd-Jones, D.; Kibbe, M.; et al. Home-Based Walking Exercise Intervention in Peripheral Artery Disease: A Randomized Clinical Trial. *JAMA* **2013**, *310*, 57–65. [CrossRef]
83. Gardner, A.W.; Parker, D.E.; Montgomery, P.S.; Blevins, S.M. Step-Monitored Home Exercise Improves Ambulation, Vascular Function, and Inflammation in Symptomatic Patients With Peripheral Artery Disease: A Randomized Controlled Trial. *J. Am. Heart Assoc.* **2014**, *3*, e001107. [CrossRef]
84. Zwierska, I.; Walker, R.D.; Choksy, S.A.; Male, J.S.; Pockley, A.G.; Saxton, J.M. Upper- vs Lower-Limb Aerobic Exercise Rehabilitation in Patients with Symptomatic Peripheral Arterial Disease: A Randomized Controlled Trial. *J. Vasc. Surg.* **2005**, *42*, 1122–1130. [CrossRef] [PubMed]
85. McDermott, M.M.; Guralnik, J.M.; Criqui, M.H.; Ferrucci, L.; Liu, K.; Spring, B.; Tian, L.; Domanchuk, K.; Kibbe, M.; Zhao, L.; et al. Unsupervised Exercise and Mobility Loss in Peripheral Artery Disease: A Randomized Controlled Trial. *J. Am. Heart Assoc.* **2015**, *4*, e001659. [CrossRef]
86. McDermott, M.M.; Guralnik, J.M.; Criqui, M.H.; Ferrucci, L.; Zhao, L.; Liu, K.; Domanchuk, K.; Spring, B.; Tian, L.; Kibbe, M.; et al. Home-Based Walking Exercise in Peripheral Artery Disease: 12-Month Follow-up of the GOALS Randomized Trial. *J. Am. Heart Assoc.* **2014**, *3*, e000711. [CrossRef] [PubMed]
87. Collins, T.C.; Lunos, S.; Carlson, T.; Henderson, K.; Lightbourne, M.; Nelson, B.; Hodges, J.S. Effects of a Home-Based Walking Intervention on Mobility and Quality of Life in People with Diabetes and Peripheral Arterial Disease: A Randomized Controlled Trial. *Diabetes Care* **2011**, *34*, 2174–2179. [CrossRef]
88. Lamberti, N.; Straudi, S.; Manfredini, R.; De Giorgi, A.; Gasbarro, V.; Zamboni, P.; Manfredini, F. Don't Stop Walking: The in-Home Rehabilitation Program for Peripheral Artery Disease Patients during the COVID-19 Pandemic. *Intern. Emerg. Med.* **2021**, *16*, 1307–1315. [CrossRef]
89. Allen, T.J. *Textbook of Work Physiology: Physiological Bases of Exercise*, 4th ed.; Human Kinetics: Champaign, IL, USA, 2004; Volume 56, p. 248. [CrossRef]
90. Bobbert, A.C. Physiological Comparison of Three Types of Ergometry. *J. Appl. Physiol.* **1960**, *15*, 1007–1014. [CrossRef]
91. Stenberg, J.; Astrand, P.O.; Ekblom, B.; Royce, J.; Saltin, B. Hemodynamic Response to Work with Different Muscle Groups, Sitting and Supine. *J. Appl. Physiol.* **1967**, *22*, 61–70. [CrossRef]
92. Treat-Jacobson, D.; McDermott, M.M.; Bronas, U.G.; Campia, U.; Collins, T.C.; Criqui, M.H.; Gardner, A.W.; Hiatt, W.R.; Regensteiner, J.G.; Rich, K.; et al. Optimal Exercise Programs for Patients With Peripheral Artery Disease: A Scientific Statement From the American Heart Association. *Circulation* **2019**, *139*, e10–e33. [CrossRef]

93. Bronas, U.G.; Treat-Jacobson, D.; Leon, A.S. Comparison of the Effect of Upper Body-Ergometry Aerobic Training vs Treadmill Training on Central Cardiorespiratory Improvement and Walking Distance in Patients with Claudication. *J. Vasc. Surg.* **2011**, *53*, 1557–1564. [CrossRef] [PubMed]
94. Tew, G.; Nawaz, S.; Zwierska, I.; Saxton, J.M. Limb-Specific and Cross-Transfer Effects of Arm-Crank Exercise Training in Patients with Symptomatic Peripheral Arterial Disease. *Clin. Sci.* **2009**, *117*, 405–413. [CrossRef] [PubMed]
95. Lauret, G.J.; Fakhry, F.; Fokkenrood, H.J.P.; Hunink, M.G.M.; Teijink, J.A.W.; Spronk, S. Modes of Exercise Training for Intermittent Claudication. *Cochrane Database Syst. Rev.* **2014**, *4*, CD009638. [CrossRef] [PubMed]
96. Walker, R.D.; Nawaz, S.; Wilkinson, C.H.; Saxton, J.M.; Pockley, A.G.; Wood, R.F.M. Influence of Upper- and Lower-Limb Exercise Training on Cardiovascular Function and Walking Distances in Patients with Intermittent Claudication. *J. Vasc. Surg.* **2000**, *31*, 662–669. [CrossRef] [PubMed]
97. McGuigan, M.R.; Bronks, R.; Newton, R.U.; Sharman, M.J.; Graham, J.C.; Cody, D.V.; Kraemer, W.J. Resistance Training in Patients with Peripheral Arterial Disease: Effects on Myosin Isoforms, Fiber Type Distribution, and Capillary Supply to Skeletal Muscle. *J. Gerontol. A Biol. Sci. Med. Sci.* **2001**, *56*, B302–B310. [CrossRef]
98. Sanderson, B.; Askew, C.; Stewart, I.; Walker, P.; Gibbs, H.; Green, S. Short-Term Effects of Cycle and Treadmill Training on Exercise Tolerance in Peripheral Arterial Disease. *J. Vasc. Surg.* **2006**, *44*, 119–127. [CrossRef] [PubMed]
99. Hiatt, W.R.; Wolfel, E.E.; Meier, R.H.; Regensteiner, J.G. Superiority of Treadmill Walking Exercise versus Strength Training for Patients with Peripheral Arterial Disease. Implications for the Mechanism of the Training Response. *Circulation* **1994**, *90*, 1866–1874. [CrossRef]
100. Ritti-Dias, R.M.; Wolosker, N.; de Moraes Forjaz, C.L.; Carvalho, C.R.F.; Cucato, G.G.; Leão, P.P.; de Fátima Nunes Marucci, M. Strength Training Increases Walking Tolerance in Intermittent Claudication Patients: Randomized Trial. *J. Vasc. Surg.* **2010**, *51*, 89–95. [CrossRef]
101. Parmenter, B.J.; Raymond, J.; Dinnen, P.; Lusby, R.J.; Fiatarone Singh, M.A. High-Intensity Progressive Resistance Training Improves Flat-Ground Walking in Older Adults with Symptomatic Peripheral Arterial Disease. *J. Am. Geriatr. Soc.* **2013**, *61*, 1964–1970. [CrossRef] [PubMed]
102. Saetre, T.; Enoksen, E.; Lyberg, T.; Stranden, E.; Jørgensen, J.J.; Sundhagen, J.O.; Hisdal, J. Supervised Exercise Training Reduces Plasma Levels of the Endothelial Inflammatory Markers E-Selectin and ICAM-I in Patients with Peripheral Arterial Disease. *Angiology* **2011**, *62*, 301–305. [CrossRef]
103. Nowak, W.; Mika, P.; Nowobilski, R.; Kusinska, K.; Bukowska-Strakova, K.; Nizankowski, R.; Jozkowicz, A.; Szczeklik, A.; Dulak, J. Exercise Training in Intermittent Claudication: Effects on Antioxidant Genes, Inflammatory Mediators and Proangiogenic Progenitor Cells. *Thromb. Haemost.* **2012**, *108*, 824–831. [CrossRef]
104. Fukase, T.; Dohi, T.; Kato, Y.; Chikata, Y.; Takahashi, N.; Endo, H.; Doi, S.; Nishiyama, H.; Okai, I.; Iwata, H.; et al. Long-Term Impact of High-Sensitivity C-Reactive Protein in Patients with Intermittent Claudication Due to Peripheral Artery Disease Following Endovascular Treatment. *Heart Vessels* **2021**, *36*, 1670–1678. [CrossRef] [PubMed]
105. Januszek, R.; Mika, P.; Konik, A.; Petriczek, T.; Nowobilski, R.; Niżankowski, R. The Effect of Treadmill Training on Endothelial Function and Walking Abilities in Patients with Peripheral Arterial Disease. *J. Cardiol.* **2014**, *64*, 145–151. [CrossRef]
106. Mika, P.; Wilk, B.; Mika, A.; Marchewka, A.; Niżankowski, R. The Effect of Pain-Free Treadmill Training on Fibrinogen, Haematocrit, and Lipid Profile in Patients with Claudication. *Eur. J. Cardiovasc. Prev. Rehabil.* **2011**, *18*, 754–760. [CrossRef] [PubMed]
107. Mika, P.; Spodaryk, K.; Cencora, A.; Mika, A. Red Blood Cell Deformability in Patients With Claudication After Pain-Free Treadmill Training. *Clin. J. Sport Med.* **2006**, *16*, 335–340. [CrossRef] [PubMed]
108. Dopheide, J.F.; Geissler, P.; Rubrech, J.; Trumpp, A.; Zeller, G.C.; Daiber, A.; Münzel, T.; Radsak, M.P.; Espinola-Klein, C. Influence of Exercise Training on Proangiogenic TIE-2 Monocytes and Circulating Angiogenic Cells in Patients with Peripheral Arterial Disease. *Clin. Res. Cardiol. Off. J. Ger. Card. Soc.* **2016**, *105*, 666–676. [CrossRef] [PubMed]
109. Jones, W.S.; Duscha, B.D.; Robbins, J.L.; Duggan, N.N.; Regensteiner, J.G.; Kraus, W.E.; Hiatt, W.R.; Dokun, A.O.; Annex, B.H. Alteration in Angiogenic and Anti-Angiogenic Forms of Vascular Endothelial Growth Factor-A in Skeletal Muscle of Patients with Intermittent Claudication Following Exercise Training. *Vasc. Med.* **2012**, *17*, 94–100. [CrossRef] [PubMed]
110. Tisi, P.V.; Hulse, M.; Chulakadabba, A.; Gosling, P.; Shearman, C.P. Exercise Training for Intermittent Claudication: Does It Adversely Affect Biochemical Markers of the Exercise-Induced Inflammatory Response? *Eur. J. Vasc. Endovasc. Surg.* **1997**, *14*, 344–350. [CrossRef]
111. Saxton, J.M.; Zwierska, I.; Blagojevic, M.; Choksy, S.A.; Nawaz, S.; Pockley, A.G. Upper- versus Lower-Limb Aerobic Exercise Training on Health-Related Quality of Life in Patients with Symptomatic Peripheral Arterial Disease. *J. Vasc. Surg.* **2011**, *53*, 1265–1273. [CrossRef] [PubMed]
112. Lin, E.; Nguyen, C.H.; Thomas, S.G. Completion and Adherence Rates to Exercise Interventions in Intermittent Claudication: Traditional Exercise versus Alternative Exercise—A Systematic Review. *Eur. J. Prev. Cardiol.* **2019**, *26*, 1625–1633. [CrossRef]
113. Delaney, C.L.; Miller, M.D.; Chataway, T.K.; Spark, J.I. A Randomised Controlled Trial of Supervised Exercise Regimens and Their Impact on Walking Performance, Skeletal Muscle Mass and Calpain Activity in Patients with Intermittent Claudication. *Eur. J. Vasc. Endovasc. Surg.* **2014**, *47*, 304–310. [CrossRef]
114. Mika, P.; Spodaryk, K.; Cencora, A.; Unnithan, V.B.; Mika, A. Experimental Model of Pain-Free Treadmill Training in Patients with Claudication. *Am. J. Phys. Med. Rehabil.* **2005**, *84*, 756–762. [CrossRef] [PubMed]

115. Barak, S.; Stopka, C.B.; Martinez, C.A.; Carmeli, E. Benefits of Low-Intensity Pain-Free Treadmill Exercise on Functional Capacity of Individuals Presenting with Intermittent Claudication Due to Peripheral Arterial Disease. *Angiology* **2009**, *60*, 477–486. [CrossRef] [PubMed]
116. Bulińska, K.; Kropielnicka, K.; Jasiński, T.; Wojcieszczyk-Latos, J.; Pilch, U.; Dąbrowska, G.; Skórkowska-Telichowska, K.; Kałka, D.; Zywar, K.; Paszkowski, R.; et al. Nordic Pole Walking Improves Walking Capacity in Patients with Intermittent Claudication: A Randomized Controlled Trial. *Disabil. Rehabil.* **2016**, *38*, 1318–1324. [CrossRef]
117. Collins, E.G.; O'Connell, S.; McBurney, C.; Jelinek, C.; Butler, J.; Reda, D.; Gerber, B.S.; Hurt, C.; Grabiner, M. Comparison of Walking With Poles and Traditional Walking for Peripheral Arterial Disease Rehabilitation. *J. Cardiopulm. Rehabil. Prev.* **2012**, *32*, 210–218. [CrossRef] [PubMed]
118. Beckitt, T.A.; Day, J.; Morgan, M.; Lamont, P.M. Calf Muscle Oxygen Saturation and the Effects of Supervised Exercise Training for Intermittent Claudication. *J. Vasc. Surg.* **2012**, *56*, 470–475. [CrossRef] [PubMed]
119. Stauber, S.; Guéra, V.; Barth, J.; Schmid, J.P.; Saner, H.; Znoj, H.; Grolimund, J.; von Känel, R. Psychosocial Outcome in Cardiovascular Rehabilitation of Peripheral Artery Disease and Coronary Artery Disease Patients. *Vasc. Med.* **2013**, *18*, 257–262. [CrossRef] [PubMed]
120. Mockford, K.A.; Gohil, R.A.; Mazari, F.; Khan, J.A.; Vanicek, N.; Coughlin, P.A.; Chetter, I.C. Effect of Supervised Exercise on Physical Function and Balance in Patients with Intermittent Claudication. *Br. J. Surg.* **2014**, *101*, 356–362. [CrossRef] [PubMed]
121. Guidon, M.; McGee, H. Exercise-Based Interventions and Health-Related Quality of Life in Intermittent Claudication: A 20-Year (1989–2008) Review. *Eur. J. Cardiovasc. Prev. Rehabil.* **2010**, *17*, 140–154. [CrossRef]
122. Golledge, J.; Leicht, A.S.; Yip, L.; Rowbotham, S.E.; Pinchbeck, J.; Jenkins, J.S.; Clapperton, R.; Dally-Watkins, M.; Fiatarone Singh, M.A.; Mavros, Y.; et al. Relationship Between Disease Specific Quality of Life Measures, Physical Performance, and Activity in People with Intermittent Claudication Caused by Peripheral Artery Disease. *Eur. J. Vasc. Endovasc. Surg.* **2020**, *59*, 957–964. [CrossRef]
123. De Donato, G.; Pasqui, E.; Alba, G.; Abu Leil, M.; Palasciano, G. The Limitations of Social Behaviour Imposed by CoVid-19 Impacted the Perception and the Evolution of Peripheral Arterial Disease Negatively. *Ann. Vasc. Surg.* **2021**, *73*, 107–113. [CrossRef] [PubMed]

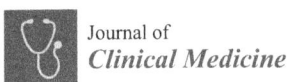

Review

TECAR Therapy Associated with High-Intensity Laser Therapy (Hilt) and Manual Therapy in the Treatment of Muscle Disorders: A Literature Review on the Theorised Effects Supporting Their Use

Dan Alexandru Szabo [1,2,*], Nicolae Neagu [1], Silvia Teodorescu [3], Corina Predescu [4], Ioan Sabin Sopa [5] and Loredana Panait [3]

1. Department of Human Movement Sciences, George Emil Palade University of Medicine, Pharmacy, Science, and Technology of Targu Mures, 540139 Targu Mures, Romania
2. Department ME1, Faculty of Medicine in English, George Emil Palade University of Medicine, Pharmacy, Science, and Technology of Targu Mures, 540139 Targu Mures, Romania
3. Department of Doctoral Studies, National University of Physical Education and Sports, 060057 Bucharest, Romania
4. Department of Special Motor and Rehabilitation Medicine, National University of Physical Education and Sports, 060057 Bucharest, Romania
5. Department of Environmental Sciences, Physics, Physical Education and Sports, "Lucian Blaga" University Sibiu, 550012 Sibiu, Romania
* Correspondence: dan-alexandru.szabo@umfst.ro

Abstract: Background: It has been estimated that between 30 and 50 per cent of all injuries that take place throughout participation in a sport are the consequence of soft tissue injuries, and muscle injuries are the primary cause of physical disability. Methods: The current literature review was designed between October 2021 and April 2022, according to the PRISMA standards, using the PubMed, Scopus, and Web of Science databases. At the screening stage, we eliminated articles that did not fit into the themes developed in all subchapters of the study ($n = 70$), articles that dealt exclusively with orthopaedics ($n = 34$), 29 articles because the articles had only the abstract visible, and 17 articles that dealt exclusively with other techniques for the treatment of musculoskeletal disorders. The initial search revealed 343 titles in the databases, from which 56 duplicate articles were automatically removed, and 2 were added from other sources. Results: The combination of these three techniques results in the following advantages: It increases joint mobility, especially in stiff joints, it increases the range of motion, accelerates tissue repair, improves tissue stability, and extensibility, and it reduces soft tissue inflammation (manual therapy). In addition, it decreases the concentration of pro-inflammatory mediators and improves capillary permeability, resulting in the total eradication of inflammation (HILT). It warms the deep tissues, stimulates vascularity, promotes the repose of tissues (particularly muscle tissue), and stimulates drainage (TECAR). Conclusions: TECAR therapy, combined with manual therapy and High-Intensity Laser therapy in treating muscle diseases, presented optimal collaboration in the recovery process of all muscle diseases.

Keywords: TECAR therapy; high-intensity laser therapy; manual therapy; muscle disorders

1. Introduction

According to the World Health Organization, rehabilitation can be defined as a set of interventions designed to optimise body functions and reduce the disabilities of people with various health problems [1]. Due to the awareness of the importance of functional rehabilitation and medical recovery, the availability of rehabilitation services is constantly increasing along with increases in chronic diseases and disabilities [2]. Medical recovery aims to increase the quality of life, ensuring, in addition to gaining functional independence, the reintegration of the individual into society, with this being one of the main objectives set at the beginning of the recovery program [3–5].

Muscle injuries are the most common cause of physical disability, especially in sports. It was calculated that 30 to 50% of all injuries that occur during the practice of a sport are the result of soft tissue injuries [6].

Although non-surgical athletes with muscle injuries have a fair prognosis after therapy [7], the severe implications of treatment failure can be dramatic for the athlete, delaying the resumption of physical exercise by weeks or even months [8].

Skeletal muscles represent about 40% of the cumulative load of the human body [9]. Its composition consists of several individual fibres grouped in a muscle spindle; this gives the skeletal muscle a striated appearance. A single muscle fibre comprises actin and myosin fibres covered by a cell membrane (sarcolemma). These fibres are the functional unit of the organ, leading to contraction and relaxation. There are two significant classifications of skeletal muscles: type I (slow oxidative) and type II (rapid contraction) [10]. The great diversity is based on their purpose; the structure of skeletal muscles causes differences in the pace and duration of contractions in distinct muscle groups [8]. Skeletal muscles endorse the skeletal system to maintain posture and control voluntary movement. Skeletal muscles also contribute to energy metabolism and storage [11]. Some muscles cross one or more joints to generate movement. Muscles with tonic or postural function are generally wide, flat, and localised muscles in a single joint, with a low rate of contraction and an ability to generate and maintain a high contractile force. They are generally located in deeper compartments [8].

Muscles crossing two joints have a higher speed of contraction and a more remarkable ability to change their length but a lower ability to withstand tension. They are generally located in superficial compartments [7].

The current classification of muscle lesions divides them into slight, mild, and severe, depending on the medical characteristics showcased [12].

Mild muscle injuries (grade I) affect only some muscle fibres, with slight oedema and embarrassment, escorted by a small or no lack of the ability or restriction of motion during muscular contraction; it is impossible to manipulate any muscle deficiency. Although the discomfort does not trigger a significant functional disability, the athlete is not recommended to continue activities due to the high risk of the magnitude of the trauma increasing.

Moderate muscle damage (grade II) causes more considerable muscle damage, with a noticeable function loss (ability to contract). A small muscular defect or gap can be palpated at the site of damage, and a minor nearby hematoma with potential bruising forms within two to four days. The progression of healing usually lasts two to three weeks, and after about a month, the convalescent might gradually resume physical exercise [11].

Injuries that extend severe injuries occur over the whole cross-section of the muscle, resulting in the total loss of muscular function and acute discomfort, regarding muscle injuries (grade III) and muscle tears, respectively. An apparent deficiency of muscle structure and bruising is usually extensive and placed at a distance from the site of the injury. The time required to heal such lesions varies between four and six weeks. This injury requires intensive rehabilitation for extended intervals (up to three or four months). Such people may experience discomfort for months following the procedure onset and treatment of the lesion.

Muscle cramps lead to continuous, involuntary, painful, and localised contractions of a whole muscle faction, a single muscle, or selected muscle fibres. In healthy persons or the presence of diseases, cramps might endure from seconds to a minute for idiopathic or recognised reasons. The palpation of the cramped muscle region reveals a knot [12].

Early mobilisation induces an increase in local vascularity in the lesion area, better regeneration of muscle fibres, and better parallel orientation of regenerated myofibrils concerning movement restrictions [13]. However, re-injury at the initial site of trauma is common if active mobilisation is started immediately after injury [14].

Muscle fatigue is one of the main factors in decreasing muscle flexibility [15]. Numerous ways have been used over time to facilitate muscle recovery from fatigue, such as stretching techniques [16], massages, active recovery [17], contrast water therapy [18], cryotherapy [19], and thermotherapy [20].

This review aims to highlight the multitude of physiotherapy procedures in treating muscle diseases in athletes and non-athletes. Due to the produced effects, manual therapy combined with HILT or TECAR therapy, or even all three therapies used in a treatment plan, can provide optimal muscle recovery in a shorter time; therefore, the use of combined and not isolated recovery procedures is a better alternative in muscle recovery.

Moreover, we aim to reintroduce manual therapy, a relatively old technique used in physical therapy, and to use it as an adjunct technique in the therapy of muscle conditions, along with new techniques used in physical therapy, such as HILT and especially TECAR therapy. Therefore, another purpose of this review is to combine the old techniques of physical therapy with the new ones to find a treatment plan that is as effective as possible in treating muscle diseases.

The novelty of this review consists of the association of these recovery procedures, specifically the association of manual therapy with HILT and TECAR therapy, which are usually used in isolation in the recovery process for the therapy of muscle diseases. TECAR therapy, in particular, produces many beneficial effects on the body and muscle tissue. As a result of the probes used in the treatment, we can obtain perfect collaboration with manual therapy techniques, such as passive mobilisations, massages, or manipulation.

2. Materials and Methods

The current literature review was developed between December 2021 and April 2022 utilising the PubMed, Scopus, and Web of Science databases in accordance with the PRISMA criteria. The search formula had the following form:

(a) PubMed: (TECAR therapy) OR (HILT Therapy) OR (Manual Therapy) OR (Muscle disorders) AND (Treatment) AND (High-frequency) OR (Electric stimulation) AND (Laser treatment) OR (Muscle pain) AND (Back) AND (Knee) OR (Therapeutic effect) OR (Ultrasound Therapy) OR (Mobilisation) OR (Physical Rehabilitation) OR (knee joint effusion) OR (elastography) OR (Hydrotherapy) OR (Electromyographic activity) OR (Musculoskeletal pain) OR (therapeutic ultrasound) OR (Pain intensity evaluation) OR (Massage therapy) OR (Capacitive and Resistive Electric Transfer).

(b) Scopus: (Therapeutic effect) OR (Ultrasound Therapy) OR (Mobilisation) OR (Physical Rehabilitation) OR (knee joint effusion) OR (elastography) OR (Hydrotherapy) OR (Electromyographic activity) OR (Musculoskeletal pain) OR (Therapeutic ultrasound) OR (Pain intensity evaluation) OR (TECAR therapy) OR (HILT therapy) OR (Manual Therapy) OR (Muscle disorders) AND (Massage therapy) OR (Capacitive and Resistive Electric Transfer).

(c) Web of Science: (Muscle pain) AND (Back) AND (Knee) OR (Therapeutic effect) OR (Ultrasound Therapy) OR (Mobilisation) OR (Physical Rehabilitation) OR (knee joint effusion) OR (elastography) (TECAR therapy) OR (HILT Therapy) OR (therapeutic ultrasound) OR (Pain intensity evaluation) OR (Massage therapy) OR (Manual Therapy) OR (Muscle disorders) AND (Treatment) AND (High-frequency) OR (Electric stimulation) AND (Laser treatment) OR (Capacitive and Resistive Electric Transfer).

The records identified from the databases using the key phrases described above were created using the reference management program EndNote (X9.3.3), and the duplicate articles were also deleted with its assistance.

After that, depending on the design of the studies, we aimed to include all articles of the following type: systematic reviews, meta-analyses, case-control studies, cross-sectional studies, literature reviews, and case reports, and we excluded expert opinions, letters to the editor, and conference reports.

A word form was used to extract the data. From each article that was selected and included for review, we extracted the information that we thought fit, according to each sub-chapter, to elaborate the present literature review.

The initial search identified 341 titles in the databases described above, of which 56 duplicate articles were automatically removed, and 2 were added from other sources. The remaining 343 articles were analysed by their titles and abstracts for relevance, resulting in another 70 studies being removed. Studies were excluded at the screening stage due to items that did not fit the themes developed in all subchapters of the study ($n = 70$) because the articles dealt exclusively with orthopaedics ($n = 34$). A total of 29 articles were excluded because the articles had only the abstract visible, and 17 articles exclusively treated other muscle disorder treatment techniques/disorders. The inclusion phase resulted in 137 articles included in the study. Figure 1 represents the complete PRISMA diagram.

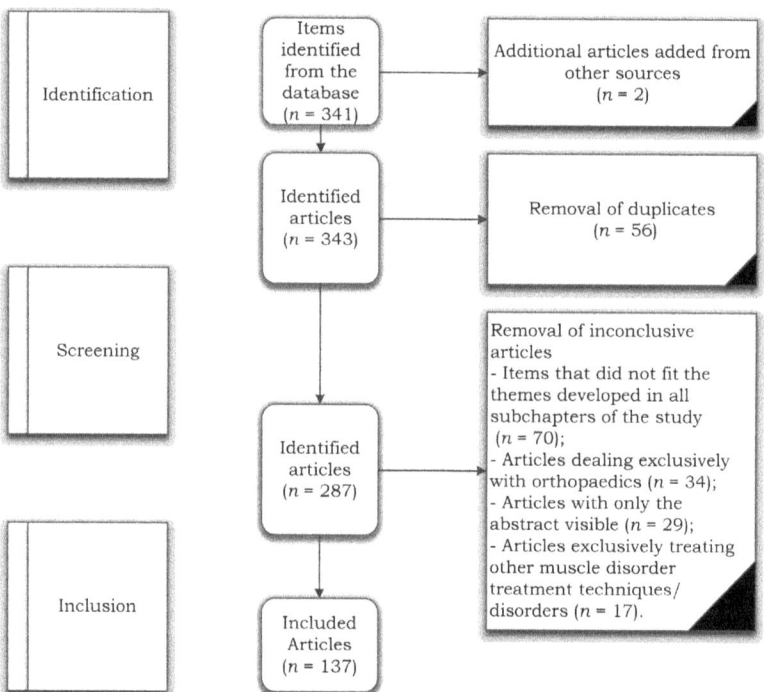

Figure 1. Study selection flowchart based on PRISMA criteria.

3. Manual Therapy vs. TECAR vs. HILT Therapy

Manual treatment is applied in treating muscle disorders in approximately every recovery program. Its effectiveness is debated, requiring much faster and more efficient recovery methods. Capacitive and resistive electrical transfer (TECAR), a type of diathermy, has recently been created as a form of deep thermotherapy and is used in sports medicine [21]. This device provides radio frequency energy, passing between an active and an inactive electrode and generating heat inside the body [22]. This therapy has shown that TECAR therapy is more efficient than a warm packet at increasing blood circulation, a conventional form of thermotherapy commonly used in clinical practice. Improving blood circulation plays an essential role in improving muscle recovery after fatigue. Thus, TECAR therapy can effectively improve muscle recovery after fatigue, which leads to maintaining and improving muscle flexibility [21].

Although manual therapy has been used to treat various muscle ailments since ancient times, for better and faster recovery of these ailments, more muscular stimulation is needed to have the desired effect (Figure 1). TECAR therapy combines manual therapy with deep thermotherapy, based on high-frequency electric currents, allowing for faster recovery of the affected muscles [23]. Due to the positive effects on muscle tissue, TECAR therapy seems to be a more helpful alternative in treating muscle disorders than conventional manual therapy, where cellular metabolism is not as strongly stimulated, and vasodilation is not as intense [24].

Laser treatment is a pain-free, non-invasive therapy that can be used to treat various clinical conditions. Laser therapy has significantly reduced acute and chronic pain, rheumatoid arthritis, chronic osteoarthritis, carpal tunnel syndrome, fibromyalgia, knee injuries, shoulder pain, and postoperative pain [25,26]. The reduction in pain after laser treatment results from its anti-inflammatory effects, the increased microcirculation and stimulation of immune processes, nerve regeneration, and the secretion of β-endorphins [26]. These properties of high-frequency laser therapy can influence the healing and regeneration of muscle tissue, which is recommended in most muscle conditions, both in athletes and non-athletes. Compared to TECAR therapy, HILT requires a much shorter treatment period, but its use with manual therapy does not seem as effective as using manual therapy with TECAR therapy because, as mentioned, the duration of treatment is short. The device does not allow a massage to be performed on the treated area. However, manipulations, massages, active or passive mobilisations, or other manual therapy techniques may be performed before or after HILT treatment (Figure 2).

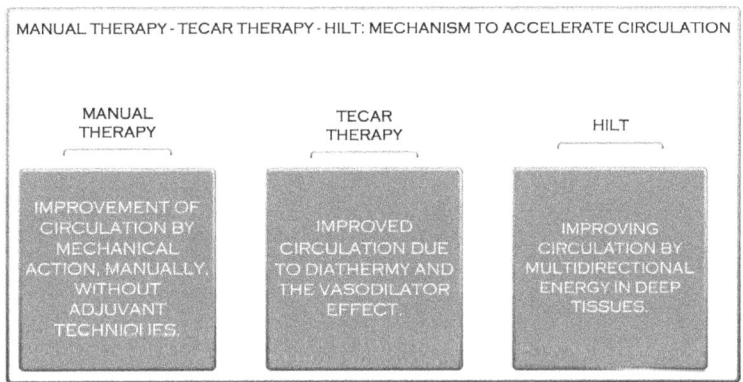

Figure 2. The acceleration mechanism of manual therapy, TECAR therapy, and HILT.

4. The Benefits of Manual Therapy in the Treatment of Muscle Diseases

Manual therapy is a technique used in physical therapy that involves using the hands to apply a force for therapeutic purposes. Manual therapy includes a wide range of therapeutic procedures such as massages, joint mobilisations/manipulations, myofascial releases, nerve manipulations, counter-stress, and acupressure (Figure 3).

Although manual therapy can be considered today as an old technique used by physical therapists, it remains one of the basic techniques of recovery used by physiotherapists in most recovery programs [27–29].

Manual therapy has been used to treat individuals suffering from various diseases since ancient times. The use of hands for healing dates back to the Old Testament and appears to have been advocated in the fifth century B.C. Hippocrates suggested the application of manual therapy, including traction prone to associated manipulation of the spine. He proved the efficiency of several manual approaches and proposed modifications to force delivery characteristics such as direction, pace, and frequency [30] (Figure 4).

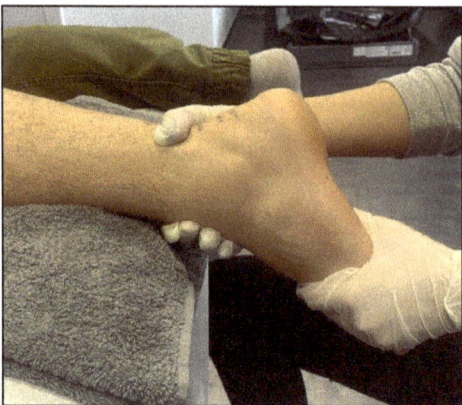

Figure 3. Manual therapy after Achilles tendinopathy.

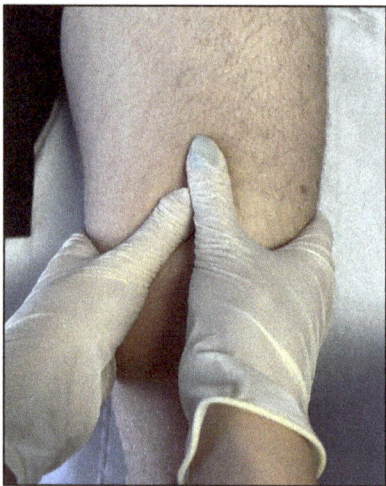

Figure 4. Relaxing massage of the thigh muscles (quadriceps).

Currently, manual treatment is applied in treating patients with various conditions, including musculoskeletal disorders, joint dysfunctions, spinal disorders, lymphedema, musculotendinous junction disorders, cystic fibrosis, and, most importantly, after immobilisation [31].

Among the essential benefits of manual therapy are modulating pain, increasing joint mobility, especially in stiff joints and increasing range of motion, accelerating tissue repair, improving tissue stability and extensibility, reducing soft tissue inflammation, reducing muscle tension, inducing relaxation, facilitating movement, and preparing segments for exercise therapy [32]

5. The Benefits of HILT Therapy in the Treatment of Muscle Disorders

As previously stated, laser treatment is a non-invasive treatment with minimal risk of adverse effects [33].

High-intensity laser treatment (HILT) is primarily employed in physio-kinetic therapy therapeutic regimens [34–36]. The primary distinction between HILT therapy and low-intensity laser therapy is that more giant beams (power > 500 mW) are irradiated to penetrate deeper, bringing a desired large amount of multidirectional energy into the deep tissues in a short time [37,38].

Moreover, the application techniques, the treatment time, and the cost of the device are different between these two generations of laser therapy [39,40]. However, High-Intensity Laser Therapy seems to have multiple benefits in the therapy of musculoskeletal disorders, precisely due to the effects produced in the tissues and also due to the reduction in recovery time [41–43].

HILT provides high tissue energy, and its optical energy forms dynamic vibrations. It then generates photochemical effects, such as increased mitochondrial oxidation, and it facilitates the formation of adenosine triphosphate (ATP) and ultimately leads to the rapid absorption of oedema and the elimination of exudates by increasing metabolism and blood circulation [44,45].

HILT has its own photomechanical, photothermal, and photochemical properties and has many therapeutic effects, including oedema reduction, analgesic effects, and physical stimulation [46]. Another benefit of HILT is its greater penetration strength and depth into deep tissues [47].

High-intensity laser treatment (HILT) has lately been applied in fundamental research and clinical rehabilitation practice with promising results (Watt-level performance) (high-intensity laser, Class IV laser) [48,49].

The high-intensity laser is usually used in two ways—pulsed and continuous [50]. Each mode impacts the tissue differently and triggers different therapeutic effects. The general therapeutic effects are bio-stimulation, pain relief, anti-inflammatory effects, superficial thermal effects, and muscle relaxation [51].

The high-intensity laser delivers energy to the cells, stimulates cellular metabolism, and promotes quicker resorption of the pro-inflammatory mediators [52].

Decreasing the concentration of pro-inflammatory mediators improves capillary permeability, resulting in the total eradication of inflammation and a speedier return to daily activities and sports. The high-intensity laser can provide extremely brief heartbeats at a maximum repetition rate [53]. This property can create real pressure. Pressure waves are transported through the tissue, stimulating the free nerve endings. According to the pain control mechanism, the mechanical stimulation of free nerve terminals causes their inhibition and, as a result, pain reduction [54]. The high-intensity laser has an immediate and long-lasting analgesic effect. The energy transferred by the continuous emission of HILT to the tissue causes superficial hyperthermia and vasodilation in the treated area [55]. As the blood perfusion increases, more blood passes through the treated area, and the muscles relax. In painful indications related to muscles, such as muscle injuries and muscle contracture, the patient feels immediate relief from discomfort triggered by muscle tension, and an amplitude of movement increases immediately [56].

Bio-stimulation means stimulating the body to help enhance healing and recovery at the cellular level. Mitochondria in cells metabolise oxygen. A cascade of respiratory enzymes processes oxygen and delivers it to ATP synthase, which synthesises the body's energy source—ATP. As a result of the quicker exchange of oxygen and metabolites caused by laser irradiation, more oxygen atoms reach the mitochondria. Mitochondria are further stimulated to synthesise ATP faster. ATP allows faster R.N.A. and D.N.A. synthesis and leads to faster recovery, faster healing, and reduced oedema in the treated area [57].

Class IV laser therapy (High-Intensity Laser Therapy) can be used to treat a range of ailments, including knee, hip, and ankle osteoarthritis; rheumatoid arthritis; shoulder pain impact syndromes [58]; hip or shoulder bursitis; lumbar disc degeneration; herniated disc sciatica; tendonitis; lateral and medial epicondylitis; plantar fasciitis; and a variety of muscle disorders [59]. Compared to other procedures used in medical recovery, high-frequency laser therapy has a limited range of contraindications, but they must be considered before starting therapy using this type of laser [60].

Pregnancy is one of the absolute contraindications of HILT therapy, and although, to date, there are no documents indicating that laser therapy is harmful to a pregnant woman or her child, to be safe and to prevent any problems, the use of this procedure in pregnancy is not recommended [61].

Another contraindication to HILT is cancer. Therefore, the use of laser therapy in a patient who has cancer or is suspected of having cancer is not recommended.

There are several relative contraindications, which each physiotherapist takes into account in the use of HILT therapy, including:

- Thyroid disorders: The thyroid is known to be sensitive to light, and although it has not yet been found to harm the thyroid gland, caution and careful dosing are recommended when using the laser [62].
- Clotting problems: Laser therapy affects blood clotting, so its use for patients with such problems should be consulted with a specialist or even replaced with another procedure [63].
- Children: Although there is no contraindication to the use of the laser for children, its dose should be adjusted according to weight [64].

6. The Benefits of TECAR Therapy in the Treatment of Muscle Diseases

TECAR treatment is a type of non-invasive electrothermal treatment classified as deep thermotherapy, based on the planning of electric tides in the field of radiofrequency, constituting a monopolar capacitive resistive radiofrequency of 448 kHz [65–68].

TECAR or capacitive-resistive electric transfer (CRet) is often used in the treatment of muscle, joint, and tendon injuries in traumatology and sports [67,69,70]. CRet is a non-invasive electrothermal treatment characterised as deep thermotherapy based on the application of electric flows in the radiofrequency range of 300 kHz to 1.2 MHz [71–73]. Unlike superficial thermotherapy, which has a relatively limited ability to penetrate muscle tissue [74,75], CRet may create heat in deep muscle tissue, hence increasing haemoglobin saturation [76]. Applying an electromagnetic field of around 0.5 MHz to the human body is responsible for this form of therapy's physiological effects. It has been discovered that an increase in blood perfusion is associated with a rise in body temperature, and other effects, such as cell proliferation, seem to be primarily connected to the current flow [77,78]. It has been demonstrated that cell growth begins at 0.00005 A per square millimetre [69,78].

TECAR therapy is characterised by its quick action and is employed in high-performance sports because it speeds up the recovery process [79,80]. Thermal changes in the neuro-motor arrangement caused by TECAR treatment generate vasodilation, minimise muscle spasms, speed up cellular metabolism, and increase the extensibility of soft tissues [81,82].

TECAR therapy is available in capacitive (C.A.P.) and resistive (R.E.S.) modes. These modes are often given with a number of immaculate medical steel probes (electrodes) that have been manufactured [83]. According to TECAR, depending on the strength of the treated tissue, the two treatment techniques generate various tissue responses. When a cushioning ceramic coating functions as a dielectric mechanism (C.A.P.) on the active electrode, energy transfer generates only heat to the superficial layers of tissue, with selective action on soft tissues with low impedance (rich in water), e.g., adipose matter, muscles, and the lymphatic system [79].

The resistive mode targets denser tissues with more fat and fibre (such as bones, ligaments, and tendons). High-frequency waves penetrate deep into tissues and cause a rise in exchange and temperature, and recent studies have shown the effects of radiofrequency on skin microcirculation and intramuscular blood flow [84,85] (Figure 5).

It should be noted that this new technology is a valuable tool in the therapy of different pathologies compared to other therapies used in recovery in terms of the presence and/or absence of specific positive effects while having distinctive features compared to conventional treatments [86]. It is guaranteed that TECAR therapy provides a balance between the therapist's manual capacity and the unique energy that this technology emanates from the tissues, thus giving therapists and patients much more satisfactory results [87]. Among its positive effects is better blood circulation, which removes inflammatory catabolites [88]. TECAR therapy also substantially improves blood circulation in the peritendinous region and increases haemoglobin saturation [89]. In addition, this therapy warms deep tissues, stimulates vascularity, promotes the repose of tissues (particularly muscle tissue), and stimulates drainage (oedema and hematoma) [90]. Based on these properties, TECAR treatment is employed in most orthopaedic pathologies before the start of rehabilitation exercises [91].

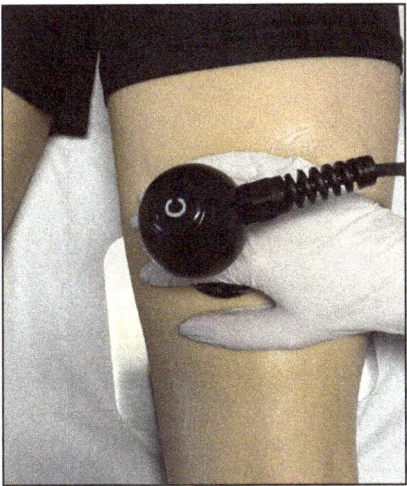

Figure 5. TECAR therapy in the treatment of hamstring muscles.

Among the physiological effects of TECAR therapy are increased extensibility of collagen tissue due to reduced viscosity; reduced discomfort because of anti-irritant behaviour or release of endorphins; reduced spasms and muscle contractions due to reduced activity of secondary efferents; faster dissociation of oxygen because of more available haemoglobin [92], accompanied by a reduction in the activation energy of important chemical and metabolic reactions; vasodilation with increased local blood flow, contributing to the replenishment of oxygen and nutrients; the elimination of catabolites; and accelerated reabsorption of hemorrhagic masses [93].

7. Manual Therapy–TECAR–HILT Therapy: Recommendations in the Treatment of Muscle Diseases

Capacitive-resistive electrical transfer therapy (TECAR) is mainly used to treat musculoskeletal injuries [93]. TECAR is a deep thermotherapy non-invasive electrothermal therapy. It uses electric currents at radio frequencies ranging from 300 kHz to 1.2 MHz [90]. This current can induce warming of deep muscle tissue, improving haemoglobin saturation, increasing deep and superficial blood flow, vasodilation, increased temperature, fluid removal, and cell proliferation [94]. Responses such as increased blood perfusion appear to be associated with increased temperature, which is generated due to a physical reaction generated by current flow (Joule effect) [95]. Increased cell escalation, nevertheless, seems to be associated with the current flow rather than increased temperature. Precisely due to these effects produced by TECAR therapy, it seems ideal for treating all muscle disorders compared to other therapies used, especially in athletes [96].

As mentioned above, TECAR therapy offers two different modes of treatment: capacitive and resistive. Different therapy methods trigger various tissue reactions relying on the treated tissue's strength [92]. A ceramic layer insulates the capacitive mode, and energy transfer creates heat in the surface tissue layer's selective action in the tissues with low impedance (rich in water). The resistive mode does not have an insulating ceramic layer; the radio frequency energy travels immediately across the physique in the orientation of the unemployed electrode, causing heat to be generated in the more profound and more resilient tissues (through lower water content) [97,98]. Given the benefits induced in part by each electrode (capacitive and resistive), the capacitive mode seems ideal in the therapy of muscle injuries, muscle cramps, spasms, contractions, and myalgias, as well as for reducing post-exercise muscle tension.

Unlike surface thermotherapy, which has a minimal ability to reach muscle tissue, TECAR therapy can generate heat in deep muscle tissue, improving haemoglobin saturation [99]. The physiological effects of this sort of therapy are caused by exposing the human body to an electromagnetic field of around 0.5 MHz. This approach has improved blood circulation, deep and surface temperatures, vasodilation, lymphatic effects, and increased cell proliferation [100]. An increase in blood strain has been noticed and is related to rising temperatures, but other effects—such as cell proliferation—seem to be mainly related to the stream of the current [101].

The mechanism of action of HILT Is not precise. It is considered to have both photochemical and photothermal effects, resulting in an anti-inflammatory, anti-edematous, analgesic, and repairing treatment. It is suspected that the analgesic influences of HILT are based on various mechanisms of action, such as slowing down the transmission of pain stimuli and increasing the production of morphine-mimetic substances in the body [102].

This treatment provides changes in blood flow and an expansion in the permeability of blood vessels and accelerates the response of cellular metabolism [103]. Furthermore, the photochemical consequences of HILT can promote collagen formation in the structure of tendons as well as enhance bloodstream and vascular resistance permeability, causing anti-inflammatory effects [104]. Thus, HILT can support the maintenance of the destroyed tissue and eliminate painful stimuli. Regarding muscle disorders, HILT is recommended in their treatment precisely because of the effects produced, initially to relieve pain and accelerate the healing process of affected muscle tissue [105].

Manual therapy appears to have been utilised in the treatment of muscle ailments since ancient times, with physio-kinetic therapists using it from the acute stages of the disease before thermotherapy and electrotherapy became widespread [106]. The manipulation of muscle tissue primarily helps to increase elasticity and prevent muscle atrophy and joint stiffness caused by trauma [107,108]. However, massages, especially in the severe phase of muscle injuries, are recommended and have many beneficial effects in the therapy of muscle contractures [109]. Passive, active, passive–active, and active–passive mobilisations are among the most used manual therapy techniques in the therapy of muscle diseases, being included in the protocol for the use of muscle diseases [110]. These techniques must be launched as quickly as necessary because, with their help, we can prevent the installation of joint stiffness and deficits [111] (Figure 6).

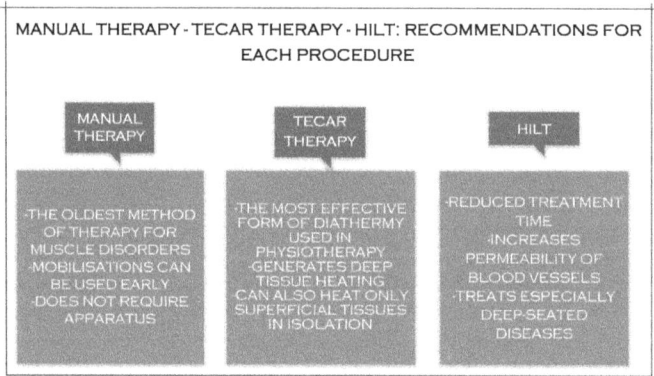

Figure 6. The advantages of recommending manual therapy, TECAR, and HILT therapy.

8. Manual Therapy–TECAR–HILT Therapy: Methods of Use in the Treatment of Muscle Diseases

Skeletal muscles allow people to move and perform daily activities. They play a crucial role in respiratory mechanics and help maintain posture and balance. They also protect vital organs in the body [112].

Various medical conditions result from abnormal skeletal muscle function [113]; these conditions include myopathies, paralysis, myasthenia gravis, urinary and/or intestinal incontinence, ataxia, weakness, tremors, and other disorders [114]. Nerve diseases can cause neuropathy and skeletal muscle dysfunction. Furthermore, skeletal muscle/tendon ruptures can occur acutely in high-level athletes or recreational sport participants and can cause a significant disability in all patients, regardless of activity status [115,116].

TECAR therapy is one of the most beneficial treatments used in muscle diseases due to the multitude of positive effects it brings to muscle tissue [117] (Figure 7).

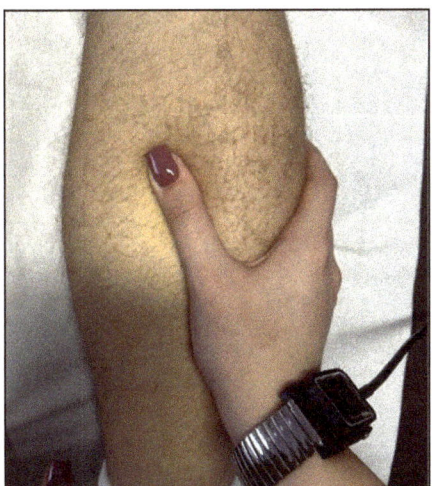

Figure 7. TECAR therapy with massaging calf muscles.

Moreover, TECAR therapy has several uses for the better healing of muscle tissue. One of these is the one used by TECAR Winback therapy, where the positive electrode consists of a bracelet that the therapist places around his or her radio-carpal joint, using his or her hand to perform the treatment. This function offers the therapist better manipulation of the muscle tissue, working passively with the patient to mobilise the joint and simultaneously combining manual therapy with TECAR therapy. TECAR therapy also has fixed applicators, which are fixed in the patient in the proximity of the disease, thus offering the therapist the possibility of performing a complex treatment, combining the advantageous influences of diathermy with manual therapy and passive therapy mobilisations.

HILT (High-Intensity Laser Therapy) is a convenient, non-invasive, and painless way that improves joint mobility [118], stimulates adequate tissue deepening [119], and offers anti-inflammatory, analgesic, and other valuable benefits in tissue healing [120]. In addition, the anti-inflammatory, anti-edematous, and analgesic effects are practical in the first treatment sessions [121]. Treatment sessions are short and recommended to be conducted daily for a faster effect. Depending on the brand of laser used, HILT can be used both in direct contact with the skin and at a distance of a few millimetres from it. The patient feels a warm sensation in the treated region, which is easily tolerated.

Another benefit of HILT, for which its use is recommended, is given by the depth at which the laser penetrates the tissue, having the ability to penetrate superficial tissues, reaching the site of the lesion to be treated [122–124].

HILT is a therapy used in isolation and in combination with other thermotherapy and electrotherapy procedures [125,126]. Moreover, in most cases, it is used in conjunction with physical therapy, playing an essential role in modulating pain [127].

Manual therapy is used in all muscle diseases, isolation, and other procedures, especially in physiotherapy [128,129]. Its method of use varies, and the physiotherapist can use his or her own hands to treat various devices/accessories specific to physical therapy. Massaging is very effective in muscle contractions, fatigue, or muscle loads [130] combined with cryotherapy. Physiotherapists also use joint mobilisation during physical therapy sessions to maintain joint mobility and to make the patient aware of the movement, especially after surgery [131].

Manual resistance physical exercises performed by the physiotherapist are also practical, especially in the early stages of recovery from muscle disorders, before the patient can perform exercises with elastic or mechanical resistance.

9. Manual Therapy–TECAR–HILT Therapy: Contraindications

Although TECAR therapy currently seems to be one of the most beneficial therapies used in recovery [132], it also has several contraindications that the therapist must consider before starting treatment with this type of therapy [133]. Among the most critical absolute contraindications of TECAR therapy are patients with pacemakers, patients with hemorrhagic gastrointestinal ulcers, patients with infusion pumps and electric cable implants, patients in the first six months of pregnancy, in the treatment of localised cancerous area/tumours, patients with allergic reactions to certain substances in the conductive cream, patients with deep-vein thrombosis, patients with uncontrolled ischemic heart disease, patients with local pulmonary embolism, patients with phlebitis, and for treating areas with bleeding or where the skin has partial or open wounds (Figure 7).

In addition to the contraindications of TECAR therapy, there are several precautions that the therapist must take into account when using this type of therapy. One of them is removing metallic materials from the patient, such as bracelets, earrings, and watches, especially from the area where the treatment is to be performed. It is also good to know that TECAR therapy is recommended for adults, as it can have adverse effects on growth cartilage, although this has not yet been demonstrated [134].

HILT also has several significant contraindications that physicians and physiotherapists should consider before recommending or performing a high-intensity laser treatment. As with TECAR therapy, pregnancy is a contraindication to high-intensity laser treatment, and although there is no evidence that laser therapy can harm the pregnant woman or the child, for safety reasons, this type of treatment is recommended in the case of pregnancy [135]. Cancer is also a contraindication in the case of HILT therapy, as it is in the case of other therapies, because the effects it can have on cancer cells are not known [136]. In some countries, however, such as France, the laser is used to treat mucosal pain (Figure 8).

Unlike other therapies, HILT is also recommended for patients with pacemakers, implants, screws and plaques and even for children [137].

Manual therapy a procedure with some of the fewest contraindications, and it can be used in almost any category of patient (Figure 8). However, it is recommended to avoid using it in patients with uncontrolled hypertension, mental problems, delirium, or epilepsy.

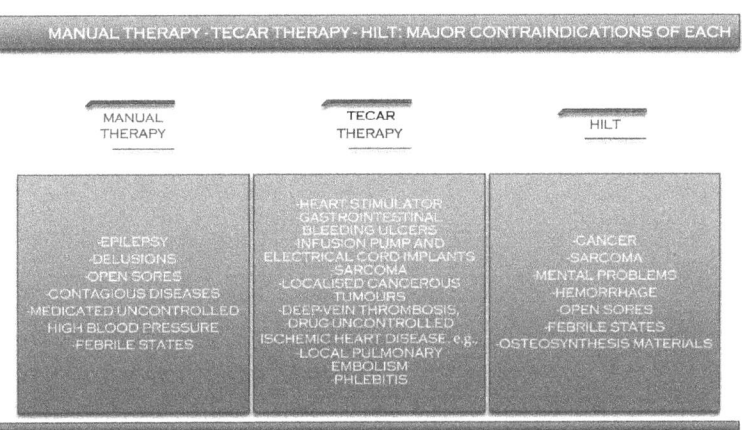

Figure 8. Contraindications of manual therapy, TECAR, and HILT therapy.

10. Limitations of the Study

This study is a description of the theoretical framework of how these techniques work rather than what has been demonstrated by research studies regarding valid research designs and reliable and valid outcome measures. Our research includes studies with various pathologies with which these therapeutic modalities are used, without going into the details of their effectiveness.

11. Conclusions

Given the many benefits that capacitive and resistive electrical transfer therapy has on muscle disorders, it should be integrated into most recovery protocols to enhance the healing process and to make rehabilitation faster and more straightforward.

However, manual therapy remains as one of the safest and most frequently used methods by physical therapists, with very few contraindications and allowing the therapist to feel and treat with his or her own hands. If combined, these therapies can have much better results, such as the effects of manual therapy (reducing muscle tension, inducing relaxation, and increasing mobility through passive movements performed by the physical therapist) along with the many effects resulting from TECAR muscle tissue therapy (increasing cellular metabolic processes, activating the body's natural repair processes, improving blood flow and improving pain), and also with the effects produced by HILT (accelerating cellular metabolism, faster resorption of pro-inflammatory mediators). HILT is also beneficial in treating muscle diseases, affecting blood circulation and cellular metabolism, thus accelerating tissue regeneration.

TECAR therapy combined with manual therapy in the management of muscle disorders provides excellent coordination in the healing process, which is beneficial for all types of muscle diseases. Through the variety of benefits of each one, more positive results can be obtained, unless used specifically with only one of the two therapies. Moreover, manual therapy combined with HILT appears to have similar effects to the previous combination but is not as pleasant for the patient. TECAR therapy with HILT and manual therapy may be ideal for treating muscle disorders to accelerate healing, maintain tissue elasticity and joint mobility, and restore the patient to pre-injury fitness.

Author Contributions: Conceptualisation, D.A.S., N.N., S.T., I.S.S., C.P. and L.P.; methodology, D.A.S., N.N. and S.T.; software, I.S.S. and C.P.; validation, D.A.S., N.N. and S.T., formal analysis, D.A.S., I.S.S., C.P. and L.P.; investigation, D.A.S., N.N. and S.T.; resources, D.A.S. and L.P.; data curation, D.A.S., N.N. and L.P.; writing—original draft preparation, D.A.S., N.N., S.T., I.S.S., C.P. and L.P.; writing—review and editing, D.A.S., N.N. and S.T.; visualisation, D.A.S. and I.S.S.; supervision, D.A.S., N.N., S.T. and I.S.S.; project administration, D.A.S., N.N., S.T., I.S.S., C.P. and L.P.; All authors have read and agreed to the published version of the manuscript.

Funding: This research received no external funding.

Institutional Review Board Statement: Not applicable.

Informed Consent Statement: Not applicable.

Data Availability Statement: Not applicable.

Conflicts of Interest: The authors declare no conflict of interest.

References

1. Nas, K.; Yazmalar, L.; Şah, V.; Aydin, A.; Öneş, K. Rehabilitation of spinal cord injuries. *World J. Orthop.* **2015**, *6*, 8. [CrossRef] [PubMed]
2. Jesus, T.S.; Landry, M.D.; Hoenig, H. Global need for physical rehabilitation: Systematic analysis from the global burden of disease study. *Int. J. Environ. Res. Public Health* **2019**, *16*, 980. [CrossRef] [PubMed]
3. Fuentes, M.M.; Wang, J.; Haarbauer-Krupa, J.; Yeates, K.O.; Durbin, D.; Zonfrillo, M.R.; Jaffe, K.M.; Temkin, N.; Tulsky, D.; Bertisch, H.; et al. Unmet rehabilitation needs after hospitalisation for traumatic brain injury. *Pediatrics* **2018**, *141*, e20172859. [CrossRef] [PubMed]
4. Kamenov, K.; Mills, J.A.; Chatterji, S.; Cieza, A. Needs and unmet needs for rehabilitation services: A scoping review. *Disabil. Rehabil.* **2019**, *41*, 1227–1237. [CrossRef] [PubMed]
5. Bright, T.; Wallace, S.; Kuper, H. A systematic review of access to rehabilitation for people with disabilities in low- and middle-income countries. *Int. J. Environ. Res. Public Health* **2018**, *15*, 2165. [CrossRef]
6. Ekstrand, J.; Hägglund, M.; Waldén, M. Epidemiology of muscle injuries in professional football (soccer). *Am. J. Sports Med.* **2011**, *39*, 1226–1232. [CrossRef]
7. Logerstedt, D.; Arundale, A.; Lynch, A.; Snyder-Mackler, L. A conceptual framework for a sports knee injury performance profile (SKIPP) and return to activity criteria (RTAC). *Braz. J. Phys. Ther.* **2015**, *19*, 340–359. [CrossRef]
8. Alessandrino, F.; Balconi, G. Complications of muscle injuries. *J. Ultrasound.* **2013**, *16*, 215–222. [CrossRef]
9. Wong, K.; Sun, F.; Trudel, G.; Sebastiani, P.; Laneuville, O. Temporal gene expression profiling of the rat knee joint capsule during immobilisation-induced joint contractures. *BMC Musculoskelet. Disord.* **2015**, *16*, 125. [CrossRef]
10. Lynch, A.D.; Logerstedt, D.S.; Axe, M.J.; Snyder-Mackler, L. Quadriceps activation failure after anterior cruciate ligament rupture is not mediated by knee joint effusion. *J. Orthop. Sports Phys. Ther.* **2012**, *42*, 502–510. [CrossRef]
11. Frontera, W.R.; Ochala, J. Skeletal muscle: A brief review of structure and function. *Calcif. Tissue Int.* **2015**, *96*, 183–195. [CrossRef] [PubMed]
12. Shieh, P.B. Muscular dystrophies and other genetic myopathies. *Neurol. Clin.* **2013**, *31*, 1009–1029. [CrossRef]
13. Mueller-Wohlfahrt, H.W.; Haensel, L.; Mithoefer, K.; Ekstrand, J.; English, B.; McNally, S.; Orchard, J.; van Dijk, C.N.; Kerkhoffs, G.M.; Schamasch, P.; et al. Terminology and classification of muscle injuries in sport: The Munich consensus statement. *Br. J. Sports Med.* **2013**, *47*, 342–350. [CrossRef] [PubMed]
14. Edouard, P.; Branco, P.; Alonso, J.M. Muscle injury is the principal injury type and hamstring muscle injury is the first injury diagnosis during top-level international athletics championships between 2007 and 2015. *Br. J. Sports Med.* **2016**, *50*, 619–630. [CrossRef] [PubMed]
15. Bordoni, B.; Sugumar, K.; Varacallo, M. *Muscle Cramps*; StatPearls Publishing: Treasure Island, FL, USA, 2021.
16. Hotfiel, T.; Carl, H.D.; Swoboda, B.; Heinrich, M.; Heiß, R.; Grim, C.; Engelhardt, M. Current conservative treatment and management strategies of skeletal muscle injuries. *Z. Orthop. Und Unf.* **2016**, *154*, 245–253.
17. Delos, D.; Maak, T.G.; Rodeo, S.A. Muscle injuries in athletes: Enhancing recovery through scientific understanding and novel therapies. *Sports Health* **2013**, *5*, 346–352. [CrossRef]
18. Yanagisawa, O.; Niitsu, M.; Kurihara, T.; Fukubayashi, T. Evaluation of human muscle hardness after dynamic exercise with ultrasound real-time tissue elastography: A feasibility study. *Clin. Radiol.* **2011**, *66*, 815–819. [CrossRef]
19. Ghasemi, M.; Bagheri, H.; Olyaei, G.; Talebian, S.; Shadmehr, A.; Jalaei, S.; Kalantari, K.K. Effects of cyclic static stretch on fatigue recovery of triceps surae in female basketball players. *Biol. Sport* **2013**, *30*, 97–102. [CrossRef]
20. Castro-Sánchez, A.M.; Matarán-Peñarrocha, G.A.; Lara-Palomo, I.; Saavedra-Hernández, M.; Arroyo-Morales, M.; Moreno-Lorenzo, C. Hydrotherapy for the treatment of pain in people with multiple sclerosis: A randomised controlled trial. *Evid. Based Complement. Altern. Med.* **2012**, *2012*, 473963. [CrossRef]

21. Elias, G.P.; Varley, M.C.; Wyckelsma, V.L.; McKenna, M.J.; Minahan, C.L.; Aughey, R.J. Effects of water immersion on post training recovery in Australian footballers. *Int. J. Sports Physiol. Perform.* **2012**, *7*, 357–366. [CrossRef]
22. Leeder, J.; Gissane, C.; van Someren, K.; Gregson, W.; Howatson, G. Cold water immersion and recovery from strenuous exercise: A meta-analysis. *Br. J. Sports Med.* **2012**, *46*, 233–240. [CrossRef] [PubMed]
23. Osti, R.; Pari, C.; Salvatori, G.; Massari, L. Tri-length laser therapy associated to TECAR therapy in the treatment of low-back pain in adults: A preliminary report of a prospective case series. *Lasers Med. Sci.* **2015**, *30*, 407–412. [CrossRef] [PubMed]
24. Pereira, W.M.; Ferreira, L.A.; Rossi, L.P.; Kerpers, I.I.; Grecco, S.L.A.; de Paula, A.R.J.; Oliveira, C.S. Influence of heat on fatigue and electromyographic activity of the biceps brachii muscle. *J. Bodyw. Mov. Ther.* **2011**, *15*, 478–484. [CrossRef]
25. Hayashi, K.; Arai, Y.C.; Ikemoto, T.; Nishihara, M.; Suzuki, S.; Hirakawa, T.; Matsuo, S.; Kobayashi, M.; Haruta, M.; Kawabata, Y.; et al. Predictive factors for the outcome of multidisciplinary treatments in chronic low back pain at the first multidisciplinary pain center of Japan. *J. Phys. Ther. Sci.* **2015**, *27*, 2901–2905. [CrossRef] [PubMed]
26. Alayat, M.S.; Atya, A.M.; Ali, M.M.; Shosha, T.M. Long-term effect of high-intensity laser therapy in the treatment of patients with chronic low back pain: A randomised blinded placebo-controlled trial. *Lasers Med. Sci.* **2014**, *29*, 1065–1073. [CrossRef] [PubMed]
27. Pillastrini, P.; Gardenghi, I.; Bonetti, F.; Capra, F.; Guccione, A.; Mugnai, R.; Violante, F.S. An updated overview of clinical guidelines for chronic low back pain management in primary care. *Jt. Bone Spine* **2012**, *79*, 176–185. [CrossRef] [PubMed]
28. Hernández-Bule, M.L.; Paíno, C.L.; Trillo, M.Á.; Úbeda, A. Electric stimulation at 448 kHz promotes proliferation of human mesenchymal stem cells. *Cell Physiol. Biochem.* **2014**, *34*, 1741–1755. [CrossRef]
29. Kato, S.; Saitoh, Y.; Miwa, N. Repressive effects of a capacitive-resistive electric transfer (CRet) hyperthermic apparatus combined with provitamin C on intracellular lipid-droplets formation in adipocytes. *Int. J. Hyperth.* **2013**, *29*, 30–37. [CrossRef]
30. Cheng, H.; Huang, Y.; Yue, H.; Fan, Y. Electrical Stimulation Promotes Stem Cell Neural Differentiation in Tissue Engineering. *Stem Cells Int.* **2021**, *2021*, 6697574. [CrossRef]
31. Oostendorp, R.A.B. Credibility of manual therapy is at stake "Where do we go from here?". *J. Man Manip. Ther.* **2018**, *26*, 189–192. [CrossRef]
32. Reid, D.; Cook, C.; Sizer, P.S. Is orthopedic manipulative physical therapy not fashionable anymore? Lessons learned from 2016 IFOMPT meeting and future directions. *J. Man Manip. Ther.* **2017**, *25*, 1–2. [CrossRef] [PubMed]
33. Babatunde, O.O.; Jordan, J.L.; Van der Windt, D.A.; Hill, J.C.; Foster, N.E.; Protheroe, J. Effective treatment options for musculoskeletal pain in primary care: A systematic overview of current evidence. *PLoS ONE* **2017**, *12*, e0178621. [CrossRef] [PubMed]
34. Kim, G.J.; Choi, J.; Lee, S.; Jeon, C.; Lee, K. The effects of high intensity laser therapy on pain and function in patients with knee osteoarthritis. *J. Phys. Ther. Sci.* **2016**, *28*, 3197–3199. [CrossRef] [PubMed]
35. Conforti, M.; Fachinetti, G.P. High power laser therapy treatment compared to simple segmental physical rehabilitation in whiplash injuries (1° and 2° grade of the Quebec Task Force classification) involving muscles and ligaments. *Muscles Ligaments Tendons J.* **2013**, *3*, 106–111. [CrossRef] [PubMed]
36. Ezzati, K.; Fekrazad, R.; Raoufi, Z. The effects of photo-biomodulation therapy on post-surgical pain. *J. Lasers Med. Sci.* **2019**, *10*, 79–85. [CrossRef] [PubMed]
37. Thabet, A.A.E.; Elsodany, A.M.; Battecha, K.H.; Alshehri, M.A.; Refaat, B. High-intensity laser therapy versus pulsed electromagnetic field in the treatment of primary dysmenorrhea. *J. Phys. Ther. Sci.* **2017**, *29*, 1742–1748. [CrossRef]
38. Thabet, A.A.E.; Mahran, H.G.; Ebid, A.A.; Alshehri, M.A. Effect of pulsed high intensity laser therapy on delayed caesarean section healing in diabetic women. *J. Phys. Ther. Sci.* **2018**, *30*, 570–575. [CrossRef]
39. Pekyavas, N.O.; Baltaci, G. Short-term effects of high-intensity laser therapy, manual therapy, and Kinesio taping in patients with subacromial impingement syndrome. *Lasers Med. Sci.* **2016**, *31*, 1133–1141. [CrossRef]
40. Ordahan, B.; Karahan, A.Y.; Kaydok, E. The effect of high-intensity versus low-level laser therapy in the management of plantar fasciitis: A randomised clinical trial. *Lasers Med. Sci.* **2018**, *33*, 1363–1369. [CrossRef]
41. Taradaj, J.; Rajfur, K.; Shay, B.; Rajfur, J.; Ptaszkowski, K.; Walewicz, K.; Dymarek, R.; Sopel, M.; Rosińczuk, J. Photo-biomodulation using high—Or low-level laser irradiations in patients with lumbar disc degenerative changes: Disappointing outcomes and remarks. *Clin. Interv. Aging* **2018**, *13*, 1445–1455. [CrossRef]
42. Song, H.J.; Seo, H.J.; Lee, Y.; Kim, S.K. Effectiveness of high-intensity laser therapy in the treatment of musculoskeletal disorders: A systematic review and meta-analysis of randomised controlled trials. *Medicine* **2018**, *97*, e13126. [CrossRef] [PubMed]
43. Thoomes, E.J.; Scholten-Peeters, W.; Koes, B.; Falla, D.; Verhagen, A.P.; Clin, J. The effectiveness of conservative treatment for patients with cervical radiculopathy: A systematic review. *Pain* **2013**, *29*, 1073–1086. [CrossRef] [PubMed]
44. Kheshie, A.R.; Alayat, M.S.; Ali, M.M. High-intensity versus low-level laser therapy in the treatment of patients with knee osteoarthritis: A randomised controlled trial. *Lasers Med. Sci.* **2014**, *29*, 1371–1376. [CrossRef] [PubMed]
45. Yıldırım, M.A.; Uçar, D.; Öneş, K. Comparison of therapeutic duration of therapeutic ultrasound in patients with knee osteoarthritis. *J. Phys. Ther. Sci.* **2015**, *27*, 3667–3670. [CrossRef] [PubMed]
46. Boyraz, I.; Yildiz, A.; Koc, B.; Sarman, H. Comparison of high-intensity laser therapy and ultrasound treatment in the patients with lumbar discopathy. *Biomed. Res. Int.* **2015**, *2015*, 304328. [CrossRef]
47. Zielińska, P.; Nicpoń, J.; Kiełbowicz, Z.; Soroko, M.; Dudek, K.; Zaborski, D. Effects of high intensity laser therapy in the treatment of tendon and ligament injuries in performance horses. *Animals* **2020**, *10*, 1327. [CrossRef] [PubMed]

48. Ezzati, K.; Laakso, E.L.; Salari, A.; Hasannejad, A.; Fekrazad, R.; Aris, A. The beneficial effects of high-intensity laser therapy and co-interventions on musculoskeletal pain management: A systematic review. *J. Lasers Med. Sci.* **2020**, *11*, 81–90. [CrossRef]
49. Abdelbasset, W.K.; Nambi, G.; Alsubaie, S.F.; Abodonya, A.M.; Saleh, A.K.; Ataalla, N.N.; Ibrahim, A.A.; Tantawy, S.A.; Kamel, D.M.; Verma, A.; et al. A randomised comparative study between high-intensity and low-level laser therapy in the treatment of chronic nonspecific low back pain. *Evid. Based Complement. Altern. Med.* **2020**, *2020*, 1350281. [CrossRef]
50. Pellegrino, R.; Paolucci, T.; Brindisino, F.; Mondardini, P.; Di Iorio, A.; Moretti, A.; Iolascon, G. Effectiveness of High-Intensity Laser Therapy Plus Ultrasound-Guided Peritendinous Hyaluronic Acid Compared to Therapeutic Exercise for Patients with Lateral Elbow Tendinopathy. *J. Clin. Med.* **2022**, *11*, 5492. [CrossRef]
51. Alayat, M.S.; El Soudany, A.M.; El Fiky, A.A. Efficacy of high—And low-level laser therapy in the treatment of Bell's palsy: A randomised double-blind placebo-controlled trial. *Lasers Med. Sci.* **2014**, *29*, 335–342. [CrossRef]
52. Alayat, M.S.; El Soudany, A.M.; Ali, M.E. Efficacy of multiwave locked system laser on pain and function in patients with chronic neck pain: A randomised placebo-controlled trial. *Photomed. Laser Surg.* **2017**, *35*, 450–455. [CrossRef] [PubMed]
53. Alayat, M.S.; Aly, T.H.A.; Elsayed, A.E.M.; Fadil, A.S.M. Efficacy of pulsed Nd:YAG laser in the treatment of patients with knee osteoarthritis: A randomised controlled trial. *Lasers Med. Sci.* **2017**, *32*, 503–511. [CrossRef] [PubMed]
54. Thabet, A.A.E.; Alshehri, M.A. Effect of pulsed high-intensity laser therapy on pain, adhesions, and quality of life in women having endometriosis: A randomized controlled trial. *Photomed. Laser Surg.* **2018**, *36*, 363–369. [CrossRef]
55. Tkocz, P.; Matusz, T.; Kosowski, Ł.; Walewicz, K.; Argier, Ł.; Kuszewski, M.; Hagner-Derengowska, M.; Ptaszkowski, K.; Dymarek, R.; Taradaj, J. A Randomised-Controlled Clinical Study Examining the Effect of High-Intensity Laser Therapy (HILT) on the Management of Painful Calcaneal Spur with Plantar Fasciitis. *J. Clin. Med.* **2021**, *10*, 4891. [CrossRef] [PubMed]
56. Alayat, M.S.M.; Abdel-Kafy, E.M.; Elsoudany, A.M.; Helal, O.F.; Alshehri, M.A. Efficacy of high intensity laser therapy in the treatment of male with osteopenia or osteoporosis: A randomised placebo-controlled trial. *J. Phys. Ther. Sci.* **2017**, *29*, 1675–1679. [CrossRef]
57. Ebid, A.A.; El-Kafy, E.M.; Alayat, M.S. Effect of pulsed Nd:YAG laser in the treatment of neuropathic foot ulcers in children with spina bifida: A randomised controlled study. *Photomed. Laser Surg.* **2013**, *31*, 565–570. [CrossRef]
58. Wyszynska, J.; Bal-Bochenska, M. Efficacy of high-intensity laser therapy in treating knee osteoarthritis: A first systematic review. *Photomed. Laser Surg.* **2018**, *36*, 343–353. [CrossRef]
59. Cotler, H.; Chow, R.T.; Hamblin, M.R.; Carroll, J. The use of low-level laser therapy (LLLT) for musculoskeletal pain. *MOJ Orthop. Rheumatol.* **2015**, *2*, 00068. [CrossRef] [PubMed]
60. Tortorici, S.; Messina, P.; Scardina, G.A. Effectiveness of low-level laser therapy on pain intensity after lower third molar extraction. *Int. J. Clin. Dent.* **2019**, *12*, 357–367.
61. Chow, R.; Armati, P.; Laakso, E.L.; Bjordal, J.M.; Baxter, G.D. Inhibitory effects of laser irradiation on peripheral mammalian nerves and relevance to analgesic effects: A systematic review. *Photomed. Laser Surg.* **2011**, *29*, 365–381. [CrossRef]
62. Holanda, V.M.; Chavantes, M.C.; Wu, X.; Anders, J.J. The mechanistic basis for photo-biomodulation therapy of neuropathic pain by near infrared laser light. *Lasers Surg. Med.* **2017**, *49*, 516–524. [PubMed]
63. Ketz, A.K.; Byrnes, K.R.; Grunberg, N.E. Characterization of macrophage/microglial activation and effect of photo-biomodulation in the spared nerve injury model of neuropathic pain. *Pain Med.* **2017**, *18*, 932–946.
64. Thabet, A.A.; Ebid, A.A.; El-Boshy, M.E.; Almuwallad, A.O.; Hudaimoor, E.A.; Alsaeedi, F.E.; Alsubhi, R.H.; Almatrook, R.H.; Aljifry, R.F.; Alotaibi, S.H.; et al. Pulsed high-intensity laser therapy versus low level laser therapy in the management of primary dysmenorrhea. *J. Phys. Ther. Sci.* **2021**, *33*, 695–699. [CrossRef] [PubMed]
65. Collins, C.K.; Masaracchio, M.; Brismée, J.-M. The future of orthopedic manual therapy: What are we missing? *J. Man Manip. Ther.* **2017**, *25*, 169–171. [CrossRef] [PubMed]
66. Coronado, R.A.; Bialosky, J.E. Manual physical therapy for chronic pain: The complex whole is greater than the sum of its parts. *J. Man Manip. Ther.* **2017**, *25*, 115–117. [CrossRef] [PubMed]
67. Duñabeitia, I.; Arrieta, H.; Torres-Unda, J.; Gil, J.; Santos-Concejero, J.; Gil, S.M.; Irazusta, J.; Bidaurrazaga-Letona, I. Effects of a capacitive-resistive electric transfer therapy on physiological and biomechanical parameters in recreational runners: A randomised controlled crossover trial. *Phys. Ther. Sport* **2018**, *32*, 227–234. [CrossRef]
68. Diego, I.M.A.; Fernández-Carnero, J.; Val, S.L.; Cano-de-la-Cuerda, R.; Calvo-Lobo, C.; Piédrola, R.M.; Oliva, L.C.L.; Rueda, F.M. Analgesic effects of a capacitive-resistive monopolar radiofrequency in patients with myofascial chronic neck pain: A pilot randomised controlled trial. *Rev. Assoc. Med. Bras.* **2019**, *65*, 156–164. [CrossRef]
69. Rodríguez-Sanz, J.; López-De-Celis, C.; Hidalgo-García, C.; Canet-Vintró, M.; Fanlo-Mazas, P.; Pérez-Bellmunt, A. Temperature and current flow effects of different electrode placement in shoulder capacitive-resistive electric transfer applications: A cadaveric study. *BMC Musculoskelet. Disord.* **2021**, *22*, 139. [CrossRef]
70. Sousa, L.D.S.-D.; Sanchez, C.T.; Maté-Muñoz, J.L.; Hernández-Lougedo, J.; Barba, M.; Lozano-Estevan, M.D.C.; Garnacho-Castaño, M.V.; García-Fernández, P. Application of Capacitive-Resistive Electric Transfer in Physiotherapeutic Clinical Practice and Sports. *Int. J. Environ. Res. Public Health* **2021**, *18*, 12446. [CrossRef]
71. Beltrame, R.; Ronconi, G.; Ferrara, P.E.; Salgovic, L.; Vercelli, S.; Solaro, C.; Ferriero, G. Capacitive and resistive electric transfer therapy in rehabilitation: A systematic review. *Int. J. Rehabil. Res.* **2020**, *43*, 291–298. [CrossRef]

72. Nakamura, M.; Sato, S.; Kiyono, R.; Yahata, K.; Yoshida, R.; Kasahara, K.; Konrad, A. The Effect of Capacitive and Resistive Electric Transfer Intervention on Delayed-Onset Muscle Soreness Induced by Eccentric Exercise. *Int. J. Environ. Res. Public Health* **2022**, *19*, 5723. [CrossRef] [PubMed]
73. López-De-Celis, C.; Hidalgo-García, C.; Pérez-Bellmunt, A.; Fanlo-Mazas, P.; González-Rueda, V.; Tricás-Moreno, J.M.; Ortiz, S.; Rodríguez-Sanz, J. Thermal and non-thermal effects off capacitive-resistive electric transfer application on the Achilles tendon and musculotendinous junction of the gastrocnemius muscle: A cadaveric study. *BMC Musculoskelet. Disord.* **2020**, *21*, 46. [CrossRef]
74. Ostrowski, J.; Herb, C.C.; Scifers, J.; Gonzalez, T.; Jennings, A.; Breton, D. Comparison of muscle temperature increases produced by moist hot pack and ThermoStim probe. *J. Sport Rehabil.* **2019**, *28*, 459–463. [CrossRef] [PubMed]
75. Martínez-Pizarro, S. Transferencia eléctrica capacitiva y resistiva para mitigar el dolor [Capacitive and resistive electrical transfer for pain mitigation]. *Rehabilitacion* **2020**, *54*, 221–222. [CrossRef] [PubMed]
76. Tashiro, Y.; Hasegawa, S.; Yokota, Y.; Nishiguchi, S.; Fukutani, N.; Shirooka, H.; Tasaka, S.; Matsushita, T.; Matsubara, K.; Nakayama, Y.; et al. Effect of capacitive and resistive electric transfer on haemoglobin saturation and tissue temperature. *Int. J. Hyperth.* **2017**, *33*, 696–702. [CrossRef]
77. Hernández-Bule, M.L.; Trillo, M.Á.; Úbeda, A. Molecular mechanisms underlying antiproliferative and differentiating responses of hepatocarcinoma cells to subthermal electric stimulation. *PLoS ONE* **2014**, *9*, e84636. [CrossRef]
78. Chen, C.; Bai, X.; Ding, Y.; Lee, I.S. Electrical stimulation as a novel tool for regulating cell behavior in tissue engineering. *Biomater. Res.* **2019**, *23*, 25. [CrossRef]
79. Paolucci, T.; Pezzi, L.; Centra, M.A.; Porreca, A.; Barbato, C.; Bellomo, R.G.; Saggini, R. Effects of capacitive and resistive electric transfer therapy in patients with painful shoulder impingement syndrome: A comparative study. *J. Int. Med. Res.* **2020**, *48*, 300060519883090. [CrossRef]
80. Bito, T.; Tashiro, Y.; Suzuki, Y.; Kajiwara, Y.; Zeidan, H.; Kawagoe, M.; Sonoda, T.; Nakayama, Y.; Yokota, Y.; Shimoura, K.; et al. Acute effects of capacitive and resistive electric transfer (CRet) on the Achilles tendon. *Electromagn. Biol. Med.* **2019**, *38*, 48–54. [CrossRef]
81. Wostyn, V. *La Tecarthérapie Appliquée a la Kinésithérapie: Evaluation de Leffet Antalgique Immédiat*; Institut de Formation on Masso-Kinésithérapie: Reims, France, 2015.
82. Clijsen, R.; Leoni, D.; Schneebeli, A.; Cescon, C.; Soldini, E.; Li, L.; Barbero, M. Does the application of TECAR therapy affect temperature and perfusion of skin and muscle microcirculation? A pilot feasibility study on healthy subjects. *J. Altern. Complement. Med.* **2020**, *26*, 147–153. [CrossRef]
83. López-de-Celis, C.; Rodríguez-Sanz, J.; Hidalgo-García, C.; Cedeño-Bermúdez, S.A.; Zegarra-Chávez, D.; Fanlo-Mazas, P.; Pérez-Bellmunt, A. Thermal and Current Flow Effects of a Capacitive-Resistive Electric Transfer Application Protocol on Chronic Elbow Tendinopathy. A Cadaveric Study. *Int. J. Environ. Res. Public Health* **2021**, *18*, 1012. [CrossRef] [PubMed]
84. Masiero, S.; Pignataro, A.; Piran, G.; Duso, M.; Mimche, P.; Ermani, M.; Del Felice, A. Short-wave diathermy in the clinical management of musculoskeletal disorders: A pilot observational study. *Int. J. Biometeorol.* **2020**, *64*, 981–988. [CrossRef]
85. Ozen, S.; Doganci, E.B.; Ozyuvali, A.; Yalcin, A.P. Effectiveness of continuous versus pulsed short-wave diathermy in the management of knee osteoarthritis: A randomised pilot study. *Casp. J. Intern. Med.* **2019**, *10*, 431–438.
86. Koller, T. Mechanosensitive Aspects of Cell Biology in Manual Scar Therapy for Deep Dermal Defects. *Int. J. Mol. Sci.* **2020**, *21*, 2055. [CrossRef] [PubMed]
87. Kumaran, B.; Watson, T. Thermal build-up, decay and retention responses to local therapeutic application of 448 kHz capacitive resistive monopolar radiofrequency: A prospective randomised crossover study in healthy adults. *Int. J. Hyperth.* **2015**, *31*, 883–895. [CrossRef] [PubMed]
88. Priego-Quesada, J.I.; De la Fuente, C.; Kunzler, M.R.; Perez-Soriano, P.; Hervás-Marín, D.; Carpes, F.P. Relationship between Skin Temperature, Electrical Manifestations of Muscle Fatigue, and Exercise-Induced Delayed Onset Muscle Soreness for Dynamic Contractions: A Preliminary Study. *Int. J. Environ. Res. Public Health* **2020**, *17*, 6817. [CrossRef]
89. Notarnicola, A.; Maccagnano, G.; Gallone, M.F.; Covelli, I.; Tafuri, S.; Moretti, B. Short term efficacy of capacitive resistive diathermy therapy in patients with low back pain: A prospective randomized controlled trial. *J. Biol. Regul. Homeost. Agents* **2017**, *31*, 509–515. [PubMed]
90. Yokota, Y.; Tashiro, Y.; Suzuki, Y. Effect of capacitive and resistive electric transfer on tissue temperature, muscle flexibility and blood circulation. *J. Nov. Physiother.* **2017**, *30*, 719–725. [CrossRef]
91. Niajalili, M.; Sedaghat, M.; Reazasoltani, A.; Akbarzade Baghban, A.R.; Naimi, S.S. Effect of Capacitive Tecar Therapy on Foot Pain and Tactile Sensation in Patients with Type 2 Diabetes. *Arch. Rehab.* **2020**, *21*, 304–319. [CrossRef]
92. Du, J.; Zhen, G.; Chen, H.; Zhang, S.; Qing, L.; Yang, X.; Lee, G.; Mao, H.Q.; Jia, X. Optimal electrical stimulation boosts stem cell therapy in nerve regeneration. *Biomaterials* **2018**, *181*, 347–359. [CrossRef]
93. Zaretsky, D.V.; Romanovsky, A.A.; Zaretskaia, M.V.; Molkov, Y.I. Tissue oxidative metabolism can increase the difference between local temperature and arterial blood temperature by up to 1.3 °C: Implications for brain, brown adipose tissue, and muscle physiology. *Temperature* **2018**, *5*, 22–35. [CrossRef] [PubMed]
94. Ganzit, G.P.; Stefanini, L.; Stesina, G. *TECAR Therapy in the Treatment of Acute and Chronic Pathologies in Sports*; FMSI (Italian Sports Medicine Federation)-CONI Institute of Sports Medicine: Torino, Italy, 2015.
95. Robinson, S.E.; Buono, M.J. Effect of continuous-wave ultrasound on blood flow in skeletal muscle. *Phys. Ther.* **1995**, *75*, 145–150. [CrossRef] [PubMed]

96. Meng, S.; Rouabhia, M.; Zhang, Z. Electrical Stimulation and Cellular Behaviors in Electric Field in Biomedical Research. *Materials* **2021**, *15*, 165. [CrossRef] [PubMed]
97. Hernández-Bule, M.L.; Martínez, M.A.; Trillo, M.Á.; Martínez, L.; Toledano-Macías, E.; Úbeda, A. Response of human cancer cells to simultaneous treatment with sorafenib and radiofrequency current. *Oncol. Lett.* **2021**, *22*, 807. [CrossRef]
98. Yokota, Y.; Sonoda, T.; Tashiro, Y.; Suzuki, Y.; Kajiwara, Y.; Zeidan, H.; Nakayama, Y.; Kawagoe, M.; Shimoura, K.; Tatsumi, M.; et al. Effect of capacitive and resistive electric transfer on changes in muscle flexibility and lumbopelvic alignment after fatiguing exercise. *J. Phys. Ther. Sci.* **2018**, *30*, 719–725. [CrossRef]
99. Castellani, J.W.; Zambraski, E.J.; Sawka, M.N.; Urso, M.L. Does high muscle temperature accentuate skeletal muscle injury from eccentric exercise? *Physiol. Rep.* **2016**, *4*, e12777. [CrossRef]
100. Giombini, A.; Di Cesare, A.; Casciello, G.; Sorrenti, D.; Dragoni, S.; Gabriele, P. Hyperthermia at 434 MHz in the treatment of overuse sport tendinopathies: A randomised controlled clinical trial. *Int. J. Sports Med.* **2002**, *23*, 207–211. [CrossRef]
101. Hawkes, A.R.; Draper, D.O.; Johnson, A.W.; Diede, M.T.; Rigby, J.H. Heating capacity of rebound shortwave diathermy and moist hot packs at superficial depths. *J. Athl. Train.* **2013**, *48*, 471–476. [CrossRef]
102. Berteau, J.P. Knee Pain from Osteoarthritis: Pathogenesis, Risk Factors, and Recent Evidence on Physical Therapy Interventions. *J. Clin. Med.* **2022**, *11*, 3252. [CrossRef]
103. Naruseviciute, D.; Raimondas, K. The effect of high-intensity versus low-level laser therapy in the management of plantar fasciitis: Randomised participant blind controlled trial. *Clin. Rehabil.* **2020**, *34*, 1072–1082. [CrossRef]
104. Mamais, I.; Konstantinos, P.; Demetris, L.; Demetrios, S. Effectiveness of low-level laser therapy (LLLT) in the treatment of Lateral elbow tendinopathy (L.E.T.): An umbrella review effectiveness of LLLT in the treatment of L.E.T.: Umbrella review. *Laser Ther.* **2018**, *27*, 174–186. [CrossRef] [PubMed]
105. Starzec-Proserpio, M.; Grigol Bardin, M.; Fradette, J.; Tu, L.M.; Bérubè-Lauzière, Y.; Paré, J.; Carroll, M.-S.; Morin, M. High-Intensity Laser Therapy (HILT) as an Emerging Treatment for Vulvodynia and Chronic Musculoskeletal Pain Disorders: A Systematic Review of Treatment Efficacy. *J. Clin. Med.* **2022**, *11*, 3701. [CrossRef] [PubMed]
106. Dunning, J.R.; Butts, R.; Mourad, F.; Young, I.; Fernandez-de-Las Peñas, C.; Hagins, M.; Stanislawski, T.; Donley, J.; Buck, D.; Hooks, T.R.; et al. Upper cervical and upper thoracic manipulation versus mobilisation and exercise in patients with cervicogenic headache: A multi-center randomised clinical trial. *BMC Musculoskelet. Dis.* **2016**, *17*, 64. [CrossRef] [PubMed]
107. Collins, C.K.; Gilden, B. A non-operative approach to the management of chronic exertional compartment syndrome in a triathlete: A case report. *Int. J. Sports Phys. Ther.* **2016**, *11*, 1160–1176.
108. Rajasekaran, S.; Hall, M.M. Nonoperative management of chronic exertional compartment syndrome: A systematic review. *Curr. Sports Med. Rep.* **2016**, *15*, 191–198. [CrossRef]
109. Masaracchio, M.; Cleland, J.A.; Hellman, M.; Hagins, M. Short-term combined effects of thoracic spine thrust manipulation and cervical spine nonthrust manipulation in individuals with mechanical neck pain: A randomised clinical trial. *J. Orthop. Sports Phys. Ther.* **2013**, *43*, 118–127. [CrossRef]
110. Takasaki, H.; Hall, T.; Jull, G. Immediate and short-term effects of mulligan's mobilisation with movement on knee pain and disability associated with knee osteoarthritis—A prospective case series. *Physiother. Theory Pract.* **2013**, *29*, 87–95. [CrossRef]
111. Delitto, A.; George, S.Z.; Van Dillen, L.; Whitman, J.M.; Sowa, G.; Shekelle, P.; Denninger, T.R.; Godges, J.J. Low back pain. *J. Orthop. Sports Phys. Ther.* **2012**, *42*, A1–A57. [CrossRef]
112. Santuzzi, C.H.; Buss, H.F.; Pedrosa, D.F.; Freire, M.O.; Nogueira, B.V.; Gonçalves, W.L. Combined use of low-level laser therapy and cyclooxygenase-2 selective inhibition on skin incisional wound reepithelialisation in mice: A preclinical study. *Bras. Dermatol.* **2011**, *86*, 278–283. [CrossRef]
113. Hernández-Bule, M.L.; Medel, E.; Colastra, C.; Roldán, R.; Úbeda, A. Response of neuroblastoma cells to RF currents as a function of the signal frequency. *BMC Cancer* **2019**, *19*, 889. [CrossRef]
114. Cheng, H.; Huang, Y.; Chen, W.; Che, J.; Liu, T.; Na, J.; Wang, R.; Fan, Y. Cyclic Strain and Electrical Co-stimulation Improve Neural Differentiation of Marrow-Derived Mesenchymal Stem Cells. *Front. Cell Dev. Biol.* **2021**, *9*, 624755. [CrossRef] [PubMed]
115. Shadrin, I.Y.; Khodabukus, A.; Bursac, N. Striated muscle function, regeneration, and repair. *Cell Mol. Life Sci.* **2016**, *73*, 4175–4202. [CrossRef] [PubMed]
116. Brozovich, F.V.; Nicholson, C.J.; Degen, C.V.; Gao, Y.Z.; Aggarwal, M.; Morgan, K.G. Mechanisms of vascular smooth muscle contraction and the basis for pharmacologic treatment of smooth muscle disorders. *Pharmacol. Rev.* **2016**, *68*, 476–532. [CrossRef] [PubMed]
117. McLoon, L.K.; Vicente, A.; Fitzpatrick, K.R.; Lindström, M.; Domellöf, F.P. Composition, architecture, and functional implications of the connective tissue network of the extraocular muscles. *Investig. Ophthalmol. Vis. Sci.* **2018**, *59*, 322–329. [CrossRef] [PubMed]
118. Tantawy, S.A.; Abdelbasset, W.K.; Kamel, D.M.; Alrawaili, S.M. A randomised controlled trial comparing helium-neon laser therapy and infrared laser therapy in patients with diabetic foot ulcer. *Lasers Med. Sci.* **2018**, *33*, 1901–1906. [CrossRef]
119. Tantawy, S.A.; Abdelbasset, W.K.; Kamel, D.M.; Alrawaili, S.M.; Alsubaie, S.F. Laser photo-biomodulation is more effective than ultrasound therapy in patients with chronic nonspecific low back pain: A comparative study. *Lasers Med. Sci.* **2019**, *34*, 793–800. [CrossRef]
120. Kaydok, E.; Ordahan, B.; Solum, S.; Karahan, A.Y. Short-term Efficacy Comparison of High-intensity and Low-intensity Laser Therapy in the Treatment of Lateral Epicondylitis: A Randomized Double-blind Clinical Study. *Arch. Rheumatol.* **2019**, *35*, 60–67. [CrossRef]

121. Furlan, A.D.; Yazdi, F.; Tsertsvadze, A.; Gross, A.; Van Tulder, M.; Santaguida, L.; Gagnier, J.; Ammendolia, C.; Dryden, T.; Doucette, S.; et al. A systematic review and meta-analysis of efficacy, cost-effectiveness, and safety of selected complementary and alternative medicine for neck and low-back pain. *Evid. Based Complement. Altern. Med.* **2012**, *2012*, 953139. [CrossRef]
122. Alayat, M.S.M.; Mohamed, A.A.; Helal, O.F.; Khaled, O.A. Efficacy of high-intensity laser therapy in the treatment of chronic neck pain: A randomised double-blind placebo-control trial. *Lasers Med. Sci.* **2016**, *31*, 687–694. [CrossRef]
123. Glazov, G.; Yelland, M.; Emery, J. Low-level laser therapy for chronic non-specific low back pain: A meta-analysis of randomised controlled trials. *Acupunct. Med.* **2016**, *34*, 328–341. [CrossRef]
124. Huang, Z.; Ma, J.; Chen, J.; Shen, B.; Pei, F.; Kraus, V.B. The effectiveness of low-level laser therapy for nonspecific chronic low back pain: A systematic review and meta-analysis. *Arthritis Res. Ther.* **2015**, *17*, 360. [CrossRef]
125. Thong, I.S.K.; Jensen, M.P.; Miró, J.; Tan, G. The validity of pain intensity measures: What do the N.R.S., VAS, V.R.S., and FPS-R measure? *Scand. J. Pain* **2018**, *18*, 99–107. [CrossRef] [PubMed]
126. Lee, C.P.; Fu, T.S.; Liu, C.Y.; Hung, C.I. Psychometric evaluation of the oswestry disability index in patients with chronic low back pain: Factor and mokken analyses. *Health Qual. Life Outcomes* **2017**, *15*, 192. [CrossRef] [PubMed]
127. Kholoosy, L.; Elyaspour, D.; Akhgari, M.R.; Razzaghi, Z.; Khodamardi, Z.; Bayat, M. Evaluation of the therapeutic effect of low-level laser in controlling low back pain: A randomised controlled trial. *J. Lasers Med. Sci.* **2020**, *11*, 120–125. [CrossRef] [PubMed]
128. Dommerholt, J.; Hooks, T.; Finnegan, M.; Grieve, R. A critical overview of the current myofascial pain literature—March 2016. *J. Bodyw. Mov. Ther.* **2016**, *20*, 397–408. [CrossRef] [PubMed]
129. Yuan, S.L.K.; Matsutani, L.A.; Marques, A.P. Effectiveness of different styles of massage therapy in fibromyalgia: A systematic review and meta-analysis. *Man Ther.* **2015**, *20*, 257–264. [CrossRef]
130. Castro-Sánchez, A.M.; Matarán-Pe-arrocha, G.A.; Granero-Molina, J.; Aguilera-Manrique, G.; Quesada-Rubio, J.M.; Moreno-Lorenzo, C. Benefits of massage-myofascial release therapy on pain, anxiety, quality of sleep, depression, and quality of life in patients with fibromyalgia. *Evid. Based Complement. Altern. Med.* **2011**, *20*, 257–264. [CrossRef]
131. Castro-Sánchez, A.M.; Matarán-Pe-arrocha, G.A.; Arroyo-Morales, M.; Saavedra-Hernández, M.; Fernández-Sola, C.; Moreno-Lorenzo, C. Effects of myofascial release techniques on pain, physical function, and postural stability in patients with fibromyalgia: A randomised controlled trial. *Clin. Rehabil.* **2011**, *25*, 800–813. [CrossRef]
132. Kim, J.H.; Park, J.H.; Yoon, H.B. Immediate effects of high-frequency diathermy on muscle architecture and flexibility in subjects with gastrocnemius tightness. *Phys. Ther. Korea* **2020**, *27*, 133–139. [CrossRef]
133. Henderson, C.A.; Gomez, C.G.; Novak, S.M.; Mi-Mi, L.; Gregorio, C.C. Overview of the muscle cytoskeleton. *Compr. Physiol.* **2017**, *18*, 891–944.
134. Shamrock, A.G.; Varacallo, M. *Achilles Tendon Rupture*; StatPearls Publishing: Treasure Island, FL, USA, 2021.
135. Arnedo, F.; Andrew, A.; Till, L.; Sendrós, S.; Hellín, S. *Radiofrecuencia Monopolar Capacitiva/Resistiva 448 kHz (Indiba Activ Therapy) en el Tratamiento Rehabilitador de Lesiones de la Musculatura Isquitibial Derivada de la Práctica Deportiva: XIV Congreso Nacional de la Federación Española de Medicina del Deporte*; Santander: Boadilla del Monte, Spain, 2012; Volume XXIX, p. 915.
136. Ezzati, K.; Laakso, E.L.; Saberi, A.; Chabok, S.Y.; Nasiri, E.; Eghbali, B.B. A comparative study of the dose-dependent effects of low level and high intensity photo-biomodulation (laser) therapy on pain and electrophysiological parameters in patients with carpal tunnel syndrome: A randomised controlled trial. *Eur. J. Phys. Rehabil. Med.* **2019**, *56*, 733–740. [CrossRef] [PubMed]
137. El-Shamy, S.M.; Alayat, M.S.M.; Abdelgalil, A.A.; Alshehri, M.A. Long-term effect of pulsed nd: YAG laser in the treatment of children with juvenile rheumatoid arthritis: A randomized controlled trial. *Photomed. Laser Surg.* **2018**, *36*, 445–451. [CrossRef] [PubMed]

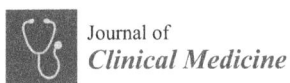

Article

Menstrual Cycle Changes Joint Laxity in Females—Differences between Eumenorrhea and Oligomenorrhea

Sae Maruyama [1], Chie Sekine [1], Mayuu Shagawa [1], Hirotake Yokota [1], Ryo Hirabayashi [1], Ryoya Togashi [1], Yuki Yamada [1], Rena Hamano [2], Atsushi Ito [2], Daisuke Sato [1] and Mutsuaki Edama [1,*]

[1] Institute for Human Movement and Medical Sciences, Niigata University of Health and Welfare, Shimami-cho 1398, Niigata City 950-3198, Japan; hpm20010@nuhw.ac.jp (S.M.); sekine@nuhw.ac.jp (C.S.); hpm21008@nuhw.ac.jp (M.S.); yokota@nuhw.ac.jp (H.Y.); hirabayashi@nuhw.ac.jp (R.H.); hpm21012@nuhw.ac.jp (R.T.); hpm21016@nuhw.ac.jp (Y.Y.); daisuke@nuhw.ac.jp (D.S.)
[2] Department of Health and Sports, Niigata University of Health and Welfare, Shimami-cho 1398, Kita-ku, Niigata City 950-3198, Japan; hamano@nuhw.ac.jp (R.H.); atsushi-ito@nuhw.ac.jp (A.I.)
* Correspondence: edama@nuhw.ac.jp; Tel./Fax: +81-25-257-4723

Abstract: The purpose of this study was to investigate the changes in anterior knee laxity (AKL), stiffness, general joint laxity (GJL), and genu recurvatum (GR) during the menstrual cycle in female non-athletes and female athletes with normal and irregular menstrual cycles. Participants were 19 female non-athletes (eumenorrhea, $n = 11$; oligomenorrhea, $n = 8$) and 15 female athletes (eumenorrhea, $n = 8$; oligomenorrhea, $n = 7$). AKL was measured as the amount of anterior tibial displacement at 67 N–133 N. Stiffness was calculated as change in (Δ)force$/\Delta$ anterior displacement. The Beighton method was used to evaluate the GJL. The GR was measured as the maximum angle of passive knee joint extension. AKL, stiffness, GJL, and GR were measured twice in four phases during the menstrual cycle. Stiffness was significantly higher in oligomenorrhea groups than in eumenorrhea groups, although no significant differences between menstrual cycle phases were evident in female non-athletes. GR was significantly higher in the late follicular, ovulation, and luteal phases than in the early follicular phase, although no significant differences between groups were seen in female athletes. Estradiol may affect the stiffness of the periarticular muscles in the knee, suggesting that GR in female athletes may change during the menstrual cycle.

Keywords: anterior knee laxity; stiffness; general joint laxity; genu recurvatum

1. Introduction

Injury to the anterior cruciate ligament (ACL) is a sports injury that occurs more frequently in women than in men [1]. Sex differences in the incidence of ACL injury are attributed in part to the influence of female hormones, the concentrations of which fluctuate during the menstrual cycle [2]. The menstrual cycle is regulated by the female hormones estradiol and progesterone, and is divided into follicular, ovulation, and luteal phases. ACL injury is reportedly more likely to occur during the follicular [3] and ovulation phases [4]. Clarifying the relationship between risk factors for ACL injury and female hormones is therefore an important step in minimizing the risk of such injury.

One potential risk factor for ACL injury in women is joint laxity. Joint laxity has been examined in terms of anterior knee laxity (AKL), general joint laxity (GJL), and genu recurvatum (GR), each of which have been reported to show associations with risk of ACL injury [5–7]. A previous study found that AKL [8,9], GJL [10], and GR [11] were all higher in women than in men. In addition, AKL, GJL, and GR may be altered by changes in the concentrations of female hormones during the menstrual cycle [9,12,13]. Previous studies therefore suggest that changes in joint laxity due to changes in female hormone concentrations may be related to differences in the timing of ACL injury during the menstrual cycle.

Some reports have suggested that AKL, which indicates the laxity of the ACL, is altered by changes in hormone levels during the menstrual cycle [9,12,14], while others have reported the AKL shows no significant change [8,15–18]. Likewise, studies have reported both that GJL changes [12,18] and that GJL remains unchanged during the menstrual cycle [17]. Such contradictory findings may be due to the fact that the timings of measurements and subjects differed between studies.

In addition, most previous studies investigating changes in joint laxity during the menstrual cycle have been conducted among women with normal menstrual cycles. Lee et al. examined the effect of oral contraceptive (OC) use on AKL and found that AKL was significantly higher in the non-OC group than in the OC group, and that AKL was increased during the ovulation and luteal phases compared with the early follicular phase [19]. Decreases in levels of female sex hormones due to OC use may thus affect AKL. In addition, it has been reported that 20–30% of Japanese female athletes reported experience menstrual irregularities [20,21] such as oligomenorrhea [22]. To investigate the effects of female hormones on joint laxity in greater detail, women with menstrual irregularities would need to be included in the study. However, to the best of our knowledge, no reports have examined changes in joint laxity during the menstrual cycle among women with menstrual irregularities. Clarification of these issues would contribute to the development of better methods for training and prevention of ACL injuries in accordance with menstrual cycle conditions.

The purpose of this study was to determine changes and differences in joint laxity (AKL, GJL, and GR) during the menstrual cycle among female athletes and non-athletes with normal and irregular menstrual cycles. We hypothesized that AKL, GJL, and GR would all change during the menstrual cycle in female athletes and non-athletes with normal menstrual cycles, and would not change during the menstrual cycle in female athletes and non-athletes with menstrual irregularities.

2. Materials and Methods

2.1. Participants

Seventy-one female non-athletes and 27 female athletes affiliated with the university were recruited between July 2020 and July 2021 and administered a questionnaire on inclusion criteria. Inclusion criteria were as follows: (1) no history of injury or surgery involving the osteochondral surfaces, ligaments, tendons, capsule, or menisci of either knee joint; and (2) no use of OCs or other hormonal medications within the 6 months preceding the first day of measurement [23]. Female non-athletes were defined as female who were physically active less than 3 times per week [17]. Non-athletes 19 people (Figure 1) and athlete 15 people (volleyball 10 people, basketball 5 people) (Figure 2) met the inclusion criteria and agreed to participate in the study. This study was approved by the ethics committee at Niigata University of Health and Welfare (approval no. 18467). This study complied with the tenets of the Declaration of Helsinki and was conducted only after obtaining written consent from potential study participants who had been fully informed (in both oral and written form) of the nature of the experiments.

2.2. Classification of the Menstrual Cycle

Participants were classified into two groups: a eumenorrhea group and an oligomenorrhea group. The eumenorrhea group was defined to include females with menstrual cycles of 25–38 days [22] for the two cycles before and during the experiment, and at least 10 menstrual cycles in the past 12 months [24]. The oligomenorrhea group was defined to include females with menstrual cycles of either less than 24 days or more than 39 days [22] in the menstrual cycle before or during the experiment, or who had nine or fewer menstrual cycles in the past 12 months [24]. The 19 female non-athletes included 11 individuals in the eumenorrhea group (mean age, 21.0 ± 0.7 years; height, 159.3 ± 4.8 cm; weight, 50.1 ± 7.4 kg; cycle length, 31.3 ± 2.1 days) and 8 individuals in the oligomenorrhea group (mean age, 21.3 ± 0.4 years; height, 158.3 ± 4.2 cm; weight, 54.7 ± 9.2 kg; cycle length, 35.4 ± 7.5 days). The 15 female athletes included 8 individuals in the eumenorrhea group (mean age, 18.8 ± 0.7 years; height, 167.2 ± 6.6 cm; weight, 65.8 ± 10.0 kg; cycle length, 31.0 ± 2.5 days) and 7 individuals in the oligomenorrhea group (mean age, 19.3 ± 0.7 years; height, 167.8 ± 5.7 cm; weight, 60.1 ± 3.6 kg; cycle length, 45.0 ± 12.0 days).

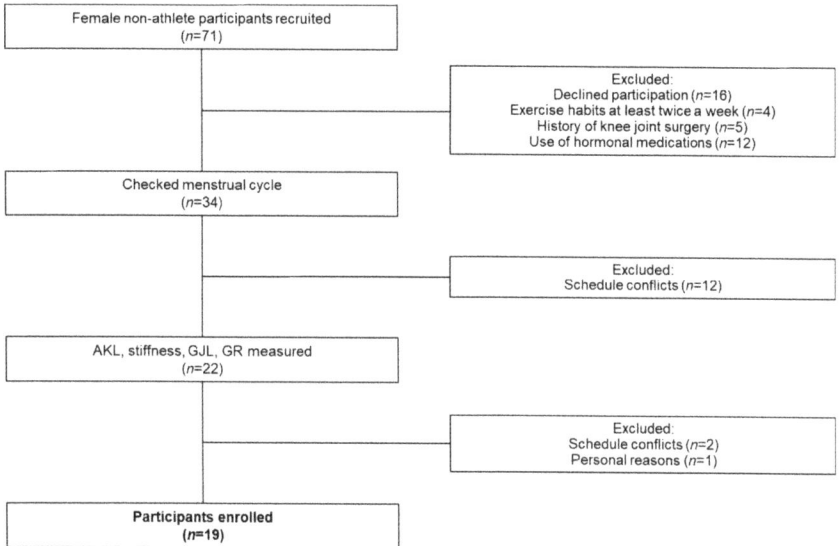

Figure 1. Flowchart for selection of female non-athlete participants. AKL, anterior knee laxity; GJL, general joint laxity; GR, genu recurvatum.

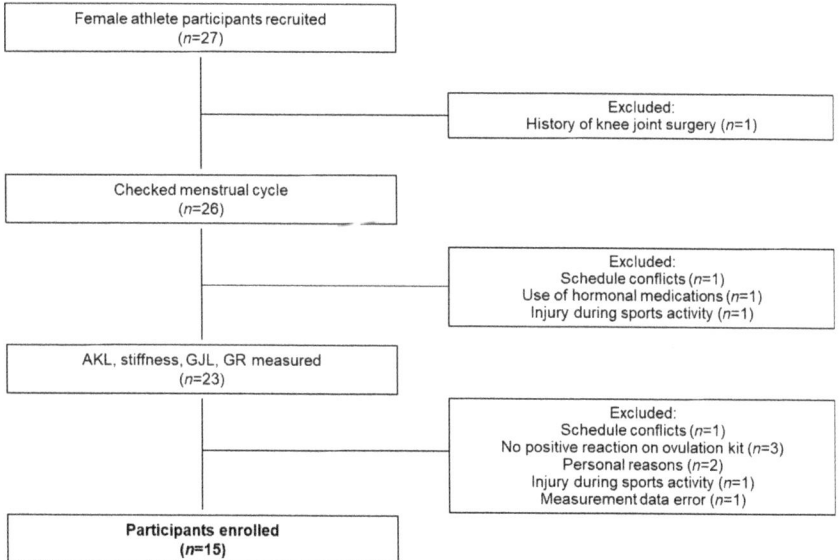

Figure 2. Flowchart for selection of female athlete participants. AKL, anterior knee laxity; GJL, general joint laxity; GR, genu recurvatum.

2.3. Menstrual Cycle Recording

Participants were asked to measure their basal body temperature (BBT) with a basal thermometer (Citizen Electronic Thermometer CTEB503L; Citizen Systems Co., Ltd., Tokyo,

Japan) every morning for 1–3 months preceding the first day of measurement. To estimate the day of ovulation, participants were given an ovulation test kit (Doctor's Choice One Step Ovulation Test Clear; Beauty and Health Research, Torrance, CA, USA) and asked to use it from the day after the end of menstruation. Participants were asked to record daily BBT, ovulation test kit results, and start and end dates of menstruation in the ONE TAP SPORTS, an athlete's condition management system (Euphoria Co., Ltd., Tokyo, Japan).

2.4. Timing of Measurements

AKL, stiffness, GJL, and GR were measured a total of eight times each on two consecutive days during each of the four phases of the menstrual cycle (early follicular, late follicular, ovulation, and luteal phases), and the average of values from those two days was used as the measurement value for each phase. Salivary hormone levels were measured only on the first day of each phase. Measurements were taken on two days between 2–4 days after the onset of menstruation in the early follicular phase, on two days between 2–4 days after the end of menstruation in the late follicular phase, on two days between 2–4 days after a positive result from the ovulation test kit day in the ovulation phase, and on two days more than 2 days after the transition to the high-temperature phase of BBT or 1 week after the first measurement in the ovulation phase in the luteal phase. In the luteal phase, if BBT during the 3 days after the estimated ovulation day was at least 0.2 °C higher than the average BBT during the first 6 days of menstruation, the BBT was considered biphasic, indicating a transition from the low- to the high-temperatures phase [25]. All measurements were performed between 07:00 and 12:00 to account for diurnal variations.

2.5. Measurement Methods

2.5.1. Hormone Level Measurement

To measure salivary concentrations of estradiol and progesterone, saliva was collected and analyzed using a saliva collection kit (SalivaBio A; Salimetrics, Carlsbad, CA, USA). Participants were asked to rinse the mouth prior to the start of the experiments, so that no food particles remained in the oral cavity. Saliva was collected at least 10 min after rinsing to prevent dilution of hormone concentrations in saliva. We also asked participants to strictly observe the following prohibitions and precautions during saliva collection: (1) no eating for at least 60 min prior to saliva collection; (2) no alcohol intake for at least 12 h prior to saliva collection; (3) no intake of sugary, acidic or caffeinated beverages prior to saliva collection; (4) no intake of dairy products for at least 20 min prior to saliva collection; (5) no tooth brushing for at least 45 min prior to saliva collection; and (6) no dental treatment within 48 h before saliva collection [26]. Saliva was collected in the mouth for 1 min, then transferred to a saliva collection container (Cryyovial; Salimetrics) using a special straw (Siva Collection Aid; Salimetrics). The saliva sample was immediately stored in a freezer at less than -80 °C. Analysis of female hormone concentrations was entrusted to Funakoshi Corporation (Tokyo, Japan). Samples were thawed at room temperature, mixed by vortexing, centrifuged at $1500\times g$ for 15 min, and analyzed by enzyme-linked immunosorbent assay using high-sensitivity salivary immunoassay kits (17β-Estradiol Enzyme Immunoassay Kit and Salivary Progesterone Enzyme Immunoassay Kit; Salimetrics). The dilution factor was uniformly 1-fold (undiluted).

2.5.2. Laxity Measurement

AKL was measured as the amount of anterior displacement of the tibia relative to the femur when loads of 67 N, 89 N, 111 N, and 133 N applied to the tibia. AKL was measured using a cruciate ligament function tester (KS Measure KSM-100; Japan Sigmax, Tokyo, Japan), and was performed only on the pivot (non-dominant) foot. Participants were placed in a supine position with the knee joint set in approximately 30° of flexion using a goniometer (Goniometer; Nishikawashinwa, Tokyo, Japan). The knee support was placed on the posterior part of the distal thigh and the foot support was placed under the foot. The position of the cruciate ligament function tester was adjusted so that the patellar contact point was at the center of the knee and the ankle fixation point was at the center of the ankle. The ankle was fixed with a lower limb fixation belt and the lower leg was fixed with a traction belt. After the participants was instructed to relax, measurement was performed by operating the load handle. Five measurements were taken and after discarding the maximum and minimum values, the average of the three remaining measurements was recorded. Measurement of knee joint angle and operation of the load handle were performed by a single researcher (S.M.). The intra-rater reliability of AKL measurement was confirmed to be higher than in our previous study [17]. Stiffness was calculated as change in (Δ)force/Δanterior displacement at 67–89 N, 89–111 N, and 111–133 N loads [17].

GJL was measured using the Beighton method [27]. Mobility was measured at five locations: fifth (little) finger, wrist, elbow, knee, and spine. Assessment criteria were as follows: (1) extension of the fifth finger greater than $90°$; (2) ability to touch the thumb to the forearm, (3) hyperextension of the elbow greater than $10°$; (4) hyperextension of the knee greater than $10°$; and (5) ability to perform forward flexion of the trunk with palm touching the floor in full extension of the knee joint. Criteria (1) to (4) were evaluated as 1 point for each side, and Criterion 5 was evaluated as 1 point, for a total of 9 points. GJL was measured using the goniometer for items based on joint angle. GJL measurements were performed by one researcher (S.M.).

GR was measured using a hyperextension apparatus (Takei Scientific Instrument Co., Niigata, Japan) to evaluate the range of motion of knee extension (Figure 3). Participants were seated in a long sitting position with the hip joint set in about $70°$ of flexion with both upper limbs behind them (Figure 3A). Knee joint extension was defined as $0°$ when the scales for seat height and foot height were the same. The distance from the knee to the heel was adjusted by placing the heel on the footrest (Figure 3B), and the right and left positions of the lower limbs were adjusted to achieve $0°$ of hip adduction (Figure 3C). The proximal patella was fixed with a knee-fixation belt, and foot width was also fixed. Participants were instructed in advance to signal just before the appearance of pain or discomfort in the knee joint, and the knee joint was extended by turning the foot elevation screw at a rate of approximately $1° \cdot s^{-1}$ or less until the signal was given. At the time the participant gave the signal, the foot was held for 10 s and the value on the scale for foot height was recorded. Maximum angle of passive knee joint extension was later calculated using the change in foot height (H) and the length from the center of the knee to the heel (L) according to the following equation:

$$GR\ [°] = Arctan\ (H/L) \times 57.2958$$

After one practice test, five measurements were taken. After discarding the maximum and minimum values, the average of the three remaining measurements was recorded. A rest period of 10 s was provided between each of the five trials. Measurements were taken only for the pivot (non-dominant) foot. GR measurements were performed by one researcher (S.M.).

2.6. Reliability of GR Measurements

The reliability of GR measurements was examined in 10 knees of 5 adult males (mean age, 23.4 ± 0.8 years; height, 168.1 ± 5.7 cm; weight, 60.9 ± 4.0 kg) and 10 knees of 5 adult females (mean age, 21 ± 0.9 years; height, 166.7 ± 8.6 cm; weight, 59.3 ± 11.9 kg) in this study, none of whom had orthopedic diseases or pain in the lower limbs. GR was measured using the methods described above, with an interval of at least 10 min between measurements by different researchers (S.M. and C.S.) to determine inter-rater reliability and an interval of at least 30 min between measurements by the same researcher (S.M.) for intra-rater reliability, on the same day. Intra- and inter-rater reliabilities were calculated using intraclass correlation coefficient (ICC) (1, 3) and (2, 3), respectively.

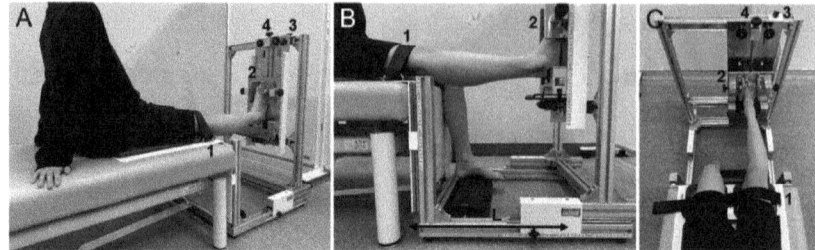

Figure 3. Position for measurement of genu recurvatum. 1: Knee-fixation belt; 2: foot width fixing part; 3: right/left adjustment of lower limbs; 4: foot elevation screw; L, length from center of knee to heel. The participant was seated on the hyperextension apparatus (Takei Scientific Instrument Co., Niigata, Japan) in a long sitting position with the hip joint set in about 70° of flexion with both upper limbs behind them (**A**). Distance from the knee to the heel was adjusted by placing the heel on the footrest (**B**), and positions of the lower limbs were adjusted to the left/right to achieve 0° of hip adduction (**C**). The proximal patella was fixed with the knee-fixation belt, and foot width was also fixed. Participants were instructed in advance to signal just before the appearance of pain or discomfort in the knee joint, and the knee joint was extended by turning the foot elevation screw at a rate of approximately $1° \cdot s^{-1}$ or less until that signal was given. At the time the signal was given, foot height was recorded. Maximum angle of passive knee joint extension was calculated later based on the result recorded.

2.7. Statistical Analysis

Statistical analyses were performed using SPSS version 27.0 (IBM Corp, Tokyo, Japan). Split-plot repeated-measures analysis of variance (ANOVA) was conducted to com-pare salivary estradiol and progesterone concentrations, AKL, stiffness, GJL, and GR menstrual cycle phases in female non-athletes and female athletes, and to compare eumenor-rhea and oligomenorrhea groups (subject factors [eumenorrhea group, oligomenorrhea group] vs. cycle phase factors [early follicular phase, late follicular phase, ovulation phase, luteal phase]). When an interaction or main effect of the subject factor or the cycle phase factor was identified, one-way repeated-measures ANOVA was used for comparison within cycle phase factors, and statistical processing was performed by the Bonferroni method as a post-test. In addition, statistical processing was performed by the independent samples *t*-test and Mann-Whitney U test as a post-test for comparison within subject factors. Probability values of 5% were considered statistically significance.

3. Results

3.1. Female Non-Athletes

In salivary estradiol, split-plot repeated-measures ANOVA showed no interactions and no main effects of subject factor, but a main effect of the cycle phase factor [$F_{(2.197, 37.343)} = 7.23$, $p = 0.002$, $\eta p2 = 0.30$]. The results of Bonferroni post hoc testing showed that salivary estradiol concentrations were significantly higher in the ovulation and luteal phases than in the early follicular phase ($p = 0.006$ and $p = 0.002$, respectively) (Table 1).

In salivary progesterone, split-plot repeated-measures ANOVA showed an interaction [$F_{(1.345, 22.872)} = 3.97$, $p = 0.048$, $\eta p2 = 0.19$]. One-way repeated-measures ANOVA and Bonferroni post hoc testing showed that salivary progesterone concentrations was significantly higher in the luteal phase than in the early follicular phase and ovulation phases in the eumenorrhea group ($p = 0.026$ and $p = 0.040$, respectively). Results from the independent sample *t*-test and post hoc Mann-Whitney U-test showed that salivary progesterone concentrations were significantly higher in the eumenorrhea group than in the oligomenorrhea group during the luteal phase ($p = 0.035$) (Table 1).

Table 1. Changes in estradiol and progesterone concentrations during the menstrual cycle.

	Early Follicular Phase	Late Follicular Phase	Ovulation Phase	Luteal Phase	Total
Estradiol [pg/mL]					
Female non-athletes (n = 19)	1.1 ± 0.3	1.3 ± 0.4	1.5 ± 0.4 [a]	1.4 ± 0.4 [b]	
Eumenorrhea group (n = 11)	1.1 ± 0.3	1.3 ± 0.4	1.5 ± 0.4	1.5 ± 0.4	1.3 ± 0.4
Oligomenorrhea group (n = 8)	1.0 ± 0.3	1.2 ± 0.4	1.5 ± 0.4	1.4 ± 0.3	1.3 ± 0.4
Female athletes (n = 15)	1.0 ± 0.3	1.0 ± 0.3	1.2 ± 0.3	1.3 ± 0.6 [f]	
Eumenorrhea group (n = 8)	0.8 ± 0.2	0.9 ± 0.3	1.2 ± 0.3	1.1 ± 0.6	1.0 ± 0.4
Oligomenorrhea group (n = 7)	1.2 ± 0.2	1.2 ± 0.3	1.1 ± 0.3	1.5 ± 0.4	1.3 ± 0.3
Progesterone [pg/mL]					
Female non-athletes (n = 19)	132.0 ± 75.3	161.1 ± 77.4	164.5 ± 94.5	343.7 ± 280.2	
Eumenorrhea group (n = 11)	146.7 ± 81.3	167.1 ± 85.4	172.1 ± 104.0	477.6 ± 324.4 [c,d,e]	233.4 ± 148.8
Oligomenorrhea group (n = 8)	111.7 ± 65.9	152.9 ± 69.7	154.1 ± 85.3	200.7 ± 105.8	154.8 ± 81.7
Female athletes (n = 15)	127.6 ± 61.0	141.2 ± 60.3	147.2 ± 73.1	231.4 ± 108.6 [g,h,i]	
Eumenorrhea group (n = 8)	101.1 ± 66.2	146.7 ± 70.3	172.1 ± 83.1	242.1 ± 128.5	165.5 ± 87.0
Oligomenorrhea group (n = 7)	157.8 ± 39.8	135.0 ± 51.3	118.8 ± 51.5	219.2 ± 89.0	157.7 ± 57.9

Values are presented as means ± SD. [a]—Statistically significant difference compared with early follicular phase in female non-athletes ($p = 0.006$). [b]—Statistically significant difference compared with early follicular phase in female non-athletes ($p = 0.002$). [c]—Statistically significant difference compared with early follicular phase in the eumenorrhea group of female non-athletes ($p = 0.026$). [d]—Statistically significant difference compared with ovulation phase in the eumenorrhea group of female non-athletes ($p = 0.040$). [e]—Statistically significant difference compared with oligomenorrhea in the luteal phase of female non-athletes ($p = 0.035$). [f]—Statistically significant difference compared with the early follicular phase in female athletes ($p = 0.039$). [g]—Statistically significant difference compared with the early follicular phase in female athletes ($p = 0.005$). [h]—Statistically significant difference compared with the late follicular phase in female athletes ($p = 0.001$). [i]—Statistically significant difference compared with the ovulation phase in female athletes ($p = 0.022$).

In AKL, the results of split-plot repeated-measures ANOVA showed no interactions or main effects of subject or cycle-phase factors at any loadings (Table 2).

Table 2. Changes in anterior knee laxity during the menstrual cycle.

		Early Follicular Phase	Late Follicular Phase	Ovulation Phase	Luteal Phase	Total
	Anterior knee laxity [mm]					
	Female non-athletes (n = 19)					
67 N	Eumenorrhea group (n = 11)	4.6 ± 1.3	4.6 ± 1.4	4.4 ± 1.2	4.2 ± 1.2	4.5 ± 1.3
	Oligomenorrhea group (n = 8)	4.5 ± 2.1	4.4 ± 1.7	4.5 ± 1.4	4.3 ± 1.5	4.4 ± 1.7
89 N	Eumenorrhea group (n = 11)	5.7 ± 1.5	5.6 ± 1.6	5.3 ± 1.3	5.2 ± 1.2	5.5 ± 1.4
	Oligomenorrhea group (n = 8)	5.4 ± 2.2	5.3 ± 1.8	5.4 ± 1.5	5.1 ± 1.4	5.3 ± 1.7
111 N	Eumenorrhea group (n = 11)	6.6 ± 1.6	6.5 ± 1.8	6.2 ± 1.4	6.0 ± 1.2	6.3 ± 1.5
	Oligomenorrhea group (n = 8)	6.0 ± 2.3	6.0 ± 1.8	6.1 ± 1.5	5.8 ± 1.5	6.0 ± 1.8
133 N	Eumenorrhea group (n = 11)	7.5 ± 1.7	7.4 ± 1.9	7.0 ± 1.5	6.8 ± 1.3	7.2 ± 1.6
	Oligomenorrhea group (n = 8)	6.7 ± 2.3	6.7 ± 1.8	6.8 ± 1.5	6.4 ± 1.5	6.6 ± 1.8
	Female athletes (n = 15)					
67 N	Eumenorrhea group (n = 8)	3.6 ± 1.2	3.8 ± 1.0	3.8 ± 1.0	3.4 ± 0.9	3.6 ± 1.0
	Oligomenorrhea group (n = 7)	4.0 ± 2.0	4.5 ± 1.3	4.0 ± 1.7	4.0 ± 1.5	4.1 ± 1.6
89 N	Eumenorrhea group (n = 8)	4.5 ± 1.4	4.7 ± 1.3	4.7 ± 1.1	4.1 ± 1.1	4.5 ± 1.2
	Oligomenorrhea group (n = 7)	4.8 ± 2.2	5.4 ± 1.6	4.8 ± 1.9	4.9 ± 1.7	5.0 ± 1.9
111 N	Eumenorrhea group (n = 8)	5.2 ± 1.5	5.4 ± 1.5	5.4 ± 1.2	4.8 ± 1.2	5.2 ± 1.4
	Oligomenorrhea group (n = 7)	5.5 ± 2.2	6.1 ± 1.8	5.5 ± 2.1	5.7 ± 2.0	5.7 ± 2.0
133 N	Eumenorrhea group (n = 8)	5.9 ± 1.6	6.0 ± 1.7	6.1 ± 1.4	5.4 ± 1.2	5.9 ± 1.5
	Oligomenorrhea group (n = 7)	6.2 ± 2.4	6.8 ± 2.0	6.1 ± 2.1	6.4 ± 2.2	6.4 ± 2.2

Values are presented as means ± SD.

In stiffness, split-plot repeated-measures ANOVA showed no interactions and no main effects of cycle-phase factors between any loadings, but a main effect of the subject factor was seen only between 89–111 N [$F(1, 17) = 6.61$, $p = 0.020$, $\eta p^2 = 0.28$] and 111–133 N [$F(1, 17) = 9.48$, $p = 0.007$, $\eta p^2 = 0.36$] loadings. The results of the Bonferroni post hoc testing showed that stiffness at 89–111 N and 111–133 N was significantly higher in the oligomenorrhea group than in the eumenorrhea group ($p = 0.020$ and $p = 0.007$, respectively) (Table 3).

Table 3. Changes in stiffness during the menstrual cycle.

		Early Follicular Phase	Late Follicular Phase	Ovulation Phase	Luteal Phase	Total
	Stiffness [N/mm]					
	Female non-athletes (n = 19)					
67–89 N	Eumenorrhea group (n = 11)	21.6 ± 4.3	23.4 ± 5.6	24.5 ± 6.3	24.6 ± 2.9	23.5 ± 4.8
	Oligomenorrhea group (n = 8)	27.5 ± 7.0	27.1 ± 5.7	25.2 ± 5.8	28.4 ± 6.0	27.1 ± 6.1
89–111 N	Eumenorrhea group (n = 11)	25.6 ± 5.5	26.5 ± 6.6	28.4 ± 7.7	27.6 ± 3.5	27.0 ± 5.8
	Oligomenorrhea group (n = 8)	34.3 ± 9.6	33.6 ± 9.0	30.6 ± 5.4	35.6 ± 3.9	33.6 ± 7.0 [a]
111–133 N	Eumenorrhea group (n = 11)	26.7 ± 6.9	27.0 ± 5.1	26.9 ± 4.5	28.1 ± 4.3	27.2 ± 5.2
	Oligomenorrhea group (n = 8)	35.5 ± 8.9	35.9 ± 10.7	32.3 ± 6.6	38.0 ± 7.4	35.4 ± 8.4 [b]
	Female athletes (n = 15)					
67–89 N	Eumenorrhea group (n = 8)	26.8 ± 8.1	28.8 ± 7.8	27.9 ± 5.1	28.3 ± 12.4	28.0 ± 0.4
	Oligomenorrhea group (n = 7)	31.5 ± 10.3	29.1 ± 12.8	31.9 ± 14.3	27.3 ± 11.4	29.9 ± 12.2
89–111 N	Eumenorrhea group (n = 8)	32.8 ± 9.0	34.2 ± 9.2	32.5 ± 7.7	36.2 ± 10.6	33.9 ± 9.1
	Oligomenorrhea group (n = 7)	33.2 ± 7.8	36.3 ± 15.7	36.7 ± 11.4	32.8 ± 14.3	34.8 ± 12.3
111–133 N	Eumenorrhea group (n = 8)	37.1 ± 11.5	38.1 ± 11.9	36.7 ± 11.5	38.0 ± 7.1	37.5 ± 10.5
	Oligomenorrhea group (n = 7)	34.6 ± 9.3	40.0 ± 21.9	43.6 ± 18.9	32.3 ± 13.1	37.7 ± 15.8

Values are presented as means ± SD. [a]—Statistically significant difference compared with the eumenorrhea group ($p = 0.020$). [b]—Statistically significant difference compared with the eumenorrhea group ($p = 0.007$).

The results of split-plot repeated-measures ANOVA about GJL and GR showed no interactions or main effects of subject or cycle-phase factors (Tables 4 and 5).

Table 4. Changes in general joint laxity during the menstrual cycle.

	Early Folliculark Phase	Late Follicular Phase	Ovulation Phase	Luteal Phase	Total
General joint laxity [points]					
Female non-athletes (n = 19)					
Eumenorrhea group (n = 11)	1.7 ± 1.4	1.6 ± 1.4	1.4 ± 1.2	1.4 ± 1.3	1.5 ± 1.3
Oligomenorrhea group (n = 8)	1.6 ± 1.3	1.6 ± 1.1	1.3 ± 1.3	1.5 ± 1.0	1.5 ± 1.2
Female athletes (n = 15)					
Eumenorrhea group (n = 8)	2.2 ± 1.7	2.3 ± 1.5	2.5 ± 1.4	2.6 ± 1.6	2.4 ± 1.5
Oligomenorrhea group (n = 7)	1.6 ± 2.5	1.9 ± 2.6	1.7 ± 2.9	1.6 ± 2.6	1.7 ± 2.6

Values are presented as means ± SD.

Table 5. Changes in genu recurvatum during the menstrual cycle.

	Early Follicular Phase	Late Follicular Phase	Ovulation Phase	Luteal Phase	Total
Genu recurvatum [°]					
Female non-athletes (n = 19)	7.0 ± 3.9	7.2 ± 3.9	7.3 ± 4.1	7.7 ± 4.1	
Eumenorrhea group (n = 11)	6.2 ± 3.9	6.3 ± 3.8	6.3 ± 3.9	6.6 ± 4.1	6.4 ± 3.9
Oligomenorrhea group (n = 8)	8.1 ± 3.9	8.4 ± 3.8	8.6 ± 4.2	9.3 ± 3.9	8.6 ± 3.9
Female athletes (n = 15)	7.7 ± 3.7	8.3 ± 3.7 [a]	8.7 ± 3.8 [b]	9.0 ± 3.8 [c]	
Eumenorrhea group (n = 8)	6.1 ± 3.7	7.0 ± 4.1	7.4 ± 4.4	7.6 ± 4.3	7.0 ± 4.1
Oligomenorrhea group (n = 7)	9.5 ± 2.8	9.8 ± 2.8	10.2 ± 2.6	10.7 ± 2.4	10.1 ± 2.6

Values are presented as means ± SD. [a]—Statistically significant difference compared with the early follicular phase in female athletes ($p = 0.050$). [b]—Statistically significant difference compared with the early follicular phase in female athletes ($p = 0.011$). [c]—Statistically significant difference compared with the early follicular phase in female athletes ($p = 0.004$).

3.2. Female Athletes

In salivary estradiol, split-plot repeated-measures ANOVA showed no interactions and no main effects of subject factor, but a main effect of the cycle-phase factor [$F(3, 39) = 5.33$, $p = 0.004$, $\eta p2 = 0.29$]. The results of Bonferroni post hoc testing showed that salivary estradiol concentrations were significantly higher in the luteal phase than in the early follicular phase ($p = 0.039$) (Table 1).

In salivary progesterone, split-plot repeated-measures ANOVA showed no interactions and no main effects of subject factor, but a main effect of the cycle-phase factor [$F(1.500, 19.502) = 14.38$, $p = 0.0004$, $\eta p2 = 0.53$]. The results of Bonferroni post hoc testing showed that salivary progesterone concentrations were significantly higher in the luteal phase than in the early follicular, late follicular, and ovulation phases ($p = 0.005$, $p = 0.001$ and $p = 0.022$, respectively) (Table 1).

The results of split-plot repeated-measures ANOVA about AKL, stiffness, and GJL showed no interactions or main effects of subject or cycle-phase factors at any loadings (Tables 2–4).

In GR, split-plot repeated-measures ANOVA showed no interactions and no main effects of the subject factor, but a main effect of the cycle-phase factor [F (1.929, 25.074) = 13.32, p = 0.0001, $\eta p2$ = 0.51]. The results of Bonferroni post hoc testing showed that GR was significantly higher in the late follicular, ovulation, and luteal phases than in the early follicular phase (p = 0.050, p = 0.011 and p = 0.004, respectively) (Table 5).

3.3. Reliability of GR Measurement

ICC (1, 3) was 0.828 and ICC (2, 3) was 0.854. According to the criteria of Landis et al. [28], reliability is considered "almost perfect" for ICCs of 0.81 or more, so the reliabilities of GR measurements in this study were considered almost perfect.

4. Discussion

To the best of our knowledge, this represents the first study to examine changes in joint laxity during the menstrual cycle among females with menstrual irregularities. The main findings of this study were that stiffness was significantly higher in the oligomenorrhea group than in the eumenorrhea group, although no significant difference in stiffness was seen between cycle phases when limited to female non-athletes. GR was significantly higher in the late follicular, ovulation, and luteal phases than in the early follicular phase, although no difference between groups was seen when limited to female athletes. No significant differences in AKL or GJL were between groups or cycle phases in either female non-athletes or female athletes.

Stiffness did not change with the menstrual cycle in female non-athletes; however, it was significantly higher in the oligomenorrhea group than the eumenorrhea. Karageanes et al. considered that repetition of the menstrual cycle (hormonal stimulation) may exert long-term effects on connective tissues, resulting in changes to estradiol receptor sensitivity or an unraveling effect in which ligaments gradually become looser [16]. In this study, the duration of exposure to estradiol may have been shorter in the oligomenorrhea group with longer menstrual cycles than in the eumenorrhea group. If the duration of exposure to estradiol affected the tensile properties of the ACL, stiffness may have been higher in the oligomenorrhea group than in the eumenorrhea group. Stiffness can be calculated and quantified from the load-displacement curve obtained from AKL measurements and has been suggested to be related to clinical end-feel [29]. Three phases are observed in the load-displacement curve: early phase: middle phase: and late phase, the late phase is considered to represent the terminal stiffness of the joint in which the ACL is fully involved in restraining tibial anterior displacement [29]. Davey et al. reported that a 1-standard deviation (SD) decrease in ACL stiffness was associated with a 2.37-fold increased risk of contralateral injury after initial ACL injury [30]. In addition, the incidence of ACL injury is reportedly higher among women with normal menstruation than among those using OCs [31]. Such considerations suggest that female non-athletes with oligomenorrhea may have fewer risk factors for ACL injury than female non-athletes with eumenorrhea.

GR in female athletes was significantly higher in the late follicular, ovulation, and luteal phases than in the early follicular phase, although no difference was evident between eumenorrhea and oligomenorrhea groups. These results support previous findings that GR changes during the menstrual cycle [12,18]. Estradiol receptors are present in the human ACL [32], myofibers of skeletal muscle and capillary endothelial cells [33]. Previous studies investigating changes in muscle stiffness during the menstrual cycle have reported that hamstring extensibility (straight leg raising angle) was higher during the ovulation phase compared to the early follicular phase [34], and muscle stiffness of the vastus medialis and semitendinosus muscles was higher during the ovulation phase compared to the luteal phase [35]. Avrillon et al. reported that the shear modulus of the semimembranosus muscle was lower among figure skaters, taekwondo practitioners, soccer players, and fencers than among non-athletes [36]. This suggests that female athletes with lower muscle stiffness may be more susceptible to changes in joint laxity than non-athletes. Therefore, it is possible that estradiol may have altered muscle stiffness, resulting in altered GR in female athletes during the menstrual cycle. The results of this study thus suggest that female athletes may be at increased risk of ACL injury from the late follicular phase to the luteal phase. In the future, a better understanding of the menstrual cycle of female athletes will be needed to develop training methods adapted to the cyclical changes in body structure and methods for preventing ACL injury.

The AKL did not change during the menstrual cycle in either female non-athletes or female athletes, and no difference was seen between eumenorrhea and oligomenorrhea groups. The results of this study support previous studies that AKL does not change during the menstrual cycle [8,15–17]. Lee et al. found that AKL was significantly higher in the non-OC group than in the OC group and that AKL changed only in the non-OC group [19]. In the present study, no difference in estradiol concentration was identified between eumenorrhea and oligomenorrhea groups, suggesting that no group differences may exist in AKL. GJL did not change during the menstrual cycle in either female non-athletes or female athletes, and no difference was apparent between eumenorrhea and oligomenorrhea groups. The results of this study differed from those of previous studies, which showed that GJL changed during the menstrual cycle [12,18]. GJL can be congenital, occurring as a part of connective tissue diseases such as Marfan's syndrome, Ehlers-Danlos syndrome, and benign joint hypermobility syndrome [37], or acquired, resulting from stretching of the capsular ligament due to repetitive microtrauma or repetitive use during sports activities [38]. GJL is thus suggested to be highly susceptible to congenital laxity or sports history, but less susceptible to female hormones during the menstrual cycle.

Several limitations to the present study must be considered when interpreting the results. First, considering the characteristics of the experimental apparatus and the safety of participants, GR was evaluated based on the subjective sensations of participants. In this study, GR was measured by extending the knee joint until just before the appearance of pain or discomfort in the knee joint, so pain or intrinsic receptive sensation may have been affected. The pain threshold reported does not change during the menstrual cycle [39], but intrinsic receptive sensation in the knee joint is reported to decrease in the early follicular phase compared to the luteal phase [40]. However, the reliability of GR measurement appeared to be high in this study, so the method of measuring GR in this study was considered to be highly valid. A second limitation was that we could not control the amount of activity of female athletes. In this study, female athletes were tested throughout a single season, because the study period was extended due to the coronavirus disease 2019 pandemic. The activity levels of female athlete participants may thus have differed between training and competition periods, which may have contributed to discrepancies in the results for AKL, GJL, and GR. Therefore, when assessing joint laxity in female athletes, consideration must be given to not only the effects of the menstrual cycle, but also the amount of activity during the season. A third limitation was the sample size. In the present study, joint laxity was measured eight times in four phases: early follicular phase, late follicular phase, ovulation phase, and luteal phase. Of the 71 female non-athletes and 27 female athletes recruited, only 19 female non-athletes and 15 female athletes completed the experiment. Some degree of caution is thus warranted when interpreting the present results. However, by measuring joint laxity at multiple time points throughout the menstrual cycle, we were able to more accurately investigate changes in joint laxity during the menstrual cycle. A fourth limitation was that the participants were limited to university students and university athletes. Previous studies have reported that age may affect the value of joint laxity [10,41]. Therefore, the results of this study may not be applicable to non-university age groups. Future studies should be conducted not only in university age group but also in middle and high school age groups.

5. Conclusions

In this study, stiffness was significantly higher in the oligomenorrhea group than in the eumenorrhea group when limited to female non-athletes. GR was significantly higher in the late follicular phase, ovulation phase, and luteal phase compared to the early follicular phase when limited to female athletes. Future studies need to clarify the effects of the menstrual cycle in female athletes and develop training methods for injury prevention that are adapted to cyclical changes in female body structure.

Author Contributions: Conceptualization, S.M. and M.E.; methodology, S.M. and M.E.; validation, S.M., C.S., M.S., H.Y., R.H. (Ryo Hirabayashi), R.T., Y.Y. and M.E.; formal analysis, S.M. and M.E. investigation, S.M., C.S., M.S. and M.E.; data curation, S.M.; writing—original draft preparation, S.M.; writing—review and editing, M.E., C.S., M.S., H.Y., R.H. (Ryo Hirabayashi), R.T., Y.Y., R.H. (Rena Hamano), A.I. and D.S.; visualization, S.M.; project administration, M.E.; funding acquisition, M.E. All authors have read and agreed to the published version of the manuscript.

Funding: This study was supported by a Grant-in-Aid for Scientific Research (19K11358) from the Japan Society for the Promotion of Science (JSPS) and commissioned by the Japan Sports Agency (Female Athletes Development and Support Projects 2020).

Institutional Review Board Statement: The study was conducted according to the guidelines of the Declaration of Helsinki and approved by the Ethics Committee of Niigata University of Health and Welfare (18467—26 August 2020).

Informed Consent Statement: Informed consent was obtained from all subjects.

Data Availability Statement: The data that support the findings of this study are available from the corresponding author.

Acknowledgments: The authors want to acknowledge and thank all female volunteers and all female college athletes who participated in this study.

Conflicts of Interest: The authors declare no conflict of interest.

References

1. Beynnon, B.D.; Vacek, P.M.; Newell, M.K.; Tourville, T.W.; Smith, H.C.; Shultz, S.J.; Slauterbeck, J.R.; Johnson, R.J. The Effects of Level of Competition, Sport, and Sex on the Incidence of First-Time Noncontact Anterior Cruciate Ligament Injury. *Am. J. Sports Med.* **2014**, *42*, 1806–1812. [CrossRef] [PubMed]
2. Hewett, T.E.; Myer, G.D.; Ford, K.R. Anterior cruciate ligament injuries in female athletes: Part 1, mechanisms and risk factors. *Am. J. Sports Med.* **2006**, *34*, 299–311. [CrossRef] [PubMed]
3. Beynnon, B.D.; Johnson, R.J.; Braun, S.; Sargent, M.; Bernstein, I.M.; Skelly, J.M.; Vacek, P.M. The relationship between menstrual cycle phase and anterior cruciate ligament injury: A case-control study of recreational alpine skiers. *Am. J. Sports Med.* **2006**, *34*, 757–764. [CrossRef] [PubMed]
4. Wojtys, E.M.; Huston, L.J.; Boynton, M.D.; Spindler, K.P.; Lindenfeld, T.N. The effect of the menstrual cycle on anterior cruciate ligament injuries in women as determined by hormone levels. *Am. J. Sports Med.* **2002**, *30*, 182–188. [CrossRef] [PubMed]
5. Vacek, P.M.; Slauterbeck, J.R.; Tourville, T.W.; Sturnick, D.R.; Holterman, L.A.; Smith, H.C.; Shultz, S.J.; Johnson, R.J.; Tourville, K.J.; Beynnon, B.D. Multivariate Analysis of the Risk Factors for First-Time Noncontact ACL Injury in High School and College Athletes: A Prospective Cohort Study With a Nested, Matched Case-Control Analysis. *Am. J. Sports Med.* **2016**, *44*, 1492–1501. [CrossRef] [PubMed]
6. Uhorchak, J.M.; Scoville, C.R.; Williams, G.N.; Arciero, R.A.; St Pierre, P.; Taylor, D.C. Risk factors associated with noncontact injury of the anterior cruciate ligament: A prospective four-year evaluation of 859 West Point cadets. *Am. J. Sports Med.* **2003**, *31*, 831–842. [CrossRef]
7. Kramer, L.C.; Denegar, C.R.; Buckley, W.E.; Hertel, J. Factors associated with anterior cruciate ligament injury: History in female athletes. *J. Sports Med. Phys. Fit.* **2007**, *47*, 446–454.
8. Beynnon, B.D.; Bernstein, I.M.; Belisle, A.; Brattbakk, B.; Devanny, P.; Risinger, R.; Durant, D. The effect of estradiol and progesterone on knee and ankle joint laxity. *Am. J. Sports Med.* **2005**, *33*, 1298–1304. [CrossRef]
9. Shultz, S.J.; Sander, T.C.; Kirk, S.E.; Perrin, D.H. Sex differences in knee joint laxity change across the female menstrual cycle. *J. Sports Med. Phys. Fit.* **2005**, *45*, 594–603.
10. Jansson, A.; Saartok, T.; Werner, S.; Renström, P. General joint laxity in 1845 Swedish school children of different ages: Age- and gender-specific distributions. *Acta Paediatr.* **2004**, *93*, 1202–1206. [CrossRef]
11. Nguyen, A.D.; Shultz, S.J. Sex differences in clinical measures of lower extremity alignment. *J. Orthop. Sports Phys. Ther.* **2007**, *37*, 389–398. [CrossRef] [PubMed]

12. Shultz, S.J.; Levine, B.J.; Nguyen, A.D.; Kim, H.; Montgomery, M.M.; Perrin, D.H. A comparison of cyclic variations in anterior knee laxity, genu recurvatum, and general joint laxity across the menstrual cycle. *J. Orthop. Res.* **2010**, *28*, 1411–1417. [CrossRef] [PubMed]
13. Shultz, S.J.; Schmitz, R.J.; Nguyen, A.D.; Levine, B.; Kim, H.; Montgomery, M.M.; Shimokochi, Y.; Beynnon, B.D.; Perrin, D.H. Knee joint laxity and its cyclic variation influence tibiofemoral motion during weight acceptance. *J. Orthop. Res.* **2011**, *43*, 287–295. [CrossRef]
14. Park, S.K.; Stefanyshyn, D.J.; Loitz-Ramage, B.; Hart, D.A.; Ronsky, J.L. Changing hormone levels during the menstrual cycle affect knee laxity and stiffness in healthy female subjects. *Am. J. Sports Med.* **2009**, *37*, 588–598. [CrossRef] [PubMed]
15. Eiling, E.; Bryant, A.L.; Petersen, W.; Murphy, A.; Hohmann, E. Effects of menstrual-cycle hormone fluctuations on musculotendinous stiffness and knee joint laxity. *Knee Surg. Sports Traumatol. Arthrosc.* **2007**, *15*, 126–132. [CrossRef] [PubMed]
16. Karageanes, S.J.; Blackburn, K.; Vangelos, Z.A. The association of the menstrual cycle with the laxity of the anterior cruciate ligament in adolescent female athletes. *Clin. J. Sport Med.* **2000**, *10*, 162–168. [CrossRef] [PubMed]
17. Maruyama, S.; Yamazaki, T.; Sato, Y.; Suzuki, Y.; Shimizu, S.; Ikezu, M.; Kaneko, F.; Matsuzawa, K.; Hirabayashi, R.; Edama, M. Relationship Between Anterior Knee Laxity and General Joint Laxity During the Menstrual Cycle. *Orthop. J. Sports Med.* **2021**, *9*, 2325967121993045. [CrossRef]
18. Shagawa, M.; Maruyama, S.; Sekine, C.; Yokota, H.; Hirabayashi, R.; Hirata, A.; Yokoyama, M.; Edama, M. Comparison of anterior knee laxity, stiffness, genu recurvatum, and general joint laxity in the late follicular phase and the ovulatory phase of the menstrual cycle. *BMC Musculoskelet. Disord.* **2021**, *22*, 886. [CrossRef]
19. Lee, H.; Petrofsky, J.S.; Daher, N.; Berk, L.; Laymon, M. Differences in anterior cruciate ligament elasticity and force for knee flexion in women: Oral contraceptive users versus non-oral contraceptive users. *Eur. J. Appl. Physiol.* **2014**, *114*, 285–294. [CrossRef]
20. Nose-Ogura, S. Advancement in female sports medicine and preventive medicine. *J. Obstet. Gynaecol. Res.* **2021**, *47*, 476–485. [CrossRef]
21. Brook, E.M.; Tenforde, A.S.; Broad, E.M.; Matzkin, E.G.; Yang, H.Y.; Collins, J.E.; Blauwet, C.A. Low energy availability, menstrual dysfunction, and impaired bone health: A survey of elite para athletes. *Scand. J. Med. Sci. Sports* **2019**, *29*, 678–685. [CrossRef] [PubMed]
22. Nose-Ogura, S.; Yoshino, O.; Dohi, M.; Kigawa, M.; Harada, M.; Hiraike, O.; Onda, T.; Osuga, Y.; Fujii, T.; Saito, S. Risk factors of stress fractures due to the female athlete triad: Differences in teens and twenties. *Scand. J. Med. Sci. Sports* **2019**, *29*, 1501–1510. [CrossRef] [PubMed]
23. Shultz, S.J.; Schmitz, R.J.; Nguyen, A.D.; Levine, B.J. Joint laxity is related to lower extremity energetics during a drop jump landing. *Med. Sci. Sports. Exerc.* **2010**, *42*, 771–780. [CrossRef] [PubMed]
24. Gibbs, J.C.; Nattiv, A.; Barrack, M.T.; Williams, N.I.; Rauh, M.J.; Nichols, J.F.; De Souza, M.J. Low bone density risk is higher in exercising women with multiple triad risk factors. *Med. Sci. Sports Exerc.* **2014**, *46*, 167–176. [CrossRef] [PubMed]
25. Moghissi, K.S. Prediction and detection of ovulation. *Fertil. Steril.* **1980**, *34*, 89–98. [CrossRef] [PubMed]
26. Salimetrics LLC.; Salivabio LLC. *Saliva Collection and Handling Advice*, 3rd ed.; Salimetrics: State College, PA, USA; Salivabio: Carlsbad, CA, USA, 2015. Available online: https://fnkprddata.blob.core.windows.net/domestic/download/pdf/SAL_handbook3.pdf (accessed on 20 December 2021).
27. Beighton, P.; Solomon, L.; Soskolne, C.L. Articular mobility in an African population. *Ann. Rheum. Dis.* **1973**, *32*, 413–418. [CrossRef]
28. Landis, J.R.; Koch, G.G. The measurement of observer agreement for categorical data. *Biometrics* **1977**, *33*, 159–174. [CrossRef]
29. Maitland, M.E.; Bell, G.D.; Mohtadi, N.G.; Herzog, W. Quantitative analysis of anterior cruciate ligament instability. *Clin. Biomech.* **1995**, *10*, 93–97. [CrossRef]
30. Davey, A.P.; Vacek, P.M.; Caldwell, R.A.; Slauterbeck, J.R.; Gardner-Morse, M.G.; Tourville, T.W.; Beynnon, B.D. Risk Factors Associated With a Noncontact Anterior Cruciate Ligament Injury to the Contralateral Knee After Unilateral Anterior Cruciate Ligament Injury in High School and College Female Athletes: A Prospective Study. *Am. J. Sports Med.* **2019**, *47*, 3347–3355. [CrossRef]
31. Herzberg, S.D.; Motu'apuaka, M.L.; Lambert, W.; Fu, R.; Brady, J.; Guise, J.M. The Effect of Menstrual Cycle and Contraceptives on ACL Injuries and Laxity: A Systematic Review and Meta-analysis. *Orthop. J. Sports Med.* **2017**, *5*, 2325967117718781. [CrossRef]
32. Liu, S.H.; Al-Shaikh, R.; Panossian, V.; Yang, R.S.; Nelson, S.D.; Soleiman, N.; Finerman, G.A.; Lane, J.M. Primary immunolocalization of estrogen and progesterone target cells in the human anterior cruciate ligament. *J. Orthop. Res.* **1996**, *14*, 526–533. [CrossRef] [PubMed]
33. Wiik, A.; Ekman, M.; Morgan, G.; Johansson, O.; Jansson, E.; Esbjörnsson, M. Oestrogen receptor beta is present in both muscle fibres and endothelial cells within human skeletal muscle tissue. *Histochem. Cell. Biol.* **2005**, *124*, 161–165. [CrossRef] [PubMed]
34. Bell, D.R.; Myrick, M.P.; Blackburn, J.T.; Shultz, S.J.; Guskiewicz, K.M.; Padua, D.A. The effect of menstrual-cycle phase on hamstring extensibility and muscle stiffness. *J. Sport. Rehabil.* **2009**, *18*, 553–563. [CrossRef] [PubMed]
35. Sung, E.S.; Kim, J.H. The difference effect of estrogen on muscle tone of medial and lateral thigh muscle during ovulation. *J. Exerc. Rehabil.* **2018**, *14*, 419–423. [CrossRef]
36. Avrillon, S.; Lacourpaille, L.; Hug, F.; Le Sant, G.; Frey, A.; Nordez, A.; Guilhem, G. Hamstring muscle elasticity differs in specialized high-performance athletes. *Scand. J. Med. Sci. Sports* **2020**, *30*, 83–91. [CrossRef]

37. Zweers, M.C.; Hakim, A.J.; Grahame, R.; Schalkwijk, J. Joint hypermobility syndromes: The pathophysiologic role of tenascin-X gene defects. *Arthritis Rheum.* **2004**, *50*, 2742–2749. [CrossRef]
38. Saccomanno, M.F.; Fodale, M.; Capasso, L.; Cazzato, G.; Milano, G. Generalized joint laxity and multidirectional instability of the shoulder. *Joints* **2013**, *1*, 171–179. [CrossRef]
39. Thompson, B.M.; Drover, K.B.; Stellmaker, R.J.; Sculley, D.V.; Janse de Jonge, X.A.K. The Effect of the Menstrual Cycle and Oral Contraceptive Cycle on Muscle Performance and Perceptual Measures. *Int. J. Environ. Res. Public Health* **2021**, *18*, 10565. [CrossRef]
40. Fouladi, R.; Rajabi, R.; Naseri, N.; Pourkazemi, F.; Geranmayeh, M. Menstrual cycle and knee joint position sense in healthy female athletes. *Knee Surg. Sports Traumatol. Arthrosc.* **2012**, *20*, 1647–1652. [CrossRef]
41. Zyroul, R.; Hossain, M.G.; Azura, M.; Abbas, A.A.; Kamarul, T. Knee laxity of Malaysian adults: Gender differentials, and association with age and anthropometric measures. *Knee* **2014**, *21*, 557–562. [CrossRef]

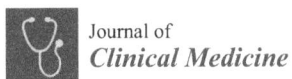

Article

Evidence-Based Surgical Treatment Algorithm for Unstable Syndesmotic Injuries

Markus Regauer [1,2,*], Gordon Mackay [3], Owen Nelson [4], Wolfgang Böcker [1] and Christian Ehrnthaller [1]

[1] Department of Orthopedics and Trauma Surgery, Musculoskeletal University Center Munich (MUM), University Hospital, LMU Munich, 81377 Munich, Germany; Wolfgang.Boecker@med.uni-muenchen.de (W.B.); Christian.Ehrnthaller@med.uni-muenchen.de (C.E.)
[2] Sportortho Rosenheim, 83022 Rosenheim, Germany
[3] Health Sciences and Sport, University of Stirling, Stirling FK9 4LA, UK; gordonmmackay@gmail.com
[4] Orthopedics and Sports Medicine, Waldo County General Hospital, Belfast, ME 04915, USA; oanelson@icloud.com
* Correspondence: Markus.Regauer@med.uni-muenchen.de; Tel.: +49-08031-900640

Abstract: Background: Surgical treatment of unstable syndesmotic injuries is not trivial, and there are no generally accepted treatment guidelines. The most common controversies regarding surgical treatment are related to screw fixation versus dynamic fixation, the use of reduction clamps, open versus closed reduction, and the role of the posterior malleolus and of the anterior inferior tibiofibular ligament (AITFL). Our aim was to draw important conclusions from the pertinent literature concerning surgical treatment of unstable syndesmotic injuries, to transform these conclusions into surgical principles supported by the literature, and finally to fuse these principles into an evidence-based surgical treatment algorithm. Methods: PubMed, Embase, Google Scholar, The Cochrane Database of Systematic Reviews, and the reference lists of systematic reviews of relevant studies dealing with the surgical treatment of unstable syndesmotic injuries were searched independently by two reviewers using specific terms and limits. Surgical principles supported by the literature were fused into an evidence-based surgical treatment algorithm. Results: A total of 171 articles were included for further considerations. Among them, 47 articles concerned syndesmotic screw fixation and 41 flexible dynamic fixations of the syndesmosis. Twenty-five studies compared screw fixation with dynamic fixations, and seven out of these comparisons were randomized controlled trials. Nineteen articles addressed the posterior malleolus, 14 the role of the AITFL, and eight the use of reduction clamps. Anatomic reduction is crucial to prevent posttraumatic osteoarthritis. Therefore, flexible dynamic stabilization techniques should be preferred whenever possible. An unstable AITFL should be repaired and augmented, as it represents an important stabilizer of external rotation of the distal fibula. Conclusions: The current literature provides sufficient arguments for the development of an evidence-based surgical treatment algorithm for unstable syndesmotic injuries.

Keywords: syndesmosis; anterior inferior tibiofibular ligament; high ankle sprain; rotational instability; posterior malleolus; stabilization; anatomic repair; syndesmotic screw; suture-button; internal bracing; treatment algorithm

Citation: Regauer, M.; Mackay, G.; Nelson, O.; Böcker, W.; Ehrnthaller, C. Evidence-Based Surgical Treatment Algorithm for Unstable Syndesmotic Injuries. *J. Clin. Med.* 2022, 11, 331. https://doi.org/10.3390/jcm11020331

Academic Editors: Antonio Frizziero and Redha Taiar

Received: 14 November 2021
Accepted: 5 January 2022
Published: 10 January 2022

Publisher's Note: MDPI stays neutral with regard to jurisdictional claims in published maps and institutional affiliations.

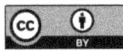

Copyright: © 2022 by the authors. Licensee MDPI, Basel, Switzerland. This article is an open access article distributed under the terms and conditions of the Creative Commons Attribution (CC BY) license (https://creativecommons.org/licenses/by/4.0/).

1. Introduction

An increasing interest in the treatment of unstable syndesmotic injuries during the last decade has led to an enormous amount of literature not easy to review [1–171]. Syndesmosis as a search term in PubMed, for example, currently revealed 1271 results as of 28 October 2021.

The ligaments stabilizing the inferior tibiofibular syndesmosis prevent excess fibular motion in multiple directions: anterior-posterior translation, lateral translation, craniocaudal translation, and internal and external rotation [6,62,63,68,79,164]. Appropriate fibular position and limited rotation are necessary for normal syndesmotic function and talar position within the ankle mortise [66]. Reconstruction of unstable syndesmotic injuries is not trivial, and there are no generally accepted treatment guidelines [18,63,80,119]. Thus, there still remain considerable controversies regarding diagnosis, classification, and treatment of unstable syndesmotic injuries [63,119,149]. The most common controversies regarding surgical treatment are related to screw fixation versus dynamic fixation, the use of reduction clamps, open versus closed reduction, and the role of the posterior malleolus and of the anterior inferior tibiofibular ligament (AITFL).

Although several studies have clearly shown serious problems concerning the use of syndesmotic screws, this method is still considered the gold standard for treatment of unstable syndesmotic injuries by the majority of orthopedic and trauma surgeons [10,12,18,19,24,27,30,39,51,53,64,70,148,159]. This controversy may be explained by an obvious lack of further education and training, by the misconception that this surgical technique is simple and easy to perform, and by the fact that syndesmotic screws still represent the cheapest solution, at least considering the short term [115].

Alternative methods for treatment of unstable syndesmotic injuries reported in literature include syndesmotic hooks or hook plates [45,160,166], transfixation bolts [162], various suture button constructs [5,8,38,94,95,106,117,120,131,132,141,142,165], ligament bracing [58,80,98,119,135,140], tendon autograft [25,56,91,98] or even allograft reconstruction [35]. During the last decades, several studies have clearly shown superior results after flexible dynamic syndesmotic stabilization compared to the use of syndesmotic screws with regard to accuracy of reduction, functional outcome, and even development of post-traumatic ankle arthritis [9,32,34,48,57,72,76,94,111,124,134,171].

Therefore, our aim was to draw important conclusions from the pertinent literature concerning surgical treatment of unstable syndesmotic injuries, to transform these conclusions into surgical principles supported by literature, and finally to fuse these principles into an evidence-based surgical treatment algorithm.

2. Materials and Methods

From 1 October 2019 to 28 October 2021, the first and senior authors (M.R. and C.E.) independently searched PubMed, Embase, Google Scholar, The Cochrane Database of Systematic Reviews, and the reference lists of systematic reviews of relevant studies dealing with the surgical treatment of unstable syndesmotic injuries. The mentioned databases were selected because they represent the prevalent and generally accepted databases used for medical research. The following search terms listed in alphabetical order were used: anatomic reduction, anatomic repair, ankle fracture, anterior inferior tibiofibular ligament (AITFL), augmentation, diastasis screw, flexible stabilization, high ankle sprain, InternalBrace, ligament bracing, positioning screw, posterior malleolus, rotational stability, suture button, syndesmo*, syndesmosis, syndesmotic screw, tibiofibular*, tightrope, and treatment algorithm. Only articles published in English, German, or Spanish language were included. Other than language, there were no further restrictions for the inclusion of articles. Letters to the editors, short comments, incomplete, or inaccessible full-text articles were excluded. Included articles were assigned to the following main topics:

- Importance of anatomic reduction
- Closed versus open reduction under direct visualization
- Role of reduction clamps
- Role of syndesmotic screws
- Role of flexible dynamic stabilization techniques
- Role of the AITFL
- Role of the posterolateral malleolus

After assessment of the scientific quality of the assigned articles, we tried to draw important conclusions from the pertinent literature concerning the surgical treatment of unstable syndesmotic injuries. Then, we transformed these conclusions into clinically relevant surgical principles supported by literature, and finally, we fused these principles into a surgical treatment algorithm.

3. Results

A total of 171 articles were included for further considerations [1–171]. Among them, 47 articles concerned syndesmotic screw fixation and 41 dynamic fixations of the syndesmosis. Twenty-five studies compared screw fixation with dynamic fixations, and seven out of these comparisons were randomized controlled trials [9,32,34,72,76,111,124]. Nineteen articles addressed the posterior malleolus, 14 the role of the AITFL, and eight the use of reduction clamps.

3.1. Importance of Anatomic Reduction

Malreduction of the distal tibiofibular syndesmosis still remains a common complication associated with the surgical management of ankle fractures [23,31]. Syndesmotic malreduction can lead to severe alterations in the biomechanics of the ankle and thereby to chronic pain and premature degenerative changes of the ankle joint [31]. Therefore, ankle fractures with need for syndesmotic stabilization are still associated with a high rate of secondary osteoarthritis [118]. As early as 1961, Willenegger stated that posttraumatic osteoarthritis of the ankle almost always is due to an incongruity between the ankle mortise and the talus and not due to an intraarticular fracture itself [162]. He reported on 31 of 32 cases that rapidly developed severe posttraumatic ankle arthritis even after only slight malreduction of the ankle mortise [162]. Several well-known studies confirmed Willenegger's early observations, and today, it is generally accepted that even a small syndesmotic displacement of less than 1 mm can have devastating consequences for the rapid development of posttraumatic ankle arthritis [1,59,62,65,100,102,111,116,123,153]. Significant increases in tibiotalar contact pressures occur when external rotation stresses are added to axial loading in an unstable tibiofibular syndesmosis. Moderate and severe syndesmotic injuries are associated with a significant increase in mean contact pressure combined with a shift in the center of pressure and rotation of the fibula and talus. In this context, simple syndesmotic injuries represent partial ruptures without signs of instability in the clinical and radiological evaluation compared to moderate and severe syndesmotic injuries. Moderate syndesmotic injuries show clinical signs of dynamic instability without static dislocation in the radiographic evaluation, and severe injuries show signs of dislocation of the fibula in the incisura tibiofibularis even in the static examinations.

Considerable changes in ankle joint kinematics and contact mechanics may explain why unstable syndesmotic injuries take longer to heal and are more likely to develop long-term dysfunction and ankle arthritis [65]. Moreover, in the long run, post-traumatic ankle osteoarthritis in known to have a large and negative impact on the patients' quality of life [172]. The single most important prognostic factor after unstable injury of the distal tibiofibular syndesmosis with or without fracture is anatomic reduction of the distal fibula and fitting into the tibial incisura [112]. Therefóre, anatomic reduction of an injured syndesmosis is crucial for an optimal long-term clinical result [7,13,31,151]. In this context, anatomic reduction is defined as complete restoration of the physiological anatomy in the first place but does also imply recovery of the physiologic tension of the repaired ligamentous structures.

Main conclusion: Anatomic reduction is crucial for the long-term results regarding functional outcome and development of posttraumatic ankle osteoarthritis.

3.2. Closed vs. Open Reduction under Direct Visualization

To reliably achieve anatomic reduction of the syndesmosis, open reduction of the AITFL under direct visualization has been advocated, as there is still a lack of appropriate examination techniques to confirm anatomic closed reduction during surgery [26,87,98,103,119,127,143,150]. Tornetta showed that the anterolateral articular surface of the distal tibia to the anteromedial fibular articular surface is an accurate visual landmark for anatomic reduction of the syndesmosis [143]. Another advantage of open reduction under direct visualization is the opportunity to avoid posttraumatic anterolateral impingement syndrome by removing torn parts of the AITFL out of the joint. And aside from that, we should remember that the main goal in the treatment of unstable syndesmotic injuries is to avoid osteoarthritis and not scars.

Main conclusion: Open reduction by direct visualization is strongly recommended.

3.3. Role of Reduction Clamps

Several studies and reports have clearly shown that it is possible and even highly likely to over-compress the syndesmosis when using reduction clamps or forceps [26,36,60,82,85,107,121,156]. In this context, over-compression is defined as any sign of displacement of the talus out of the mortise due to compression of the fibula against the tibia even in correct position of the fibula within the incisura. Haynes et al. demonstrated a significant correlation between increased clamp forces and syndesmotic over-compression and determined objective forces that lead to over-compression of the syndesmosis [60]. Another study by Miller demonstrated that intraoperative clamping and fixation can cause statistically significant malreduction of the syndesmosis [85]. This should alert clinicians that clamp and screw placement can cause iatrogenic malreduction of the syndesmosis. These dangers occur with specific clamp and screw angles in particular. Mahapatra reported that over-compression of the syndesmosis can even cause significant subluxation of the talus [82]. Therefore, care should be taken to avoid over-compression by use of reduction clamps, as this may affect ankle motion and functional outcomes. Cadaver experiments by Phisitkul et al. showed that clamp placement in the neutral anatomical axis reduced the syndesmosis most accurately, but nevertheless, over-compression was frequently observed. Placing the clamp obliquely malreduced the unstable syndesmosis [107]. Furthermore, based on the results of his recent cadaveric study, Rushing stated that inherent variabilities in the applied clamp force by surgeons appear to contribute to the unacceptably high coronal syndesmotic malreduction rate [121]. Goetz et al. have shown that Achilles tension mitigates fibular malalignment measured in cadaveric studies of syndesmotic clamping [53].

In our experience, it seems to depend on the stability of the posterior malleolus and the medial and lateral collateral ankle ligaments if significant over-compression with consecutive dislocation of the talus is possible or not, but this theory has not been proven so far. Cherney described that a stable posterior malleolus does not have a protective effect against over-compression [26]. In our opinion, this might be due to unrecognized additional injuries to the collateral ankle ligaments. Additionally, from an anatomic point of view, there is no physiologic dynamic force leading to displacement of the syndesmosis and therefore needing neutralization by a reduction clamp. As early as 1953, Costigan stated that reduction of diastasis of the ankle mortise is a very simple procedure, not requiring a reducer or any other form of mechanical device [37]. Therefore, at least in acute cases, the surgeon should prefer to analyze the real reasons preventing easy reduction of the syndesmosis instead of increasing the force of reduction clamps.

Main conclusions: There is a high risk for over-compression and malreduction of the syndesmosis by use of reduction clamps or forceps. Therefore, at least in acute cases, the use of reduction clamps or forceps should be avoided whenever possible.

3.4. Role of Syndesmotic Screws

Syndesmotic screws, also referred to as diastasis screws, situational screws, transfixation screws, trans-syndesmotic screws, or positioning screws, have been used at least since 1947 [37]. Therefore, surgical treatment with syndesmotic screw fixation has been performed for several decades now, and this method is still considered the gold standard of treatment of unstable syndesmotic injuries by the majority of orthopedic and trauma surgeons [5,61,67,125,151,159,162,163,169,170]. However, there is still an ongoing discussion concerning ideal reference points and anatomic landmarks for optimal positioning of syndesmotic screws [74,75]. The risk of malpositioning of syndesmotic screws is very high, and a lack of standard radiological or physical references for accurate syndesmotic screw placement is a potential contributing factor in syndesmotic screw malpositioning [75].

Furthermore, several studies have clearly shown serious problems concerning the use of syndesmotic screws due to malreduction of the ankle mortise or high complication rates after syndesmotic screw removal, for example, [10,12,24,39,51,54,70,100,123,148]. Ovaska analyzed patients with malreduced ankle fractures undergoing re-operation and showed that the most common indication for re-operation was syndesmotic malreduction in 59% of cases [100]. In another series of 160 consecutive patients who underwent syndesmosis screw fixation, 13 patients needed revision surgery. Among them, the incidence of recurrent diastasis of the ankle mortise was 92% [12]. Gardner evaluated twenty-five patients with ankle fractures and syndesmotic instability who had open reduction and syndesmotic fixation [51]. A total of 52% of syndesmoses were malreduced on CT scan but went undetected by plain radiographs. Radiographic measurements did not accurately reflect the status of the distal tibiofibular joint in this series of ankle fractures. Furthermore, post-reduction radiographic measurements were inaccurate for assessing the quality of the reduction [51]. In a prospective randomized controlled multicenter trial with 103 patients, the rate of malreduction using screw fixation was 39% [124]. Therefore, especially due to the repeatedly reported high risk of malreduction, the first-line use of syndesmotic screws as a gold standard for the treatment of unstable syndesmotic injuries should be reconsidered.

Main conclusions: The first-line use of syndesmotic screws as a gold standard for the treatment of unstable syndesmotic injuries should be reconsidered. Syndesmotic screws should be used only as a salvage procedure.

3.5. Role of Flexible Dynamic Stabilization Techniques

The currently emerging surgical techniques for flexible dynamic stabilization of the syndesmosis are not new regarding their principles, but the available implants provided by industry enabling low-risk and straightforward surgery have significantly improved over the past two decades [5,8,9,33,95,139].

As early as 1961, Willenegger already stated that the preservation of the natural elasticity of the syndesmosis is of greatest importance not only for the final results but also for the initial postsurgical treatment. Accordingly, he refused the use of the rigid transfixation bolt [162]. However, at that time, there was a lack of suitable alternative implants. In 1955, Schumann developed a kind of early precursor of suture-button constructs consisting of two steel plates placed over the medial and lateral malleolus connected via a transmalleolar tensioning wire bolt [131]. This indicates that even at that early time, surgeons were searching for flexible alternatives to the rigid screw or bolt fixations. Some decades later, in 1991, Seitz et al. reported on the repair of the tibiofibular syndesmosis with a flexible implant consisting of a double thickness of No. 5 braided polyester suture tied over polyethylene buttons situated medially and laterally [132].

The currently most widely-used flexible dynamic stabilization device is the knotless syndesmosis TightRope® implant system produced by Arthrex (Naples, FL, USA). Recently, this device has attracted a great deal of even public attention due to an extremely accelerated return to play in high-level athletes after surgical stabilization of high ankle sprains [104]. Tightrope surgeries have been brought into the spotlight known as "Tua surgery" by the circumstances of the Alabama Crimson Tide's 2018 football season. Starting quarterback Tua Tagovailoa suffered a high ankle sprain on 1 December 2018, and the following day, his injured right ankle was stabilized by Norman Waldrop using two knotless syndesmosis TightRope® implant systems. Tagovailoa returned to play just 27 days after surgery to lead the Alabama Crimson Tide football team to a win over Oklahoma in the College Football Playoff semifinal on 29 December 2018.

During the last decades, several studies have clearly shown superior results after flexible dynamic syndesmotic stabilization compared to the use of syndesmotic screws with regard to accuracy of reduction, functional outcome, and even development of posttraumatic ankle arthritis [9,29,32,34,48,49,55,57,69,71,72,76,83,94,102,111,115,124,125,129,130,132,138,171]. Seven of these comparisons were randomized controlled trials [9,32,34,72,76,111,124]. In 2019, for example, Sanders showed that the rate of malreduction using screw fixation was

39% compared with 15% using TightRope® fixation, and the reoperation rate was much higher in the screw group compared with TightRope® (30% vs. 4%, $p = 0.02$) with the difference driven by the rate of implant removal [124]. With deliberate malreduction in a cadaver model, Westermann reported that suture-button fixation of the syndesmosis results in less post-fixation displacement compared with screw fixation. The suture button's ability to allow for natural correction of deliberate malreduction was greatest with posterior off-axis clamping [161]. Therefore, dynamic syndesmotic fixation may even mitigate clamp-induced malreduction. A systematic review of suture-button versus syndesmotic screw in the treatment of distal tibiofibular syndesmosis injury by Zhang et al. showed that the suture-button device could lead to better objective range of motion measurements and earlier return to work. Besides, the suture-button fixation group had lower rates of implant removal, implant failure, and malreduction [171].

A randomized trial by Anderson et al. comparing suture-button with single syndesmotic screw for syndesmosis injury attested that patients treated with a suture-button device had higher AOFAS scores, OMA scores, and EQ-5D Index scores as well as better VAS scores for pain during walking and pain during rest. Moreover, the suture-button group had less widening seen radiographically at two years than did the patients in the syndesmotic screw group [9]. Five years after syndesmotic injury treated with either suture-button or syndesmotic screw within a randomized controlled trial, Ræder et al. found better AOFAS and OMA scores and even lower incidence of ankle osteoarthritis in the suture-button group [111].

These long-term results clearly favor the use of suture-button devices when treating an acute syndesmotic injury. In a recent meta-analysis performed by Shimozono, the suture-button technique resulted in improved functional outcomes as well as lower rates of broken implant and joint malreduction. Based on these findings, the suture-button technique warrants a grade A recommendation by comparison with the syndesmotic screw technique for the treatment of syndesmosis injuries [134].

Main conclusion: Use flexible dynamic stabilization techniques for treatment of unstable syndesmotic injuries whenever possible.

3.6. Role of the AITFL

According to the aforementioned literature, it is possible to achieve very good results in the treatment of unstable syndesmotic injuries using suture-button devices in most cases. However, a study by Clanton recently showed that in some cases, it might not be possible to sufficiently stabilize sagittal translation of the distal fibula by one TightRope® and especially rotary instability even by use of two such flexible dynamic suture-button devices [29]. These observations were confirmed in a biomechanical study by Goetz et al., who reported that flexible trans-syndesmotic fixation alone was found to be insufficient for restoring rotational stability to the ankle or preventing sagittal plane displacement of the distal fibula, and thus, repairs to simulate anatomic structures disrupted during a syndesmosis injury were required to restore rotational stability [55]. Moreover, Clanton showed that isolated injuries to the AITFL resulted in the most substantial reduction of resistance to external rotation and that even isolated injuries to the AITFL alone may lead to significant external rotary instability of the ankle mortise [29]. Recently, these findings were confirmed by a cadaveric robotic study by Patel, who showed that ankle instability is similar after both isolated AITFL and complete syndesmosis injury and can persist after suture-button fixation in the sagittal plane in response to an inversion stress [105].

We have also experienced these problems clinically, and therefore, we started to augment our repairs of the AITFL by use of an *Internal*Brace™ (Arthrex, Naples, FL, USA) in 2013 [119]. Shoji, Teramoto, and Hajewski published a similar surgical technique for ligament augmentation of the AITFL in 2018 and 2019, respectively [58,135,140].

Even earlier, Nelson reported in 2006 on the importance of the AITFL and described two methods for an anatomic repair or reconstruction of the AITFL [98]. However, at that time, there were no suitable implants available, so that this technique was not widely adopted. This article by Nelson was a report of 50 unselected consecutive unstable ankle fractures in which he specifically visually examined the injured AITFL and described a technique of direct visual reduction and flexible repair of the syndesmotic disruption using autograft or sutures secured to bone with traditional screws. Syndesmotic screw fixation of transmalleolar ankle fractures was not necessary in any of the 50 cases when the AITFL was repaired directly by the techniques described. In this unselected consecutive series of patients, Nelson documented a 100% incidence of injury of the AITFL independent of the fracture classification (Weber A, B, and C fractures were included in the study) [98]. The total incidence of bony avulsions of the AITFL was 26%, consisting of an 18% incidence of fibular avulsions (Wagstaffe fragments) and an 8% incidence of tibial avulsions (Tubercule de Chaput fragments). Based upon that clinical experience and continuing interest in the syndesmotic ligaments, it was Nelson's conviction that the AITFL is ruptured in virtually 100% of unstable ankle fractures and that direct visual reduction and repair of ligament disruptions and bone avulsions results in reliable restoration of ankle anatomy and stability. Consequently, Littlechild advocated that consideration should also be given to reconstruction of the AITFL to augment the syndesmosis fixation, which may provide a stronger restoration of ankle stability compared to repairing the posterior inferior tibiofibular ligament (PITFL) in isolation, for example, by fixation of a posterior malleolus avulsion fracture [77]. In total, we found 13 publications recommending open repair and augmentation of the AITFL [2,11,20,28,58,77,80,98,119,135,140,167,170].

Main conclusions: The AITFL is an important stabilizer, especially for rotary stability, and even isolated injuries to the AITFL alone may lead to significant external rotary instability of the ankle mortise. Therefore, an unstable AITFL should be repaired and augmented. Bony avulsion fragments can obstruct anatomic reduction of the distal tibiofibular joint but when reduced anatomically can serve as landmarks for reduction.

3.7. Role of the Posterior Malleolus

Sir Astley Cooper, in 1822, first described fractures of the ankle with involvement of the posterior lip of the tibia [97]. The posterior lip of the distal tibia was entitled the "posterior malleolus" by Destot in 1911, and Henderson and Stuck, in 1935, suggested the term "trimalleolar" for ankle fractures involving the medial and lateral malleolus and the posterior lip of the tibia [97]. In 1922, Lounsberry and Metz discussed trimalleolar fractures as well as those with involvement of the anterior tibial lip, and they were the first to advocate open reduction and internal fixation of displaced posterior and anterior tibial fragments [97].

The posterior malleolus is affected in around 40% of ankle fractures [146]. Anatomical reduction of the articular surface and fibular notch are essential for ankle stability and functional outcomes. To address the posterior malleolus when treating ankle fractures, surgeons should choose the most adequate approach based on the fracture pattern and their own experience [3,14–17,99,146,152,154,155]. Anatomical reduction and stable fixation of the posterior malleolus are critical to improve outcomes [1,3,14–17,21,43,46,50,84,86,99,144,146,153,154].

It was Gardner who first observed, in 2006, that syndesmotic stability may be obtained more effectively by fixation of the posterior malleolus rather than by using a syndesmotic screw [50]. This observation was later confirmed by several authors [17,84,86,144].

Tosun et al. compared posterior malleolus versus syndesmotic screw fixation in trimalleolar ankle fractures. The results of this study demonstrate that posterior malleolar fracture fixation is closely related to successful radiological and functional outcomes after trimalleolar fractures. Syndesmotic screw fixation may not be needed in cases in which the posterior malleolar fracture has been fixated. For these reasons, the authors recommended that all posterior malleolar fractures have to be fixed regardless of size [144].

Furthermore, according to Verhage, the posterior fragment size is not a clear indication for its fixation [153]. A step-off, however, seems to be an important indicator for developing posttraumatic osteoarthritis and worse functional outcome [1,21,43,153]. Therefore, displaced posterior fragments involving the intra-articular surface need to be reduced and fixated to prevent postoperative persisting step-off [153]. Furthermore, direct fixation of the posterior malleolus via an open posterolateral approach seems superior to percutaneous anterior-to-posterior fixation [15–17,84,99,154,155].

When posterior malleolus fractures occur with syndesmotic injury, anatomic fracture reduction and fixation are paramount, as they can affect syndesmotic reduction, especially with larger fragments [46]. Therefore, in any case of a displaced fracture of the posterior malleolus with a bone fragment big enough for screw or plate fixation and with an intact PITFL, the posterior malleolus should be considered the key for anatomic reduction of the syndesmosis [46]. After fixation of the posterior malleolus in an anatomic position, the further surgical steps for complete reduction and stabilization of the syndesmosis will be easy to perform. Therefore, open reduction and direct fixation of the posterior malleolus should be performed as the first step [84,97]. This surgical order has the additional advantage that fluoroscopic control of reduction quality is not limited by other implants, such as a fibular plate. In case of fixation of the posterolateral malleolus in malposition, anatomic reduction of the syndesmosis will not be possible anymore due to ligamentotaxis. Therefore, in cases where it is very difficult or even impossible to fix the posterior malleolus in an anatomic position, it might be better not to fix the posterior malleolus than to fix it in malposition.

Main conclusions: A step-off of the posterior malleolus is an important indicator for developing posttraumatic osteoarthritis and worse functional outcome. Therefore, displaced posterior malleolar fractures have to be fixed regardless of size. Fix the posterior malleolus directly from posterior whenever possible. When fixing the posterior malleolus, start with this procedure, as the posterior malleolus is the key for anatomic reduction of the syndesmosis.

As a kind of summary of our investigations, we formulated the following principles for the surgical treatment of unstable syndesmotic injuries, which can be considered supported by varying degrees of evidence in literature:

3.8. Recommended Principles for the Surgical Treatment of Unstable Syndesmotic Injuries

- Anatomic reduction is crucial for the long-term results;
- Open reduction by direct visualization is strongly recommended;
- Repair what is injured;
- Bony avulsion fragments must be identified and reduced (when big enough) and can serve as landmarks for anatomic reduction;
- The use of reduction clamps or forceps should be avoided whenever possible;
- Fix the posterolateral malleolus directly from posterior whenever possible;
- When fixing the posterolateral malleolus, start with this procedure;
- The AITFL is an important stabilizer especially for rotational stability;
- An unstable AITFL should be repaired and augmented;
- Use flexible dynamic stabilization techniques whenever possible; and
- Use syndesmotic screws only as a salvage procedure.

These recommended main principles for the surgical treatment of unstable syndesmotic injuries were fused into the following evidence-based surgical treatment algorithm (Figure 1). Practicability of this algorithm is additionally based on the clinical experience of the first author (M.R.), who has performed more than 300 flexible dynamic syndesmotic stabilizations using an *Internal*Brace™ since 16 December 2013. Corresponding clinical and radiological outcome studies are currently running.

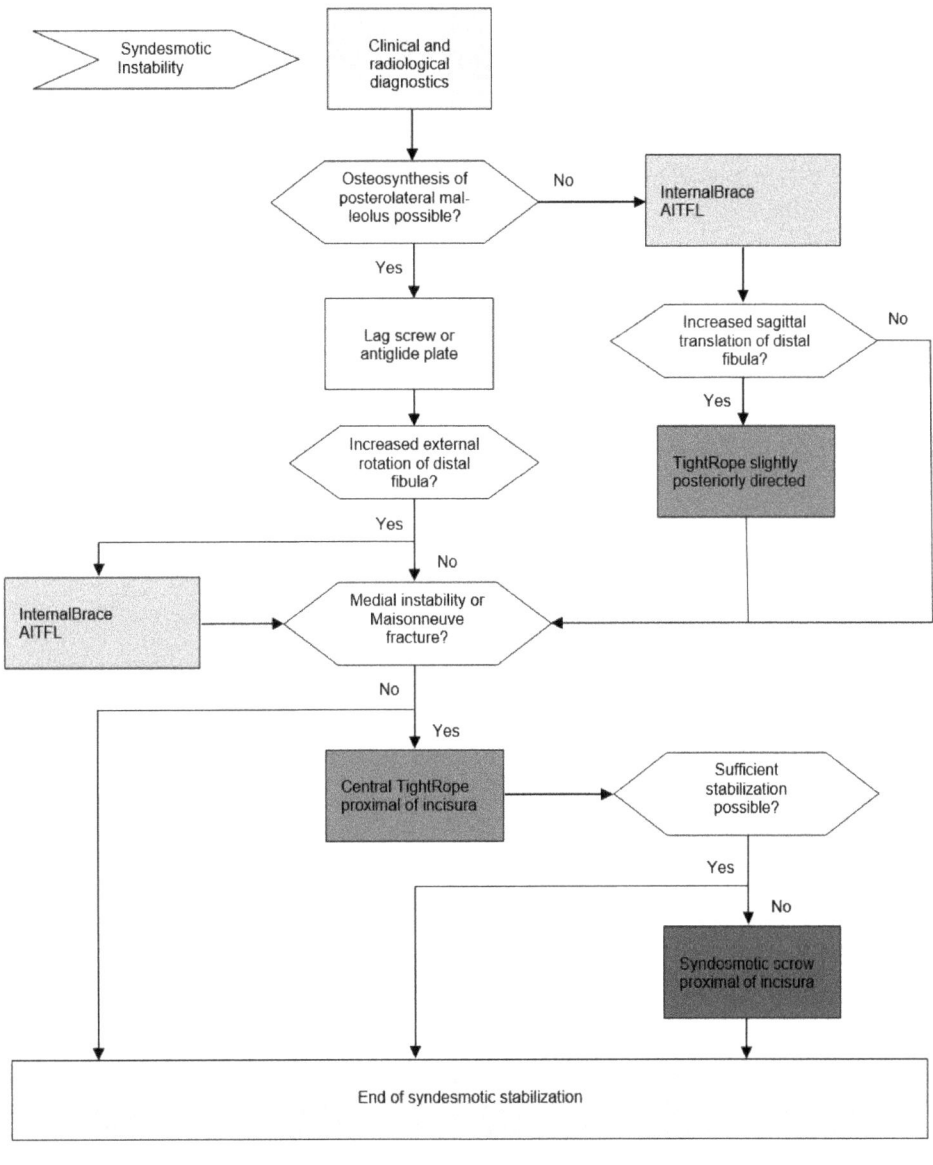

(A)

Figure 1. Cont.

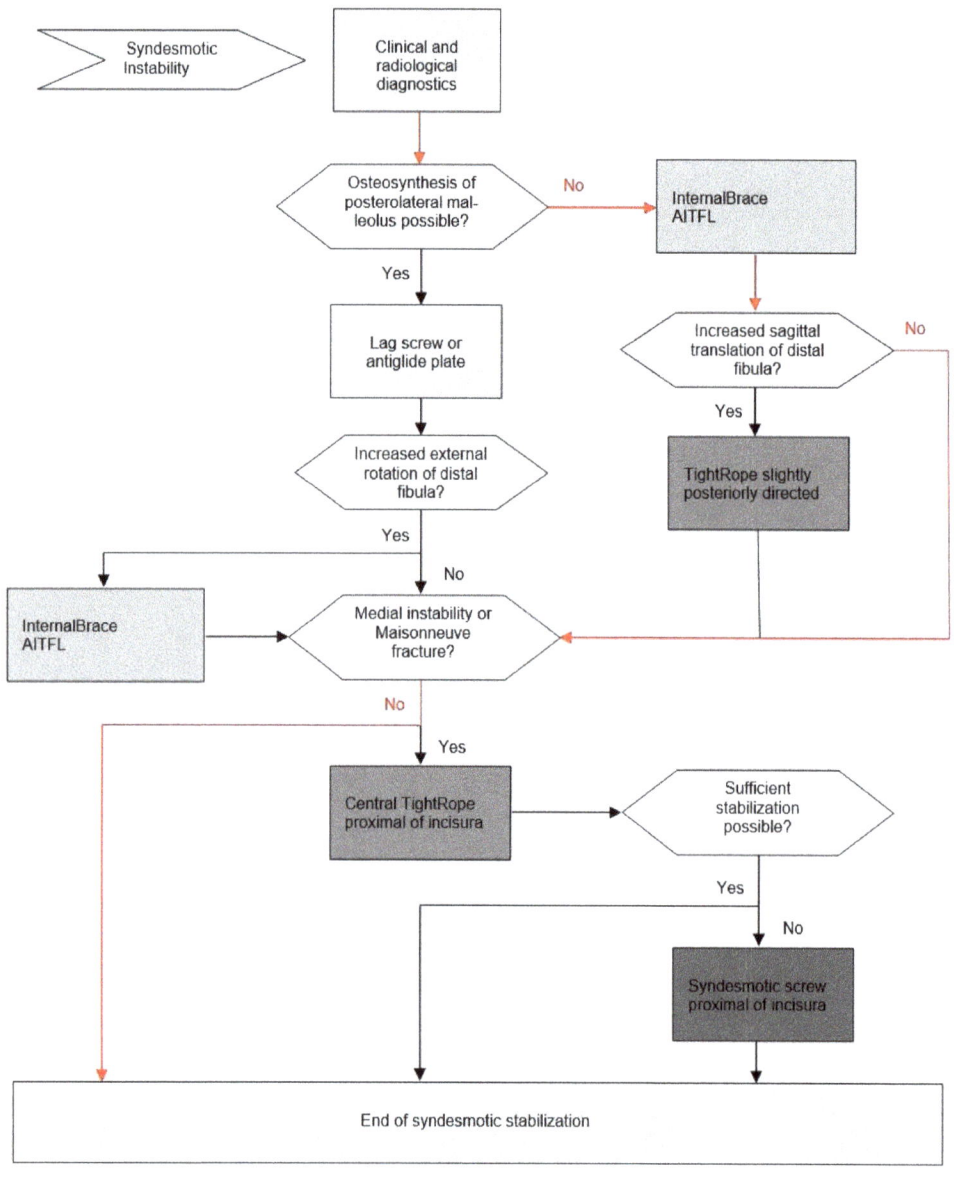

(B)

Figure 1. *Cont.*

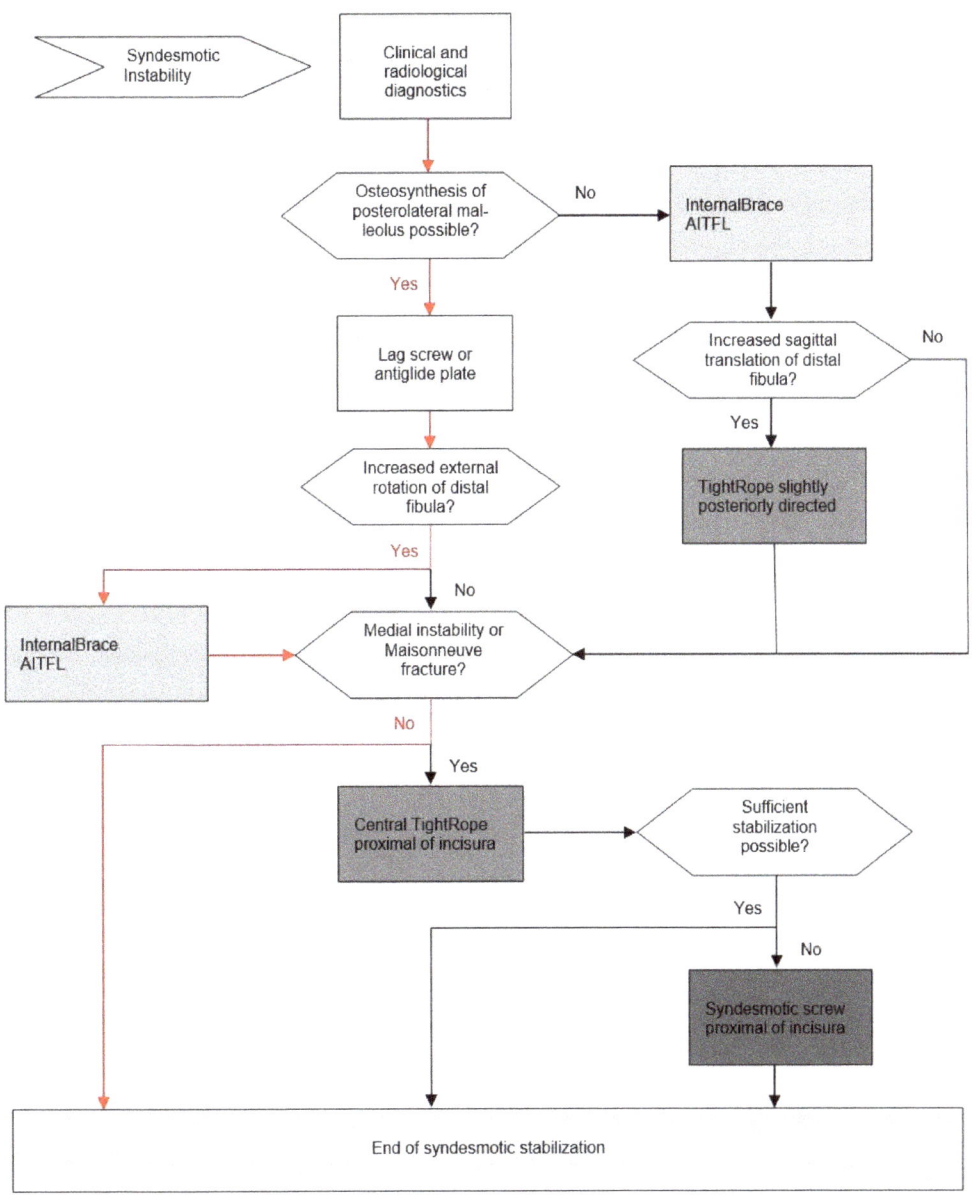

(C)

Figure 1. Cont.

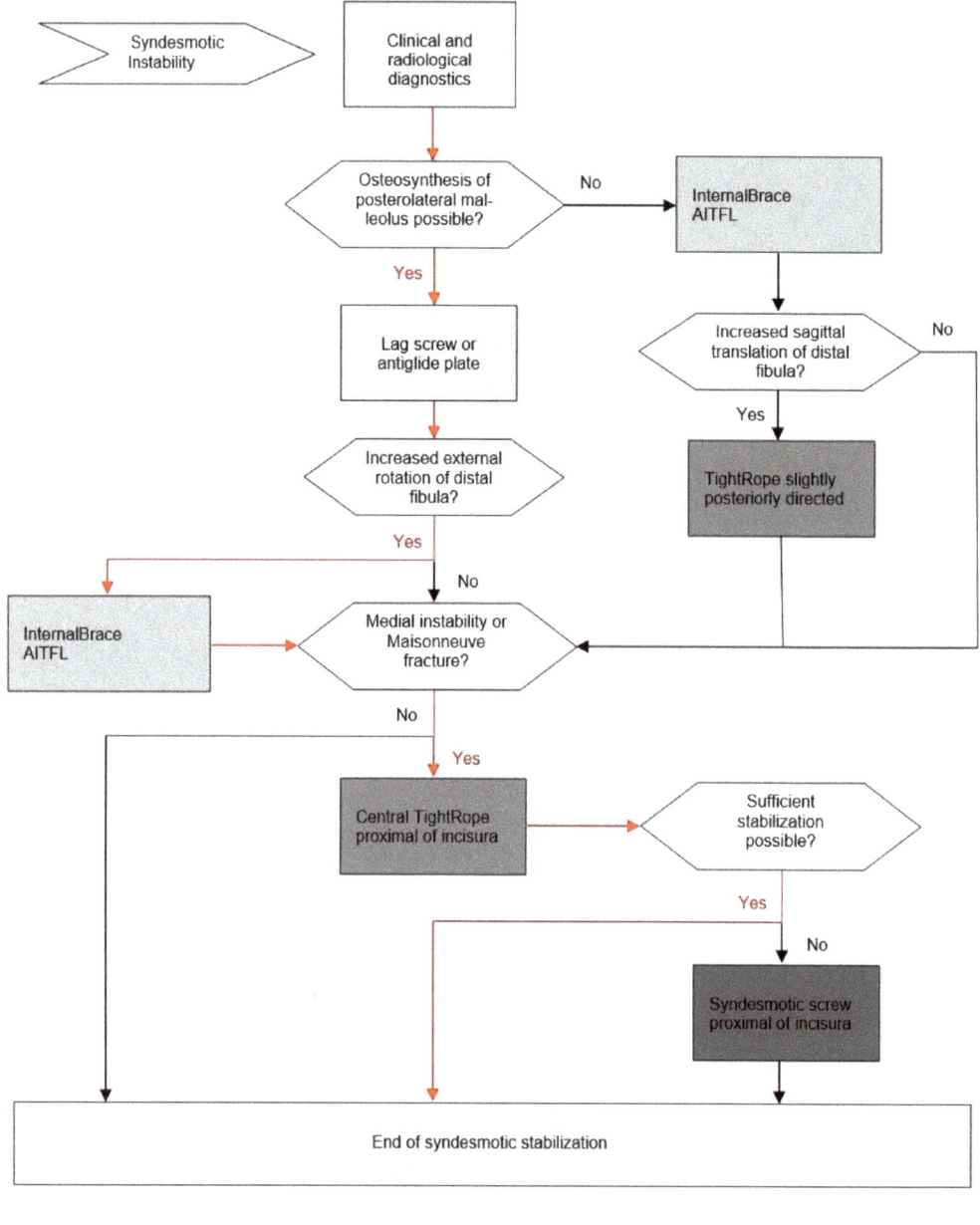

(D)

Figure 1. (**A**) Evidence-based surgical treatment algorithm for unstable syndesmotic injuries. (**B**) Evidence-based surgical treatment algorithm for unstable syndesmotic injuries. Exemplary treatment path for grade 1 injuries. (**C**) Evidence-based surgical treatment algorithm for unstable syndesmotic injuries. Exemplary treatment path for grade 2 injuries. (**D**) Evidence-based surgical treatment algorithm for unstable syndesmotic injuries. Exemplary treatment path for grade 3 injuries.

3.9. Evidence-Based Surgical Treatment Algorithm for Unstable Syndesmotic Injuries

For the first decision before starting surgery, the surgeon has to evaluate if there is a displaced posterior malleolar fragment amenable to open anatomic reduction and direct fixation with a lag screw or an anti-glide plate (Figure 1A). If so, this procedure should be performed as the first step of surgery due to the following three reasons: (1) direct fixation provides excellent primary stability of the posterior syndesmosis. (2) After anatomic reduction and direct fixation of the posterolateral malleolus, the following surgical steps will be quite easy to perform. (3) Fluoroscopic control of reduction quality is not limited by other implants like a fibular plate.

The next step after direct fixation of the posterior malleolus, or the first step in case of an intact posterior malleolus, is direct visualization of the AITFL and an intraoperative grading of the injury pattern under direct view (Figure 2). The surgeon should be aware that only grade 3 injuries would be detected by the well-known Cotton test or its hook test modifications [22,90,101,103]. Increased external rotation and posterior sagittal translation indicates an isolated tear or bony avulsion of the AITFL, representing a grade 1 injury (Figure 2A); increased anterior sagittal translation indicates an additional tear or bony avulsion of the PITFL, representing a grade 2 injury (Figure 2B); and increased lateral translation indicates additional medial instability, representing a grade 3 injury (Figure 2C). Further treatment strategy should be according to the detected individual injury pattern:

- Grade 1: Single anterior stabilization with an *Internal*Brace™ (Figure 1B);
- Grade 2: Double stabilization = anterior and posterior stabilization (Figure 1C); and
- Grade 3: Triple stabilization = double stabilization + central tightrope or syndesmotic screw (Figure 1D).

We have already exemplified in detail how to perform these stabilization techniques in 2017 [119]. In our experience, the most common procedure is anterior stabilization with an *Internal*Brace™, either as single anterior stabilization or as double stabilization in combination with direct refixation of the posterior malleolus or a slightly posteriorly directed suture-button device in order to indirectly stabilize an injured PITFL. As a promising alternative to an indirect posterior stabilization by use of a suture-button device, recently, some surgeons have also been performing a direct stabilization of the PITFL with an additional *Internal*Brace™ to an increasing degree. However, to the best of our knowledge, this technique has only been described in a cadaver model so far [119]. Triple stabilization by use of an additional central suture-button device or a syndesmotic screw proximal of the incisura is rarely necessary in our hands. As a suture-button-device, we have used the knotless syndesmotic TightRope® implant system provided by Arthrex in our own cases, as this implant, to the best of our knowledge, represents the most frequently used and most investigated suture-button-device. However, alternative implant systems provided by other manufacturers are currently available as well.

A clinical example of a single anterior stabilization in a type B ankle fracture with displaced bony tibial avulsion of the AITFL (Figure 3A) is shown in Figure 3. After secure radiological and clinical exclusion of any unstable injury to the PITFL or the posterior malleolus, the distal fibular fracture was fixed with a special anatomically shaped titanium distal fibular plate with eyelets for tape augmentation of the AITFL and PITFL (Arthrex, Naples, FL, USA). The bony AITFL avulsion fragment was anatomically reduced under direct visualization and fixed with a 3.5-mm headless compression screw (Figure 3B). Due to its size, the bony fragment was not amenable to fixation with a stronger screw. Therefore, a FiberTape® (Arthrex, Naples, FL, USA) for augmentation of the AITFL was pulled through the anterior eyelets of the plate (Figure 3C) and fixed to the distal tibia exactly in line with the course of the uninjured AITFL with a 4.75-mm SwiveLock® (Arthrex, Naples, FL, USA). Figure 3 D shows the final result after osteosynthesis of the distal fibula with a titanium plate, refixation of the bony avulsion fragment with a compression screw, and augmentation of the AITFL with an *Internal*Brace™ (Arthrex, Naples, FL, USA).

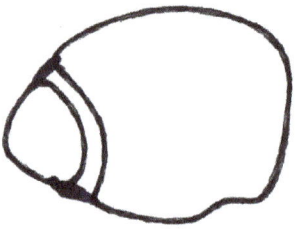
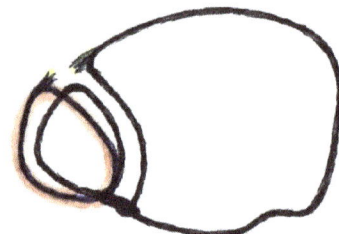

- Isolated injury of the AITFL
- Increased external rotation of the distal fibula (Frick test)
- Increased posterior translation of the distal fibula

(**A**)

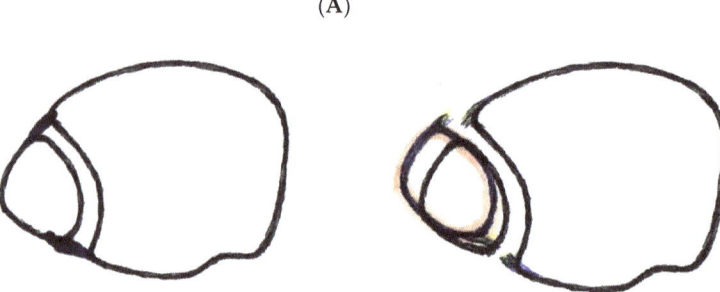

- Injury of the AITFL and the PITFL
- Increased anterior translation of the distal fibula
- Increased sagittal translation of the distal fibula

(**B**)

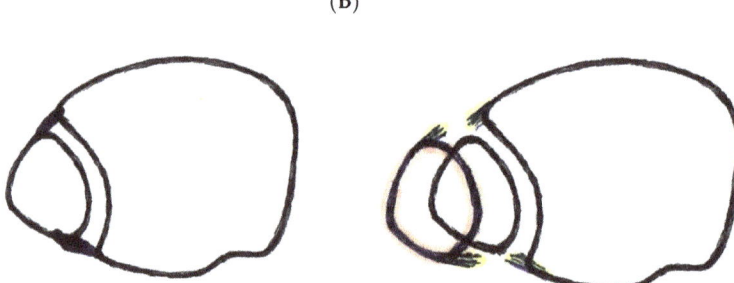

- Additional medial instability or Maisonneuve fracture
- Increased lateral translation of the distal fibula (Hook test)
- Increased sagittal translation of the distal fibula

(**C**)

Figure 2. (**A**) Intraoperative assessment of a grade 1 injury. (**B**) Intraoperative assessment of a grade 2 injury. (**C**) Intraoperative assessment of a grade 3 injury.

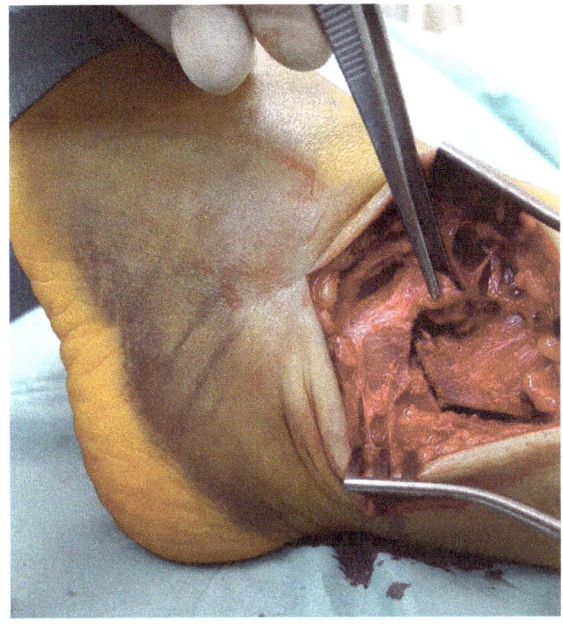

(A)

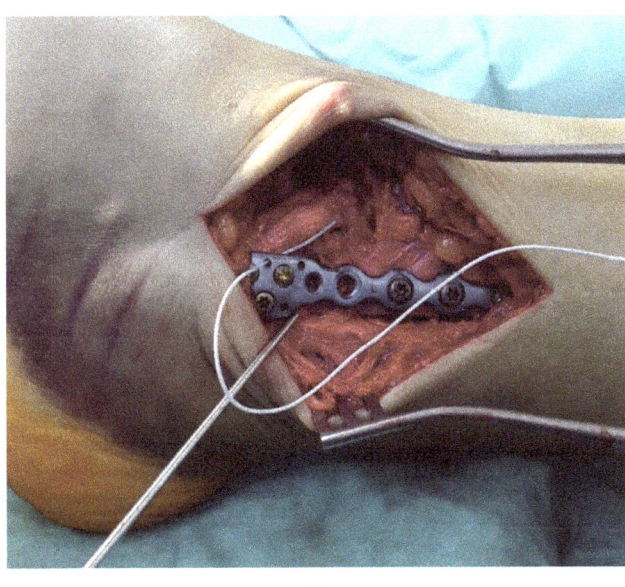

(B)

Figure 3. *Cont.*

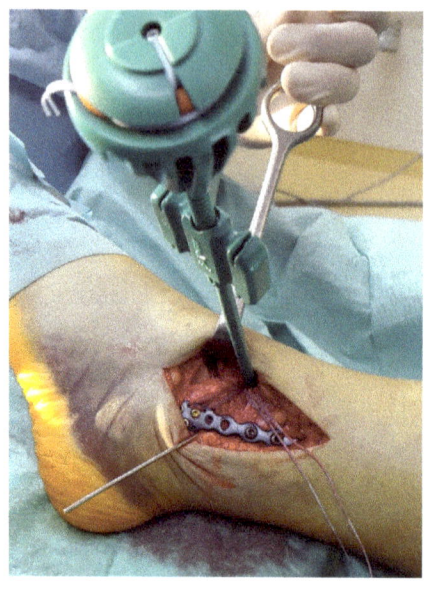

(C)

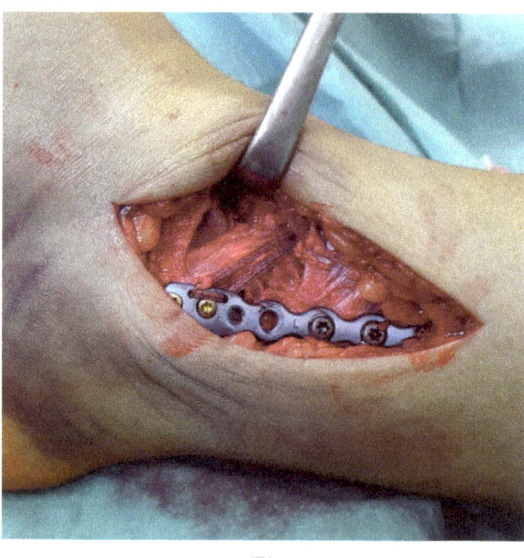

(D)

Figure 3. (**A**) Type B ankle fracture with displaced tibial bony avulsion of the AITFL. (**B**) Type B ankle fracture with displaced bony avulsion of the AITFL. The distal fibular fracture was fixed with a special anatomically shaped titanium distal fibular plate with eyelets for tape augmentation of the AITFL and PITFL (Arthrex, Naples, FL, USA). The bony AITFL avulsion fragment was anatomically reduced and fixed with a 3.5-mm headless compression screw. (**C**) Type B ankle fracture with displaced bony avulsion of the AITFL. A FiberTape® (Arthrex, Naples, FL, USA) for augmentation of the AITFL has been pulled through the anterior eyelets of the plate and fixed to the distal tibia with a 4.75-mm SwiveLock® (Arthrex, Naples, FL, USA). (**D**) Type B ankle fracture with displaced bony avulsion of the AITFL. Final result after osteosynthesis of the distal fibula with a titanium plate, refixation of the bony avulsion fragment with a compression screw, and augmentation of the AITFL with an *Internal*Brace™ (Arthrex, Naples, FL, USA).

4. Discussion

Our aim was to provide the currently best available evidence for surgical treatment of unstable syndesmotic injuries. Therefore, we searched PubMed, Embase, Google Scholar, The Cochrane Database of Systematic Reviews, and the reference lists of systematic reviews of relevant studies dealing with the surgical treatment of unstable syndesmotic injuries. Then we tried to draw important conclusions from the pertinent literature concerning surgical treatment of unstable syndesmotic injuries, to transform these conclusions into surgical principles supported by the literature, and finally to fuse these principles into an evidence-based surgical treatment algorithm. In our hands, this surgical treatment algorithm has been working well for more than seven years now.

A total of 171 articles were analyzed, and to summarize our results, we found the following main principles for surgical treatment of unstable syndesmotic injuries: (1) anatomic reduction is crucial for the long-term results; (2) open reduction by direct visualization is strongly recommended; (3) repair what is injured; (4) bony avulsion fragments must be identified and reduced and can serve as landmarks for anatomic reduction; (5) the use of reduction clamps or forceps should be avoided whenever possible; (6) fix the posterolateral malleolus directly from posterior whenever possible; (7) when fixing the posterolateral malleolus, start with this procedure; (8) the AITFL is an important stabilizer especially for rotational stability; (9) an unstable AITFL should be repaired and augmented; (10) use flexible dynamic stabilization techniques whenever possible; and (11) use syndesmotic screws only as a salvage procedure.

However, there are some limitations to our study. Our study was not a systematic review designed according to the Preferred Reporting Items for Systematic Reviews and Meta-Analyses (PRISMA) guidelines, and study quality of the cited references was not assessed based on any quality appraisal scales. Moreover, due to our language selection criteria, there might be additional important studies not considered in our work.

Furthermore, our aim was to develop the best available solution for unstable syndesmotic injuries with regard to medical and not economic issues, and we are aware of the fact that our approach for treating unstable syndesmotic injuries is quite expensive compared to the simple and cheap syndesmotic screws, for example [115]. However, regarding the well-known severe consequences of failed syndesmotic repairs, we strongly recommend treating unstable syndesmotic injuries using the best implants available. In the long run, it does not seem reasonable to save money in the primary care for unstable syndesmotic injuries because the consequence might be very high costs for the treatment of ankle osteoarthritis.

5. Conclusions

Current literature provides sufficient arguments for the development of an evidence-based surgical treatment algorithm for unstable syndesmotic injuries. Anatomic reduction is crucial to prevent posttraumatic osteoarthritis. Therefore, flexible dynamic stabilization techniques should be preferred whenever possible. An unstable AITFL should be repaired and augmented, as it represents an important stabilizer of external rotation of the distal fibula.

Author Contributions: Conceptualization, M.R.; methodology, M.R. and C.E.; investigation, M.R. and C.E.; resources, M.R., G.M. and O.N.; data curation, M.R. and O.N.; writing—original draft preparation, M.R.; writing—review and editing, G.M., O.N., W.B. and C.E.; visualization, M.R. and C.E.; supervision, W.B. All authors have read and agreed to the published version of the manuscript.

Funding: This research received no external funding.

Institutional Review Board Statement: Not applicable.

Informed Consent Statement: Not applicable.

Data Availability Statement: Not applicable.

Acknowledgments: In these extraordinary times, we would like to thank the medical staff all around the world for fighting against the COVID-19 pandemic.

Conflicts of Interest: Markus Regauer and Gordon Mackay are paid consultants of and receive royalties from Arthrex (Naples, FL, USA). The funder had no role in the design of the study; in the collection, analyses, or interpretation of data; in the writing of the manuscript; or in the decision to publish the results. The remaining authors declare no conflict of interest.

References

1. Abarquero-Diezhandino, A.; Luengo-Alonso, G.; Alonso-Tejero, D.; Sánchez-Morata, E.J.; Olaya-Gonzalez, C.; Vilá Y Rico, J. Study of the relation between the posterior malleolus fracture and the development of osteoarthritis. *Rev. Esp. Cir. Ortop. Traumatol.* **2020**, *64*, 41–49. [CrossRef]
2. Akoh, C.C.; Phisitkul, P. Anatomic Ligament Repairs of Syndesmotic Injuries. *Orthop. Clin. N. Am.* **2019**, *50*, 401–414. [CrossRef] [PubMed]
3. Alonso-Rasgado, T.; Jimenez-Cruz, D.; Karski, M. 3-D computer modelling of malunited posterior malleolar fractures: Effect of fragment size and offset on ankle stability, contact pressure and pattern. *J. Foot Ankle Res.* **2017**, *10*, 13. [CrossRef] [PubMed]
4. Amendola, A.; Williams, G.; Foster, D. Evidence-based approach to treatment of acute traumatic syndesmosis (high ankle) sprains. *Sports Med. Arthrosc. Rev.* **2006**, *14*, 232–236. [CrossRef]
5. Anand, A.; Wei, R.; Patel, A.; Vedi, V.; Allardice, G.; Anand, B.S. Tightrope fixation of syndesmotic injuries in Weber C ankle fractures: A multicentre case series. *Eur. J. Orthop. Surg. Traumatol.* **2017**, *27*, 461–467. [CrossRef]
6. Anand, P.A. Anatomy of Ankle Syndesmotic Ligaments: A Systematic Review of Cadaveric Studies. *Foot Ankle Spec.* **2020**, *13*, 341–350. [CrossRef]
7. Andersen, M.R.; Diep, L.M.; Frihagen, F.; Castberg Hellund, J.; Madsen, J.E.; Figved, W. Importance of Syndesmotic Reduction on Clinical Outcome After Syndesmosis Injuries. *J. Orthop. Trauma* **2019**, *33*, 397–403. [CrossRef]
8. Andersen, M.R.; Figved, W. Use of Suture Button in the Treatment of Syndesmosis Injuries. *JBJS Essent. Surg. Tech.* **2018**, *8*, e13. [CrossRef]
9. Andersen, M.R.; Frihagen, F.; Hellund, J.C.; Madsen, J.E.; Figved, W. Randomized Trial Comparing Suture Button with Single Syndesmotic Screw for Syndesmosis Injury. *J. Bone Jt. Surg. Am.* **2018**, *100*, 2–12. [CrossRef]
10. Andersen, M.R.; Frihagen, F.; Madsen, J.E.; Figved, W. High complication rate after syndesmotic screw removal. *Injury* **2015**, *46*, 2283–2287. [CrossRef]
11. Bae, K.J.; Kang, S.B.; Kim, J.; Lee, J.; Go, T.W. Reduction and fixation of anterior inferior tibiofibular ligament avulsion fracture without syndesmotic screw fixation in rotational ankle fracture. *J. Int. Med. Res.* **2020**, *48*, 300060519882550. [CrossRef]
12. Bafna, K.R.; Jordan, R.; Yatsonsky, D., 2nd; Dick, S.; Liu, J.; Ebraheim, N.A. Revision of Syndesmosis Screw Fixation. *Foot Ankle Spec.* **2020**, *13*, 138–143. [CrossRef]
13. Bai, L.; Zhang, W.; Guan, S.; Liu, J.; Chen, P. Syndesmotic malreduction may decrease fixation stability: A biomechanical study. *J. Orthop. Surg. Res.* **2020**, *15*, 64. [CrossRef]
14. Bartoníček, J.; Rammelt, S.; Kostlivý, K.; Vaněček, V.; Klika, D.; Trešl, I. Anatomy and classification of the posterior tibial fragment in ankle fractures. *Arch. Orthop. Trauma Surg.* **2015**, *135*, 505–516. [CrossRef]
15. Bartoníček, J.; Rammelt, S.; Tuček, M. Posterior Malleolar Fractures: Changing Concepts and Recent Developments. *Foot Ankle Clin.* **2017**, *22*, 125–145. [CrossRef]
16. Baumbach, S.F.; Böcker, W.; Polzer, H. Arthroscopically assisted fracture treatment and open reduction of the posterior malleolus: New strategies for management of complex ankle fractures. *Unfallchirurg* **2020**, *123*, 330–338. [CrossRef]
17. Baumbach, S.F.; Herterich, V.; Damblemont, A.; Hieber, F.; Böcker, W.; Polzer, H. Open reduction and internal fixation of the posterior malleolus fragment frequently restores syndesmotic stability. *Injury* **2019**, *50*, 564–570. [CrossRef]
18. Bava, E.; Charlton, T.; Thordarson, D. Ankle fracture syndesmosis fixation and management: The current practice of orthopedic surgeons. *Am. J. Orthop. (Belle Mead NJ)* **2010**, *39*, 242–246.
19. Best, R.; Mauch, F.; Bauer, G. Evidence for treatment of acute syndesmosis injuries in sports. *Unfallchirurg* **2013**, *116*, 504–511. [CrossRef]
20. Birnie, M.F.N.; van Schilt, K.L.J.; Sanders, F.R.K.; Kloen, P.; Schepers, T. Anterior inferior tibiofibular ligament avulsion fractures in operatively treated ankle fractures: A retrospective analysis. *Arch. Orthop. Trauma Surg.* **2019**, *139*, 787–793. [CrossRef]
21. Blom, R.P.; Meijer, D.T.; de Muinck Keizer, R.O.; Stufkens, S.A.S.; Sierevelt, I.N.; Schepers, T.; Kerkhoffs, G.M.M.J.; Goslings, J.C.; Doornberg, J.N. Posterior malleolar fracture morphology determines outcome in rotational type ankle fractures. *Injury* **2019**, *50*, 1392–1397. [CrossRef]
22. Candal-Couto, J.J.; Burrow, D.; Bromage, S.; Briggs, P.J. Instability of the tibio-fibular syndesmosis: Have we been pulling in the wrong direction? *Injury* **2004**, *35*, 814–818. [CrossRef]
23. Cassinelli, S.J.; Harris, T.G.; Giza, E.; Kreulen, C.; Matheny, L.M.; Robbins, C.M.; Clanton, T.O. Use of Anatomical Landmarks in Ankle Arthroscopy to Determine Accuracy of Syndesmotic Reduction: A Cadaveric Study. *Foot Ankle Spec.* **2020**, *13*, 219–227. [CrossRef]

24. Castro-Guerrero, D.E.; Rosas-Medina, J.A. Residual ankle instability in patients with syndesmosis lesions without fracture treated with situational screws. *Acta Ortop. Mex.* **2019**, *33*, 292–296. [CrossRef]
25. Che, J.; Li, C.; Gao, Z.; Qi, W.; Ji, B.; Liu, Y.; Liow, M.H.L. Novel anatomical reconstruction of distal tibiofibular ligaments restores syndesmotic biomechanics. *Knee Surg. Sports Traumatol. Arthrosc.* **2017**, *25*, 1866–1872. [CrossRef] [PubMed]
26. Cherney, S.M.; Haynes, J.A.; Spraggs-Hughes, A.G.; McAndrew, C.M.; Ricci, W.M.; Gardner, M.J. In Vivo Syndesmotic Overcompression After Fixation of Ankle Fractures With a Syndesmotic Injury. *J. Orthop. Trauma* **2015**, *29*, 414–419. [CrossRef]
27. Chissell, H.R.; Jones, J. The influence of a diastasis screw on the outcome of Weber type-C ankle fractures. *J. Bone Jt. Surg. Br.* **1995**, *77*, 435–438. [CrossRef]
28. Clanton, T.O.; Williams, B.T.; Backus, J.D.; Dornan, G.J.; Liechti, D.J.; Whitlow, S.R.; Saroki, A.J.; Turnbull, T.L.; LaPrade, R.F. Biomechanical Analysis of the Individual Ligament Contributions to Syndesmotic Stability. *Foot Ankle Int.* **2017**, *38*, 66–75. [CrossRef] [PubMed]
29. Clanton, T.O.; Whitlow, S.R.; Williams, B.T.; Liechti, D.J.; Backus, J.D.; Dornan, G.J.; Saroki, A.J.; Turnbull, T.L.; LaPrade, R.F. Biomechanical Comparison of 3 Current Ankle Syndesmosis Repair Techniques. *Foot Ankle Int.* **2017**, *38*, 200–207. [CrossRef] [PubMed]
30. Clanton, T.O.; Paul, P. Syndesmosis injuries in athletes. *Foot Ankle Clin.* **2002**, *7*, 529–549. [CrossRef]
31. Clare, M.P.; Berkowitz, M.J. Revision Open Reduction and Internal Fixation of Ankle and Syndesmosis Malunions. *Instr. Course Lect.* **2019**, *68*, 265–274.
32. Coetzee, J.; Ebeling, P. Treatment of syndesmoses disruptions: A prospective, randomized study comparing conventional screw fixation vs TightRope fiber wire fixation—Medium term results. *S. Afr. Orthop. J.* **2009**, *8*, 32–37.
33. Coetzee, J.; Ebeling, P. Treatment of syndesmosis disruptions with TightRope fixation. *Tech. Foot Ankle Surg.* **2008**, *7*, 196–202. [CrossRef]
34. Colcuc, C.; Blank, M.; Stein, T.; Raimann, F.; Weber-Spickschen, S.; Fischer, S.; Hoffmann, R. Lower complication rate and faster return to sports in patients with acute syndesmotic rupture treated with a new knotless suture button device. *Knee Surg. Sports Traumatol. Arthrosc.* **2018**, *26*, 3156–3164. [CrossRef]
35. Connors, J.C.; Grossman, J.P.; Zulauf, E.E.; Coyer, M.A. Syndesmotic Ligament Allograft Reconstruction for Treatment of Chronic Diastasis. *J. Foot Ankle Surg.* **2020**, *59*, 835–840. [CrossRef]
36. Cosgrove, C.T.; Putnam, S.M.; Cherney, S.M.; Ricci, W.M.; Spraggs-Hughes, A.; McAndrew, C.M.; Gardner, M.J. Medial Clamp Tine Positioning Affects Ankle Syndesmosis Malreduction. *J. Orthop. Trauma* **2017**, *31*, 440–446. [CrossRef]
37. Costigan, P.G. Treatment of true widening ankle mortise. *Can. Med. Assoc. J.* **1953**, *69*, 310–313.
38. Cottom, J.M.; Hyer, C.F.; Philbin, T.M.; Berlet, G.C. Treatment of syndesmotic disruptions with the Arthrex Tightrope: A report of 25 cases. *Foot Ankle Int.* **2008**, *29*, 773–780. [CrossRef]
39. De-Las-Heras Romero, J.; Alvarez, A.M.L.; Sanchez, F.M.; Garcia, A.P.; Porcel, P.A.G.; Sarabia, R.V.; Torralba, M.H. Management of syndesmotic injuries of the ankle. *EFORT Open Rev.* **2017**, *2*, 403–409. [CrossRef]
40. D'Hooghe, P.; Cruz, F.; Alkhelaifi, K. Return to Play After a Lateral Ligament Ankle Sprain. *Curr. Rev. Musculoskelet. Med.* **2020**, *13*, 281–288. [CrossRef]
41. D'Hooghe, P.; Grassi, A.; Alkhelaifi, K.; Calder, J.; Baltes, T.P.A.; Zaffagnini, S.; Ekstrand, J. Return to play after surgery for isolated unstable syndesmotic ankle injuries (West Point grade IIB and III) in 110 male professional football players: A retrospective cohort study. *Br. J. Sports Med.* **2020**, *54*, 1168–1173. [CrossRef]
42. D'Hooghe, P.; York, P.J.; Kaux, J.F.; Hunt, K.J. Fixation Techniques in Lower Extremity Syndesmotic Injuries. *Foot Ankle Int.* **2017**, *38*, 1278–1288. [CrossRef]
43. Drijfhout van Hooff, C.C.; Verhage, S.M.; Hoogendoorn, J.M. Influence of fragment size and postoperative joint congruency on long-term outcome of posterior malleolar fractures. *Foot Ankle Int.* **2015**, *36*, 673–678. [CrossRef]
44. Egol, K.A.; Pahk, B.; Walsh, M.; Tejwani, N.C.; Davidovitch, R.I.; Koval, K.J. Outcome after unstable ankle fracture: Effect of syndesmotic stabilization. *J. Orthop. Trauma* **2010**, *24*, 7–11. [CrossRef] [PubMed]
45. Engelbrecht, E. Treatment of tibio-fibular syndesmosis rupture using the syndesmosis hook. *Chirurg* **1971**, *42*, 92–94. [PubMed]
46. Fitzpatrick, E.; Goetz, J.E.; Sittapairoj, T.; Hosuru Siddappa, V.; Femino, J.E.; Phisitkul, P. Effect of Posterior Malleolus Fracture on Syndesmotic Reduction: A Cadaveric Study. *J. Bone Jt. Surg. Am.* **2018**, *100*, 243–248. [CrossRef]
47. Förschner, P.F.; Beitzel, K.; Imhoff, A.B.; Buchmann, S.; Feuerriegel, G.; Hofmann, F.; Karampinos, D.C.; Jungmann, P.; Pogorzelski, J. Five-Year Outcomes After Treatment for Acute Instability of the Tibiofibular Syndesmosis Using a Suture-Button Fixation System. *Orthop. J. Sports Med.* **2017**, *5*, 2325967117702854. [CrossRef]
48. Gan, K.; Xu, D.; Hu, K.; Wu, W.; Shen, Y. Dynamic fixation is superior in terms of clinical outcomes to static fixation in managing distal tibiofibular syndesmosis injury. *Knee Surg. Sports Traumatol. Arthrosc.* **2020**, *28*, 270–280. [CrossRef]
49. Gan, K.; Zhou, K.; Hu, K.; Lu, L.; Gu, S.; Shen, Y. Dynamic Fixation Versus Static Fixation for Distal Tibiofibular Syndesmosis Injuries: A Meta-Analysis. *Med. Sci. Monit.* **2019**, *25*, 1314–1322. [CrossRef]
50. Gardner, M.J.; Brodsky, A.; Briggs, S.M.; Nielson, J.H.; Lorich, D.G. Fixation of posterior malleolar fractures provides greater syndesmotic stability. *Clin. Orthop. Relat. Res.* **2006**, *447*, 165–171. [CrossRef]
51. Gardner, M.J.; Demetrakopoulos, D.; Briggs, S.M.; Helfet, D.L.; Lorich, D.G. Malreduction of the tibiofibular syndesmosis in ankle fractures. *Foot Ankle Int.* **2006**, *27*, 788–792. [CrossRef] [PubMed]

52. Gardner, M.J.; Graves, M.L.; Higgins, T.F.; Nork, S.E. Technical Considerations in the Treatment of Syndesmotic Injuries Associated With Ankle Fractures. *J. Am. Acad. Orthop. Surg.* **2015**, *23*, 510–518. [CrossRef]
53. Goetz, J.E.; Szabo, N.; Rudert, M.J.; Karam, M.D.; Phisitkul, P. Achilles Tension Mitigates Fibular Malalignment Measured in Cadaveric Studies of Syndesmotic Clamping. *Foot Ankle Int.* **2019**, *40*, 465–474. [CrossRef] [PubMed]
54. Goetz, J.E.; Rungprai, C.; Rudert, M.J.; Warth, L.C.; Phisitkul, P. Screw fixation of the syndesmosis alters joint contact characteristics in an axially loaded cadaveric model. *Foot Ankle Surg.* **2019**, *25*, 594–600. [CrossRef]
55. Goetz, J.E.; Davidson, N.P.; Rudert, M.J.; Szabo, N.; Karam, M.D.; Phisitkul, P. Biomechanical Comparison of Syndesmotic Repair Techniques During External Rotation Stress. *Foot Ankle Int.* **2018**, *39*, 1345–1354. [CrossRef]
56. Grass, R.; Rammelt, S.; Biewener, A.; Zwipp, H. Peroneus longus ligamentoplasty for chronic instability of the distal tibiofibular syndesmosis. *Foot Ankle Int.* **2003**, *24*, 392–397. [CrossRef]
57. Grassi, A.; Samuelsson, K.; D'Hooghe, P.; Romagnoli, M.; Mosca, M.; Zaffagnini, S.; Amendola, A. Dynamic Stabilization of Syndesmosis Injuries Reduces Complications and Reoperations as Compared With Screw Fixation: A Meta-analysis of Randomized Controlled Trials. *Am. J. Sports Med.* **2020**, *48*, 1000–1013. [CrossRef]
58. Hajewski, C.J.; Duchman, K.; Goetz, J.; Femino, J. Anatomic Syndesmotic and Deltoid Ligament Reconstruction with Flexible Implants: A Technique Description. *Iowa Orthop. J.* **2019**, *39*, 21–27.
59. Harris, J.; Fallat, L. Effects of isolated Weber B fibular fractures on the tibiotalar contact area. *J. Foot Ankle Surg.* **2004**, *43*, 3–9. [CrossRef]
60. Haynes, J.; Cherney, S.; Spraggs-Hughes, A.; McAndrew, C.M.; Ricci, W.M.; Gardner, M.J. Increased Reduction Clamp Force Associated With Syndesmotic Overcompression. *Foot Ankle Int.* **2016**, *37*, 722–729. [CrossRef]
61. Henkemeyer, H.; Püschel, R.; Burri, C. Experimental studies on the biomechanics of syndesmosis. *Langenbecks Arch. Chir.* **1975**, 369–371.
62. Hermans, J.J.; Beumer, A.; de Jong, T.A.; Kleinrensink, G.J. Anatomy of the distal tibiofibular syndesmosis in adults: A pictorial essay with a multimodality approach. *J. Anat.* **2010**, *217*, 633–645. [CrossRef]
63. Hunt, K.J. Syndesmosis injuries. *Curr. Rev. Musculoskelet. Med.* **2013**, *6*, 304–312. [CrossRef]
64. Hunt, K.J.; Phisitkul, P.; Pirolo, J.; Amendola, A. High Ankle Sprains and Syndesmotic Injuries in Athletes. *J. Am. Acad. Orthop. Surg.* **2015**, *23*, 661–673. [CrossRef]
65. Hunt, K.J.; Goeb, Y.; Behn, A.W.; Criswell, B.; Chou, L. Ankle Joint Contact Loads and Displacement with Progressive Syndesmotic Injury. *Foot Ankle Int.* **2015**, *36*, 1095–1103. [CrossRef]
66. Jelinek, J.A.; Porter, D.A. Management of unstable ankle fractures and syndesmosis injuries in athletes. *Foot Ankle Clin.* **2009**, *14*, 277–298. [CrossRef]
67. Kaye, R.A. Stabilization of ankle syndesmosis injuries with a syndesmosis screw. *Foot Ankle* **1989**, *9*, 290–293. [CrossRef]
68. Kikuchi, S.; Tajima, G.; Sugawara, A.; Yan, J.; Maruyama, M.; Oikawa, S.; Saigo, T.; Oikawa, R.; Doita, M. Characteristic features of the insertions of the distal tibiofibular ligaments on three-dimensional computed tomography- cadaveric study. *J. Exp. Orthop.* **2020**, *7*, 3. [CrossRef]
69. Klitzman, R.; Zhao, H.; Zhang, L.Q.; Strohmeyer, G.; Vora, A. Suture-button versus screw fixation of the syndesmosis: A biomechanical analysis. *Foot Ankle Int.* **2010**, *31*, 69–75. [CrossRef]
70. Knops, S.P.; Kohn, M.A.; Hansen, E.N.; Matityahu, A.; Marmor, M. Rotational malreduction of the syndesmosis: Reliability and accuracy of computed tomography measurement methods. *Foot Ankle Int.* **2013**, *34*, 1403–1410. [CrossRef]
71. Kocadal, O.; Yucel, M.; Pepe, M.; Aksahin, E.; Aktekin, C.N. Evaluation of Reduction Accuracy of Suture-Button and Screw Fixation Techniques for Syndesmotic Injuries. *Foot Ankle Int.* **2016**, *37*, 1317–1325. [CrossRef] [PubMed]
72. Kortekangas, T.; Savola, O.; Flinkkilä, T.; Lepojärvi, S.; Nortunen, S.; Ohtonen, P.; Katisko, J.; Pakarinen, H. A prospective randomised study comparing TightRope and syndesmotic screw fixation for accuracy and maintenance of syndesmotic reduction assessed with bilateral computed tomography. *Injury* **2015**, *46*, 1119–1126. [CrossRef] [PubMed]
73. Krähenbühl, N.; Weinberg, M.W.; Hintermann, B.; Haller, J.M.; Saltzman, C.L.; Barg, A. Surgical outcome in chronic syndesmotic injury: A systematic literature review. *Foot Ankle Surg.* **2019**, *25*, 691–697. [CrossRef] [PubMed]
74. Kumar, A.; Goel, L.; Chouhan, D.; Agnihotri, A.; Chauhan, S.; Passey, J. Malleolar tips as reference points for positioning of syndesmotic screw: A preliminary CT based analysis. *J. Clin. Orthop. Trauma* **2020**, *11*, 438–441. [CrossRef]
75. Kumar, A.; Passey, J.; Goel, L.; Chouhan, D.; Agnihotri, A.; Chauhan, S.; Gupta, S.; Khan, R. New landmarks for ideal positioning of syndesmotic screw: A computerised tomography based analysis and radiographic simulation. *Int. Orthop.* **2020**, *44*, 665–675. [CrossRef]
76. Laflamme, M.; Belzile, E.L.; Bédard, L.; van den Bekerom, M.P.; Glazebrook, M.; Pelet, S. A prospective randomized multicenter trial comparing clinical outcomes of patients treated surgically with a static or dynamic implant for acute ankle syndesmosis rupture. *J. Orthop. Trauma* **2015**, *29*, 216–223. [CrossRef]
77. Littlechild, J.; Mayne, A.; Harrold, F.; Chami, G. A cadaveric study investigating the role of the anterior inferior tibio-fibular ligament and the posterior inferior tibio-fibular ligament in ankle fracture syndesmosis stability. *Foot Ankle Surg.* **2020**, *26*, 547–550. [CrossRef]
78. Liu, G.; Chen, L.; Gong, M.; Xing, F.; Xiang, Z. Clinical Evidence for Treatment of Distal Tibiofibular Syndesmosis Injury: A Systematic Review of Clinical Studies. *J. Foot Ankle Surg.* **2019**, *58*, 1245–1250. [CrossRef]

79. Liu, G.T.; Ryan, E.; Gustafson, E.; VanPelt, M.D.; Raspovic, K.M.; Lalli, T.; Wukich, D.K.; Xi, Y.; Chhabra, A. Three-Dimensional Computed Tomographic Characterization of Normal Anatomic Morphology and Variations of the Distal Tibiofibular Syndesmosis. *J. Foot Ankle Surg.* **2018**, *57*, 1130–1136. [CrossRef]
80. Mackay, G.M.; Blyth, M.J.; Anthony, I.; Hopper, G.P.; Ribbans, W.J. A review of ligament augmentation with the InternalBrace™: The surgical principle is described for the lateral ankle ligament and ACL repair in particular, and a comprehensive review of other surgical applications and techniques is presented. *Surg. Technol. Int.* **2015**, *26*, 239–255.
81. Magan, A.; Golano, P.; Maffulli, N.; Khanduja, V. Evaluation and management of injuries of the tibiofibular syndesmosis. *Br. Med. Bull.* **2014**, *111*, 101–115. [CrossRef]
82. Mahapatra, P.; Rudge, B.; Whittingham-Jones, P. Is It Possible to Overcompress the Syndesmosis? *J. Foot Ankle Surg.* **2018**, *57*, 1005–1009. [CrossRef]
83. McKenzie, A.C.; Hesselholt, K.E.; Larsen, M.S.; Schmal, H. A Systematic Review and Meta-Analysis on Treatment of Ankle Fractures With Syndesmotic Rupture: Suture-Button Fixation Versus Cortical Screw Fixation. *J. Foot Ankle Surg.* **2019**, *58*, 946–953. [CrossRef]
84. Miller, M.A.; McDonald, T.C.; Graves, M.L.; Spitler, C.A.; Russell, G.V.; Jones, L.C.; Replogle, W.; Wise, J.A.; Hydrick, J.; Bergin, P.F. Stability of the Syndesmosis After Posterior Malleolar Fracture Fixation. *Foot Ankle Int.* **2018**, *39*, 99–104. [CrossRef]
85. Miller, A.N.; Barei, D.P.; Iaquinto, J.M.; Ledoux, W.R.; Beingessner, D.M. Iatrogenic syndesmosis malreduction via clamp and screw placement. *J. Orthop. Trauma* **2013**, *27*, 100–106. [CrossRef]
86. Miller, A.N.; Carroll, E.A.; Parker, R.J.; Helfet, D.L.; Lorich, D.G. Posterior malleolar stabilization of syndesmotic injuries is equivalent to screw fixation. *Clin. Orthop. Relat. Res.* **2010**, *468*, 1129–1135. [CrossRef]
87. Miller, A.N.; Carroll, E.A.; Parker, R.J.; Boraiah, S.; Helfet, D.L.; Lorich, D.G. Direct visualization for syndesmotic stabilization of ankle fractures. *Foot Ankle Int.* **2009**, *30*, 419–426. [CrossRef]
88. Miller, T.L.; Skalak, T. Evaluation and treatment recommendations for acute injuries to the ankle syndesmosis without associated fracture. *Sports Med.* **2014**, *44*, 179–188. [CrossRef]
89. Miyamoto, W.; Takao, M. Management of chronic disruption of the distal tibiofibular syndesmosis. *World J. Orthop.* **2011**, *2*, 1–6. [CrossRef]
90. Mizel, M.S. Technique tip: A revised method of the Cotton test for intra-operative evaluation of syndesmotic injuries. *Foot Ankle Int.* **2003**, *24*, 86–87. [CrossRef]
91. Morris, M.W.; Rice, P.; Schneider, T.E. Distal tibiofibular syndesmosis reconstruction using a free hamstring autograft. *Foot Ankle Int.* **2009**, *30*, 506–511. [CrossRef] [PubMed]
92. Mukhopadhyay, S.; Metcalfe, A.; Guha, A.R.; Mohanty, K.; Hemmadi, S.; Lyons, K.; O'Doherty, D. Malreduction of—Are we considering the anatomical variation? *Injury* **2011**, *42*, 1073–1076. [CrossRef] [PubMed]
93. Mulcahey, M.K.; Bernhardson, A.S.; Murphy, C.P.; Chang, A.; Zajac, T.; Sanchez, G.; Sanchez, A.; Whalen, J.M.; Price, M.D.; Clanton, T.O.; et al. The Epidemiology of Ankle Injuries Identified at the National Football League Combine, 2009–2015. *Orthop. J. Sports Med.* **2018**, *6*, 2325967118786227. [CrossRef] [PubMed]
94. Naqvi, G.A.; Cunningham, P.; Lynch, B.; Galvin, R.; Awan, N. Fixation of ankle syndesmotic injuries: Comparison of tightrope fixation and syndesmotic screw fixation for accuracy of syndesmotic reduction. *Am. J. Sports Med.* **2012**, *40*, 2828–2835. [CrossRef]
95. Naqvi, G.A.; Shafqat, A.; Awan, N. Tightrope fixation of ankle syndesmosis injuries: Clinical outcome, complications and technique modification. *Injury* **2012**, *43*, 838–842. [CrossRef]
96. Nault, M.L.; Gascon, L.; Hébert-Davies, J.; Leduc, S.; Laflamme, G.Y.; Kramer, D. Modification of Distal Tibiofibular Relationship After a Mild Syndesmotic Injury. *Foot Ankle Spec.* **2017**, *10*, 133–138. [CrossRef]
97. Nelson, M.C.; Jensen, M.K. The treatment of trimalleolar fractures of the ankle. *Surg. Gynecol. Obstet.* **1940**, *71*, 509–514.
98. Nelson, O.A. Examination and repair of the AITFL in transmalleolar fractures. *J. Orthop. Trauma* **2006**, *20*, 637–643. [CrossRef]
99. O'Connor, T.J.; Mueller, B.; Ly, T.V.; Jacobson, A.R.; Nelson, E.R.; Cole, P.A. "A to p" screw versus posterolateral plate for posterior malleolus fixation in trimalleolar ankle fractures. *J. Orthop. Trauma* **2015**, *29*, e151–e156. [CrossRef]
100. Ovaska, M.T.; Mäkinen, T.J.; Madanat, R.; Kiljunen, V.; Lindahl, J. A comprehensive analysis of patients with malreduced ankle fractures undergoing re-operation. *Int. Orthop.* **2014**, *38*, 83–88. [CrossRef]
101. Pakarinen, H.; Flinkkilä, T.; Ohtonen, P.; Hyvönen, P.; Lakovaara, M.; Leppilahti, J.; Ristiniemi, J. Intraoperative assessment of the stability of the distal tibiofibular joint in supination-external rotation injuries of the ankle: Sensitivity, specificity, and reliability of two clinical tests. *J. Bone Jt. Surg. Am.* **2011**, *93*, 2057–2061. [CrossRef]
102. Pang, E.Q.; Bedigrew, K.; Palanca, A.; Behn, A.W.; Hunt, K.J.; Chou, L. Ankle joint contact loads and displacement in syndesmosis injuries repaired with Tightropes compared to screw fixation in a static model. *Injury* **2019**, *50*, 1901–1907. [CrossRef]
103. Pang, E.Q.; Coughlan, M.; Bonaretti, S.; Finlay, A.; Bellino, M.; Bishop, J.A.; Gardner, M.J. Assessment of Open Syndesmosis Reduction Techniques in an Unbroken Fibula Model: Visualization Versus Palpation. *J. Orthop. Trauma* **2019**, *33*, e14–e18. [CrossRef]
104. Park, J.S. Surgical Stabilization of Syndesmotic Injuries With Accelerated Return to Play in High-Level Athletes. *Foot Ankle Int.* **2020**, *41*, 497–498. [CrossRef]
105. Patel, N.K.; Murphy, C.I.; Pfeiffer, T.R.; Naendrup, J.H.; Zlotnicki, J.P.; Debski, R.E.; Hogan, M.V.; Musahl, V. Sagittal instability with inversion is important to evaluate after syndesmosis injury and repair: A cadaveric robotic study. *J. Exp. Orthop.* **2020**, *7*, 18. [CrossRef]

106. Peterson, K.S.; Chapman, W.D.; Hyer, C.F.; Berlet, G.C. Maintenance of reduction with suture button fixation devices for ankle syndesmosis repair. *Foot Ankle Int.* **2015**, *36*, 679–684. [CrossRef]
107. Phisitkul, P.; Ebinger, T.; Goetz, J.; Vaseenon, T.; Marsh, J.L. Forceps reduction of the syndesmosis in rotational ankle fractures: A cadaveric study. *J. Bone Jt. Surg. Am.* **2012**, *94*, 2256–2261. [CrossRef]
108. Porter, D.A.; Jaggers, R.R.; Barnes, A.F.; Rund, A.M. Optimal management of ankle syndesmosis injuries. *Open Access J. Sports Med.* **2014**, *5*, 173–182. [CrossRef]
109. Press, C.M.; Gupta, A.; Hutchinson, M.R. Management of ankle syndesmosis injuries in the athlete. *Curr. Sports Med. Rep.* **2009**, *8*, 228–233. [CrossRef]
110. Qamar, F.; Kadakia, A.; Venkateswaran, B. An anatomical way of treating ankle syndesmotic injuries. *J. Foot Ankle Surg.* **2011**, *50*, 762–765. [CrossRef]
111. Ræder, B.W.; Figved, W.; Madsen, J.E.; Frihagen, F.; Jacobsen, S.B.; Andersen, M.R. Better outcome for suture button compared with single syndesmotic screw for syndesmosis injury: Five-year results of a randomized controlled trial. *Bone Jt. J.* **2020**, *102-B*, 212–219. [CrossRef]
112. Rammelt, S.; Manke, E. Syndesmosis injuries at the ankle. *Unfallchirurg* **2018**, *121*, 693–703. [CrossRef]
113. Rammelt, S.; Obruba, P. An update on the evaluation and treatment of syndesmotic injuries. *Eur. J. Trauma Emerg. Surg.* **2015**, *41*, 601–614. [CrossRef]
114. Rammelt, S.; Zwipp, H.; Grass, R. Injuries to the distal tibiofibular syndesmosis: An evidence-based approach to acute and chronic lesions. *Foot Ankle Clin.* **2008**, *13*, 611–633. [CrossRef] [PubMed]
115. Ramsey, D.C.; Friess, D.M. Cost-Effectiveness Analysis of Syndesmotic Screw versus Suture Button Fixation in Tibiofibular Syndesmotic Injuries. *J. Orthop. Trauma* **2018**, *32*, e198–e203. [CrossRef]
116. Ramsey, P.L.; Hamilton, W. Changes in tibiotalar area of contact caused by lateral talar shift. *J. Bone Jt. Surg. Am.* **1976**, *58*, 356–357. [CrossRef]
117. Raspovic, K.M.; Anigian, K.; Kapilow, J.; Tisano, B. Flexible Fixation in Foot and Ankle Surgery. *Clin. Podiatr. Med. Surg.* **2019**, *36*, 553–562. [CrossRef] [PubMed]
118. Ray, R.; Koohnejad, N.; Clement, N.D.; Keenan, G.F. Ankle fractures with syndesmotic stabilisation are associated with a high rate of secondary osteoarthritis. *Foot Ankle Surg.* **2019**, *25*, 180–185. [CrossRef]
119. Regauer, M.; Mackay, G.; Lange, M.; Kammerlander, C.; Böcker, W. Syndesmotic InternalBrace™ for anatomic distal tibiofibular ligament augmentation. *World J. Orthop.* **2017**, *8*, 301–309. [CrossRef] [PubMed]
120. Rigby, R.B.; Cottom, J.M. Does the Arthrex TightRope® provide maintenance of the distal tibiofibular syndesmosis? A 2-year follow-up of 64 TightRopes® in 37 patients. *J. Foot Ankle Surg.* **2013**, *52*, 563–567. [CrossRef]
121. Rushing, C.J.; Spinner, S.M.; Armstrong, A.V., Jr.; Hardigan, P. Comparison of Different Magnitudes of Applied Syndesmotic Clamp Force: A Cadaveric Study. *J. Foot Ankle Surg.* **2020**, *59*, 452–456. [CrossRef]
122. Rustenburg, C.; Blom, R.; Stufkens, S.; Kerkhoffs, G.; Emanuel, K. Invisible injuries in ankle fractures: A biomechanical analysis of the ankle syndesmosis. *Orthop. Proc.* **2018**, *100-B*, 26.
123. Sagi, H.C.; Shah, A.R.; Sanders, R.W. The functional consequence of syndesmotic joint malreduction at a minimum 2-year follow-up. *J. Orthop. Trauma* **2012**, *26*, 439–443. [CrossRef]
124. Sanders, D.; Schneider, P.; Taylor, M.; Tieszer, C.; Lawendy, A.R.; Canadian Orthopaedic Trauma Society. Improved Reduction of the Tibiofibular Syndesmosis With TightRope Compared with Screw Fixation: Results of a Randomized Controlled Study. *J. Orthop. Trauma* **2019**, *33*, 531–537. [CrossRef]
125. Schepers, T. Acute distal tibiofibular syndesmosis injury: A systematic review of suture-button versus syndesmotic screw repair. *Int. Orthop.* **2012**, *36*, 1199–1206. [CrossRef]
126. Schnetzke, M.; Vetter, S.Y.; Beisemann, N.; Swartman, B.; Grützner, P.A.; Franke, J. Management of syndesmotic injuries: What is the evidence? *World J. Orthop.* **2016**, *7*, 718–725. [CrossRef]
127. Schon, J.M.; Brady, A.W.; Krob, J.J.; Lockard, C.A.; Marchetti, D.C.; Dornan, G.J.; Clanton, T.O. Defining the three most responsive and specific CT measurements of ankle syndesmotic malreduction. *Knee Surg. Sports Traumatol. Arthrosc.* **2019**, *27*, 2863–2876. [CrossRef]
128. Schon, J.M.; Mikula, J.D.; Backus, J.D.; Venderley, M.B.; Dornan, G.J.; LaPrade, R.F.; Clanton, T.O. 3D Model Analysis of Ankle Flexion on Anatomic Reduction of a Syndesmotic Injury. *Foot Ankle Int.* **2017**, *38*, 436–442. [CrossRef]
129. Schon, J.M.; Williams, B.T.; Venderley, M.B.; Dornan, G.J.; Backus, J.D.; Turnbull, T.L.; LaPrade, R.F.; Clanton, T.O. A 3-D CT Analysis of Screw and Suture-Button Fixation of the Syndesmosis. *Foot Ankle Int.* **2017**, *38*, 208–214. [CrossRef]
130. Schottel, P.C.; Baxter, J.; Gilbert, S.; Garner, M.R.; Lorich, D.G. Anatomic Ligament Repair Restores Ankle and Syndesmotic Rotational Stability as Much as Syndesmotic Screw Fixation. *J. Orthop. Trauma* **2016**, *30*, e36–e40. [CrossRef]
131. Schumann, G. Surgical treatment of ankle fractures with comminuted supramalleolar fracture. *Zentralbl. Chir.* **1955**, *80*, 542–546.
132. Seitz, W.H., Jr.; Bachner, E.J.; Abram, L.J.; Postak, P.; Polando, G.; Brooks, D.B.; Greenwald, A.S. Repair of the tibiofibular syndesmosis with a flexible implant. *J. Orthop. Trauma* **1991**, *5*, 78–82. [CrossRef]
133. Seyhan, M.; Donmez, F.; Mahirogullari, M.; Cakmak, S.; Mutlu, S.; Guler, O. Comparison of screw fixation with elastic fixation methods in the treatment of syndesmosis injuries in ankle fractures. *Injury* **2015**, *46* (Suppl. 2), S19–S23. [CrossRef]
134. Shimozono, Y.; Hurley, E.T.; Myerson, C.L.; Murawski, C.D.; Kennedy, J.G. Suture Button Versus Syndesmotic Screw for Syndesmosis Injuries: A Meta-analysis of Randomized Controlled Trials. *Am. J. Sports Med.* **2019**, *47*, 2764–2771. [CrossRef]

135. Shoji, H.; Teramoto, A.; Suzuki, D.; Okada, Y.; Sakakibara, Y.; Matsumura, T.; Suzuki, T.; Watanabe, K.; Yamashita, T. Suture-button fixation and anterior inferior tibiofibular ligament augmentation with suture-tape for syndesmosis injury: A biomechanical cadaveric study. *Clin. Biomech.* **2018**, *60*, 121–126. [CrossRef] [PubMed]
136. Shou, K.; Adhikary, R.; Zou, L.; Yao, H.; Yang, H.; Adhikary, K.; Yang, Y.; Bao, T. The Assessment of the Reduction Algorithm in the Treatment for "Logsplitter" Injury. *Biomed Res. Int.* **2020**, *2020*, 4139028. [CrossRef] [PubMed]
137. Sman, A.D.; Hiller, C.E.; Rae, K.; Linklater, J.; Black, D.A.; Refshauge, K.M. Prognosis of ankle syndesmosis injury. *Med. Sci. Sports Exerc.* **2014**, *46*, 671–677. [CrossRef] [PubMed]
138. Solan, M.C.; Davies, M.S.; Sakellariou, A. Syndesmosis Stabilisation: Screws Versus Flexible Fixation. *Foot Ankle Clin.* **2017**, *22*, 35–63. [CrossRef] [PubMed]
139. Soreide, E.; Denbeigh, J.M.; Lewallen, E.A.; Thaler, R.; Xu, W.; Berglund, L.; Yao, J.J.; Martinez, A.; Nordsletten, L.; van Wijnen, A.J.; et al. In vivo assessment of high-molecular-weight polyethylene core suture tape for intra-articular ligament reconstruction: An animal study. *Bone Jt. J.* **2019**, *101-B*, 1238–1247. [CrossRef]
140. Teramoto, A.; Shoji, H.; Sakakibara, Y.; Suzuki, T.; Watanabe, K.; Yamashita, T. Suture-Button Fixation and Mini-Open Anterior Inferior Tibiofibular Ligament Augmentation Using Suture Tape for Tibiofibular Syndesmosis Injuries. *J. Foot Ankle Surg.* **2018**, *57*, 159–161. [CrossRef]
141. Teramoto, A.; Suzuki, D.; Kamiya, T.; Chikenji, T.; Watanabe, K.; Yamashita, T. Comparison of different fixation methods of the suture-button implant for tibiofibular syndesmosis injuries. *Am. J. Sports Med.* **2011**, *39*, 2226–2232. [CrossRef]
142. Thornes, B.; Shannon, F.; Guiney, A.M.; Hession, P.; Masterson, E. Suture-button syndesmosis fixation: Accelerated rehabilitation and improved outcomes. *Clin. Orthop. Relat. Res.* **2005**, *431*, 207–212. [CrossRef]
143. Tornetta, P., 3rd; Yakavonis, M.; Veltre, D.; Shah, A. Reducing the Syndesmosis Under Direct Vision: Where Should I Look? *J. Orthop. Trauma* **2019**, *33*, 450–454. [CrossRef]
144. Tosun, B.; Selek, O.; Gok, U.; Ceylan, H. Posterior Malleolus Fractures in Trimalleolar Ankle Fractures: Malleolus versus Transyndesmal Fixation. *Indian J. Orthop.* **2018**, *52*, 309–314. [CrossRef]
145. Tourné, Y.; Molinier, F.; Andrieu, M.; Porta, J.; Barbier, G. Diagnosis and treatment of tibiofibular syndesmosis lesions. *Orthop. Traumatol. Surg. Res.* **2019**, *105*, S275–S286. [CrossRef]
146. Vacas-Sánchez, E.; Olaya-González, C.; Abarquero-Diezhandino, A.; Sánchez-Morata, E.; Vilá-Rico, J. How to address the posterior malleolus in ankle fractures? A decision-making model based on the computerised tomography findings. *Int. Orthop.* **2020**, *44*, 1177–1185. [CrossRef]
147. Vance, N.G.; Vance, R.C.; Chandler, W.T.; Panchbhavi, V.K. Can Syndesmosis Screws Displace the Distal Fibula? *Foot Ankle Spec.* **2021**, *14*, 201–205. [CrossRef]
148. Van den Bekerom, M.P.; Kloen, P.; Luitse, J.S.; Raaymakers, E.L. Complications of distal tibiofibular syndesmotic screw stabilization: Analysis of 236 patients. *J. Foot Ankle Surg.* **2013**, *52*, 456–459. [CrossRef]
149. Van den Bekerom, M.P. Diagnosing syndesmotic instability in ankle fractures. *World J. Orthop.* **2011**, *2*, 51–56. [CrossRef]
150. Van den Heuvel, S.B.; Dingemans, S.A.; Gardenbroek, T.J.; Schepers, T. Assessing Quality of Syndesmotic Reduction in Surgically Treated Acute Syndesmotic Injuries: A Systematic Review. *J. Foot Ankle Surg.* **2019**, *58*, 144–150. [CrossRef]
151. Van Vlijmen, N.; Denk, K.; van Kampen, A.; Jaarsma, R.L. Long-term Results After Ankle Syndesmosis Injuries. *Orthopedics* **2015**, *38*, e1001–e1006. [CrossRef]
152. Von Rüden, C.; Hackl, S.; Woltmann, A.; Friederichs, J.; Bühren, V.; Hierholzer, C. The Postero-Lateral Approach—An Alternative to Closed Anterior-Posterior Screw Fixation of a Dislocated Postero-Lateral Fragment of the Distal Tibia in Complex Ankle Fractures. *Z. Orthop. Unfall.* **2015**, *153*, 289–295. [CrossRef]
153. Verhage, S.M.; Krijnen, P.; Schipper, I.B.; Hoogendoorn, J.M. Persistent postoperative step-off of the posterior malleolus leads to higher incidence of post-traumatic osteoarthritis in trimalleolar fractures. *Arch. Orthop. Trauma Surg.* **2019**, *139*, 323–329. [CrossRef]
154. Verhage, S.M.; Hoogendoorn, J.M.; Krijnen, P.; Schipper, I.B. When and how to operate the posterior malleolus fragment in trimalleolar fractures: A systematic literature review. *Arch. Orthop. Trauma Surg.* **2018**, *138*, 1213–1222. [CrossRef]
155. Verhage, S.M.; Boot, F.; Schipper, I.B.; Hoogendoorn, J.M. Open reduction and internal fixation of posterior malleolar fractures using the posterolateral approach. *Bone Jt. J.* **2016**, *98-B*, 812–817. [CrossRef]
156. Vetter, S.Y.; Beisemann, N.; Keil, H.; Schnetzke, M.; Swartman, B.; Franke, J.; Grützner, P.A.; Privalov, M. Comparison of three different reduction methods of the ankle mortise in unstable syndesmotic injuries. *Sci. Rep.* **2019**, *9*, 15445. [CrossRef]
157. Vopat, M.L.; Vopat, B.G.; Lubberts, B.; DiGiovanni, C.W. Current trends in the diagnosis and management of syndesmotic injury. *Curr. Rev. Musculoskelet. Med.* **2017**, *10*, 94–103. [CrossRef]
158. Wake, J.; Martin, K.D. Syndesmosis Injury from Diagnosis to Repair: Physical Examination, Diagnosis, and Arthroscopic-assisted Reduction. *J. Am. Acad. Orthop. Surg.* **2020**, *28*, 517–527. [CrossRef]
159. Weening, B.; Bhandari, M. Predictors of functional outcome following transsyndesmotic screw fixation of ankle fractures. *J. Orthop. Trauma* **2005**, *19*, 102–108. [CrossRef] [PubMed]
160. Weng, Q.; Lin, C.; Liu, Y.; Dai, G.; Lutchooman, V.; Hong, J. Biomechanical Analysis of a Novel Syndesmotic Plate Compared With Traditional Screw and Suture Button Fixation. *J. Foot Ankle Surg.* **2020**, *59*, 522–528. [CrossRef]
161. Westermann, R.W.; Rungprai, C.; Goetz, J.E.; Femino, J.; Amendola, A.; Phisitkul, P. The effect of suture-button fixation on simulated syndesmotic malreduction: A cadaveric study. *J. Bone Jt. Surg. Am.* **2014**, *96*, 1732–1738. [CrossRef] [PubMed]

162. Willenegger, H. Treatment of luxation fractures of the tibiotarsal joint according to biomechanical viewpoints. *Helv. Chir. Acta* **1961**, *28*, 225–239. [PubMed]
163. Willenegger, H.; Weber, G.B. Malleolar fractures. *Langenbecks Arch. Klin. Chir.* **1965**, *313*, 489–502. [CrossRef]
164. Williams, B.T.; Ahrberg, A.B.; Goldsmith, M.T.; Campbell, K.J.; Shirley, L.; Wijdicks, C.A.; LaPrade, R.F.; Clanton, T.O. Ankle syndesmosis: A qualitative and quantitative anatomic analysis. *Am. J. Sports Med.* **2015**, *43*, 88–97. [CrossRef]
165. Wood, A.R.; Arshad, S.A.; Kim, H.; Stewart, D. Kinematic Analysis of Combined Suture-Button and Suture Anchor Augment Constructs for Ankle Syndesmosis Injuries. *Foot Ankle Int.* **2020**, *41*, 463–472. [CrossRef]
166. Xian, H.; Miao, J.; Zhou, Q.; Lian, K.; Zhai, W.; Liu, Q. Novel Elastic Syndesmosis Hook Plate Fixation versus Routine Screw Fixation for Syndesmosis Injury. *J. Foot Ankle Surg.* **2018**, *57*, 65–68. [CrossRef]
167. Yasui, Y.; Takao, M.; Miyamoto, W.; Innami, K.; Matsushita, T. Anatomical reconstruction of the anterior inferior tibiofibular ligament for chronic disruption of the distal tibiofibular syndesmosis. *Knee Surg. Sports Traumatol. Arthrosc.* **2011**, *19*, 691–695. [CrossRef]
168. Yin, Z.; Wang, Z.; Ge, D.; Yan, J.; Jiang, C.; Liang, B. Treatment of a high-energy transsyndesmotic ankle fracture: A case report of "logsplitter injury". *Medicine* **2020**, *99*, e19380. [CrossRef]
169. Yu, G.S.; Lin, Y.B.; Xiong, G.S.; Xu, H.B.; Liu, Y.Y. Diagnosis and treatment of ankle syndesmosis injuries with associated interosseous membrane injury: A current concept review. *Int. Orthop.* **2019**, *43*, 2539–2547. [CrossRef]
170. Zhan, Y.; Yan, X.; Xia, R.; Cheng, T.; Luo, C. Anterior-inferior tibiofibular ligament anatomical repair and augmentation versus trans-syndesmosis screw fixation for the syndesmotic instability in external-rotation type ankle fracture with posterior malleolus involvement: A prospective and comparative study. *Injury* **2016**, *47*, 1574–1580. [CrossRef]
171. Zhang, P.; Liang, Y.; He, J.; Fang, Y.; Chen, P.; Wang, J. A systematic review of suture-button versus syndesmotic screw in the treatment of distal tibiofibular syndesmosis injury. *BMC Musculoskelet. Disord.* **2017**, *18*, 286. [CrossRef]
172. D'Ambrosi, R.; Di Silvestri, C.; Manzi, L.; Indino, C.; Maccario, C.; Usuelli, F.G. Post-traumatic ankle osteoarthritis: Quality of life, frequency and associated factors. *Muscles Ligaments Tendons J.* **2019**, *9*, 363–371. [CrossRef]

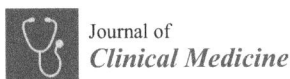

Article

Can a Single Trial of a Thoracolumbar Myofascial Release Technique Reduce Pain and Disability in Chronic Low Back Pain? A Randomized Balanced Crossover Study

Luana Rocha Paulo [1,2,3], Ana Cristina Rodrigues Lacerda [1,4], Fábio Luiz Mendonça Martins [1,4], José Sebastião Cunha Fernandes [4], Leonardo Sette Vieira [2], Cristiano Queiroz Guimarães [2], Sílvia de Simoni Guedes Ballesteros [2], Marco Túlio Saldanha dos Anjos [5], Patrícia Aparecida Tavares [3], Sueli Ferreira da Fonseca [4], Murilo Xavier Oliveira [1,4], Mário Bernardo-Filho [6], Danúbia da Cunha de Sá-Caputo [6], Vanessa Amaral Mendonça [1,4] and Redha Taiar [7,*]

1 Postgraduate Program of Rehabilitation and Functional Performance (PPGReab), Federal University of Jequitinhonha and Mucuri Valleys (UFVJM), Diamantina 39803-371, Brazil; luana.r.p@hotmail.com (L.R.P.); lacerdaacr@gmail.com (A.C.R.L.); fmartins.ufvjm@gmail.com (F.L.M.M.); muriloxavier@gmail.com (M.X.O.); vaafisio@hotmail.com (V.A.M.)
2 Academia Brasileira de Fascias, Juatuba 35675-000, Brazil; leosettefisio@gmail.com (L.S.V.); cristiano_fisioterapia@yahoo.com.br (C.Q.G.); guedesilvia@gmail.com (S.d.S.G.B.)
3 Physiotherapy Departament, Una University Center, Divinópolis 35500-017, Brazil; tavaresaguiar@yahoo.com.br
4 Physiotherapy Departament, Federal University of Jequitinhonha and Mucuri Valleys, Diamantina 39803-371, Brazil; jscf1912@gmail.com (J.S.C.F.); suffonseca@hotmail.com (S.F.d.F.)
5 Dinâmica Soluções em Saúde, Belo Horizonte 30210-590, Brazil; msaldanhadosanjos@yahoo.com.br
6 Laboratory of Mechanical Vibrations and Integrative Practices, State University of Rio de Janeiro, Rio de Janeiro 20550-013, Brazil; bernardofilhom@gmail.com (M.B.-F.); dradanubia@gmail.com (D.d.C.d.S.-C.)
7 MATériaux et Ingénierie Mécanique (MATIM), Université de Reims Champagne-Ardenne, 51100 Reims, France
* Correspondence: redha.taiar@univ-reims.fr

Abstract: Although manual therapy for pain relief has been used as an adjunct in treatments for chronic low back pain (CLBP), there is still the belief that a single session of myofascial release would be effective. This study was a crossover clinical trial aimed to investigate whether a single session of a specific myofascial release technique reduces pain and disability in subjects with CLBP. 41 participants over 18 years old were randomly enrolled into 3 situations in a balanced and crossover manner: experimental, placebo, and control. The subjects underwent a single session of myofascial release on thoracolumbar fascia and the results were compared with the control and placebo groups. The outcomes, pain and functionality, were evaluated using the numerical pain rating scale (NPRS), pressure pain threshold (PPT), and Oswestry Disability Index (ODI). There were no effects between-tests, within-tests, nor for interaction of all the outcomes, i.e., NPRS ($\eta^2 = 0.32$, F = 0.48, $p = 0.61$), PPT ($\eta^2 = 0.73$, F = 2.80, $p = 0.06$), ODI ($\eta^2 = 0.02$, F = 0.02, $p = 0.97$). A single trial of a thoracolumbar myofascial release technique was not enough to reduce pain intensity and disability in subjects with CLBP.

Keywords: fascia; chronic low back pain; myofascial release

1. Introduction

Chronic non-specific low back pain (CLBP) is a condition characterized by pain, stiffness, and/or muscular tension [1] and is an important health problem throughout the world [2]. In CLBP, pain processing and modulation by the central nervous system may be altered. Manual therapy (MT) is a conservative intervention for treatment of

CLBP [1,3,4]. Myofascial release is a form of MT, which involves the application of low-load and long-duration stretches to the myofascial complex. Although the mechanisms of action and effectiveness in individuals with CLBP are still unclear, myofascial release techniques are widely used by physical therapists in the management of CLBP, with the intent to restore the optimal length of the fasciae tissue, decrease pain intensity, and improve functionality [1,4–9]. Previous reports point to the effects of stabilization or global physical exercise in pain relief in subjects with CLBP with few studies for manual techniques alone or as an adjunct therapy [10–14].

Considering that previous studies recommended the adoption of interventions focused on the soft-tissues for the management of CLBP, there is still the belief among clinicians that an isolated session of MT, e.g., myofascial release, is effective in reducing pain intensity and disability [9,15]. As far as we know, only one study investigated the effects of an isolated myofascial release protocol on pain intensity and disability in patients with CLBP. Although the authors did not show clearly whether the improvement in pain intensity and disability was clinically relevant, they suggested the myofascial protocol that was used reduced these outcomes [4]. In this investigation, one of the areas chosen for intervention was the thoracolumbar fascia (TLF), which contains a great proportion of post-ganglionic sympathetic fibers and is densely innervated by free nerve endings, as low-threshold-mechanosensitive C fibers, which are responsive to MT [5,16] with repeated mechanical or biochemical stimulation.

The anatomical distribution of TLF layers, the aforementioned specificities of this tissue, and the support of the literature on the potential nociceptive function of TLF in the etiology of low back pain [17], allow for the inference that active movement of the trunk, such as flexion-extension, will increase the shear of the tissue and contribute to pain reduction and function [7,18–25]. Therefore, the present study aimed to verify if there is an immediate effect of a specific myofascial release technique on the TLF of individuals with CLBP, measured by pain intensity and disability, in comparison with that of control and placebo situations [23,25].

2. Materials and Methods

2.1. Study Design

This was a crossover open clinical trial performed between February and June 2019. The trial was registered with the Clinical Trials Government Identifier (ReBEC—reference number 8197). The current study conformed to the Consolidated Standards of Reporting Trials statement for reporting clinical trial studies. All subjects provided written informed consent to participate in this study, which was conducted in accordance with ethical principles for research involving humans (principles of the Declaration of Helsinki) and received approval from the Ethics and Research Committee of the Federal University of Jequitinhonha and Mucuri Valleys (reference number 3.435.537).

All the participants underwent three situations in a randomized and balanced order. The sequence of situations was randomized using a website (www.random.org, accessed on 8 July 2019). A familiarization with the experimental procedures was performed, followed by anamnesis (age, sex, and level of physical activity) and evaluation of the prognosis or risk profile using the STarT Back Screening Tool (SBST) questionnaire, which consists of nine items divided into physical and psychosocial subscales [26].

2.2. Study Populations

Subjects were recruited in the city of Diamantina, Minas Gerais, Brazil. Inclusion requirements and eligibility were men and women over 18 years old, with a medical diagnosis of CLBP or low back pain for more than 3 months, who obtained a minimum cut-off value of 2 points of pain by the Numerical Pain Rating Scale (NPRS) during data collection. Exclusion criteria were previous or scheduled surgeries in the torso or limbs; those with suspicion of severe fractures or pathologies (tumor, inflammation, infection, rheumatological disorder, aortic aneurysm); diagnosis of radiculopathy or neuropathy (with or without spinal canal stenosis with proof of magnetic resonance imaging—MRI); structural deformity in the spinal column; spondyloarthropathy, disabling pain and physical disability that would make it impossible to perform the study procedures; use of painkillers or anti-inflammatory medicines 48 h before the first test phase or during the study; neurological or psychiatric disorder; and presence or suspicion of pregnancy. In addition, the subjects that self-reported physical activity levels equal to or greater than those recommended by the American College of Sports Medicine (ACSM) were excluded [27–29].

2.3. Sample Size Calculation

The sample size was estimated by the GPower® program (Franz Faul, Universität Kiel, Kiel, Germany), version 3.1.9.2. For this, we used a priori analysis, with ANOVA for comparisons between groups for the variable NPRS [30]. The effect size was calculated from the difference in the means with standard deviation within each group of 0.9. Thus, considering an effect size of 0.42, power of 0.80%, and alpha error 5%, the sample size was estimated at 41 volunteers. There were no withdrawals, so there was no need to analyze the data with the intention to treat.

A total of 52 subjects agreed to participate, of them, 10 individuals gave up or did not attend the test site on the scheduled date and 1 individual did not meet the described inclusion criteria. Therefore, 41 subjects participated in all stages of the research (Figure 1). Of the 41 individuals, 61% were women and 56% declared themselves sedentary. In addition, the median age was 36 years and the self-reported pain averaged 3.4 to 3.7 points. Among the subjects, 56% were classified in terms of poor prognosis in the SBST as low risk (Table 1).

Table 1. Characteristics of the participants at baseline.

Characteristics	Subjects (n = 41) Mean (95% CI *) or %
Age (years)	36 (22–50)
Gender, women (%)	60.98
Sedentary (%)	56.09
NRPS [1] baseline (0–10)	3.68 (1.39–5.97)
PPT [2] (N/cm^2)	34 (16.57–51.43)
FTF [3] (cm)	13 (2–24)
SBST [4]—prognosis (%)	
• Low risk	56.1
• Medium risk	24.4
• High risk	19.5

* CI: confidence interval; [1] NRPS: visual numeric pain scale; [2] PPT: pain pressure threshold; [3] FTF: fingertip-to-floor; [4] SBST: STarT Back Screening Tool.

2.4. Outcome Measures

The measurements of pain were the primary outcome. We used the Pressure Pain Threshold (PPT) and NPRS as the instruments to measure pain. As a secondary outcome, the Oswestry Disability Index questionnaire (ODI—version 2.0, Department of Nursing, Faculty of Medical Sciences, State University of Campinas, Campinas, SP, Brazil) evaluated the prognosis and functionality of the subjects. All analyses were performed to compare the results before (pre-test) and immediately after (follow-up) each experimental situation.

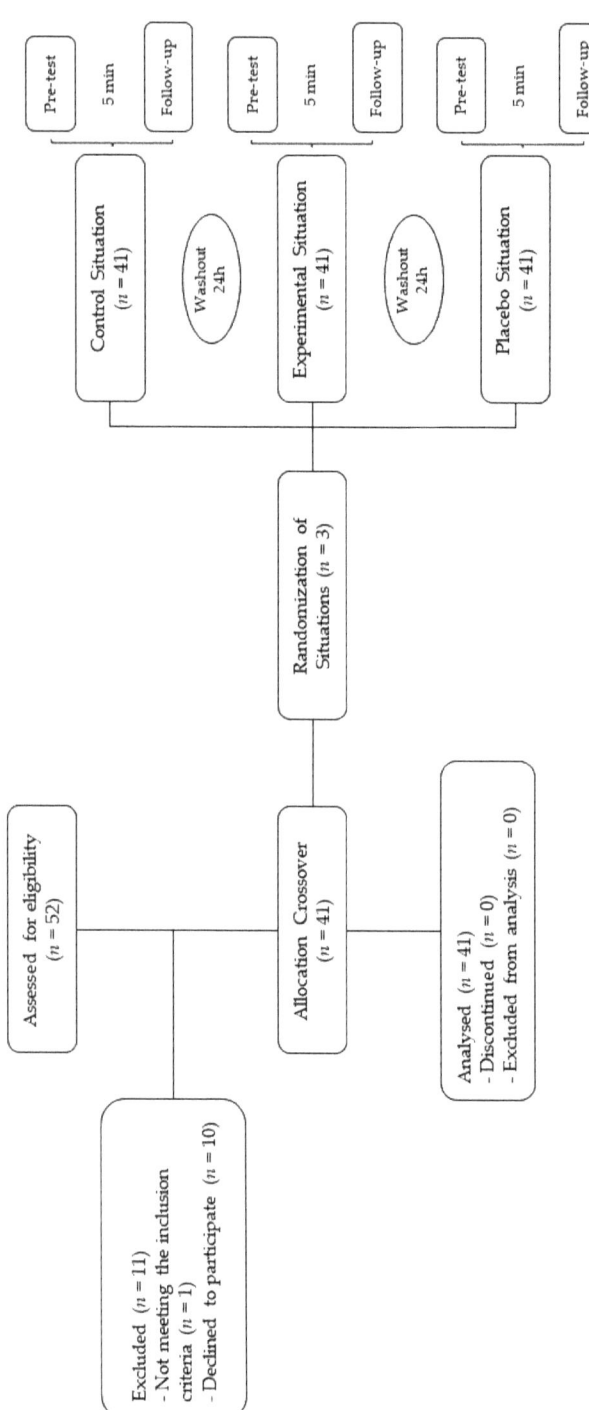

Figure 1. Flow of participants throughout in all stages of the research.

For pain measurements, the NPRS was used to quantify the intensity of pain in all areas of the study, ranging from 0 to 10, with 0 classified as no pain and 10 as the worst pain imaginable. This instrument is proven to be a competing and valid predictor of pain intensity [31]. The pain threshold was assessed using a PPT device (FDX Series Force Gage, Wagner Instruments, Greenwich, CT, USA), with a graduation capacity of 50×0.05 lbf, 800×0.5 ozf, 25×0.02 kgf and 250×0.2 N, and a 1 cm^2 plunger connected to a mechanical force gauge that indicates the pressure applied at the marked location. The plunger of the device was positioned perpendicularly to the paravertebral muscles, respecting the proximity of 2 cm laterally to the midline between the L3–L4 spinous process. The pressure was applied progressively and perpendicular to the skin, with an average of 1 kg/cm^2/s, until the volunteer signaled the onset of pain or discomfort. After signaling, the device was removed from contact with the individual's body and the Newton's quantification was noted [32,33]. Initially, a familiarization was performed on the anterior muscles of the forearm. For the assessment, after the participants were positioned for the interventions, the point for assessed was marked with a pen and three measurements were taken at the same site (pre-test and follow-up), with a 30 s interval between them. The mean of the three measurements was used for analysis [1,34].

The ODI Version 2.0 questionnaire [35] was used to quantify the disability caused by low back pain in daily activities. Scores were given from 0% (no dysfunction; independence) to 100% (lowest level of functionality; total dependence), divided into 5 levels, where the first described no limitation and the others described limitation or inability to function. The total score is the percentage value calculated by the following equation: Total score = (Σ item score/50) $\times$ 100. With all 10 questions answered, the total score was divided by 50 (10×5). The published minimally clinically important difference (MCID) values for ODI is 12.88 (sensitivity 88%, specificity 85%) [36]. It must be taken into consideration that the ODI is a questionnaire with a one-dimensional factorial structure. Important psychometric properties and internal consistency, and their ability to measure functional limitations were considered to be very accurate according to the actual level of severity of the dysfunction experienced by the assessed subjects [37].

2.5. Intervention

Forty-one of the fifty-two volunteers were selected after the initial screening and exclusion through the eligibility criteria. All were enrolled in the three situations: (1) control (C), (2) experimental (Exp), and (3) placebo (Plac). In our work, a single trained and experienced therapist, a member of the Brazilian Academy of Fasciae (ABSFascias), applied the technique in all situations. Due to the design of our study, only the assessor was blinded. However, all the subjects performed the three situations on consecutive days respecting a minimum interval of 24 h in order to minimize the potential bias due to the high level of adaptability of the connective tissue [3].

2.5.1. Control

The subjects were instructed to remain in the supine position for five minutes on a stretcher to minimize the effects of tension forces or stimuli on the tissue, without making movements, to mimic the time spent in the act of performing the intervention.

2.5.2. Experimental

The subjects underwent a single session of the new approach to be tested to release the TLF in a sedestation position with feet supported and the thoracolumbar region properly undressed. The trunk flexion goniometry of each participant was performed and the value of 30° was marked with a barrier to limit the necessary movement during the technique. The trained researcher positioned their hands on all participants without sliding over the skin or forcing the tissue, with the cranial hand close to the last rib and at the T12–L1 level on the right side of the individual's body and the caudal hand on the ipsilateral side between the iliac crest and the sacrum. Then, the researcher caused a slight traction in the tissues by moving their hands away from each other in a longitudinal direction. Then, the participant was instructed to perform five repetitions of active trunk flexion-extension (30°), while the researcher followed the movement with both hands simultaneously positioned, without losing the initial tissue traction and position (Figure 2). The same technique and the same number of repetitions of active trunk flexion-extension were repeated with the researcher's hands positioned on the opposite sides. This technique lasted approximately five minutes [3,38,39].

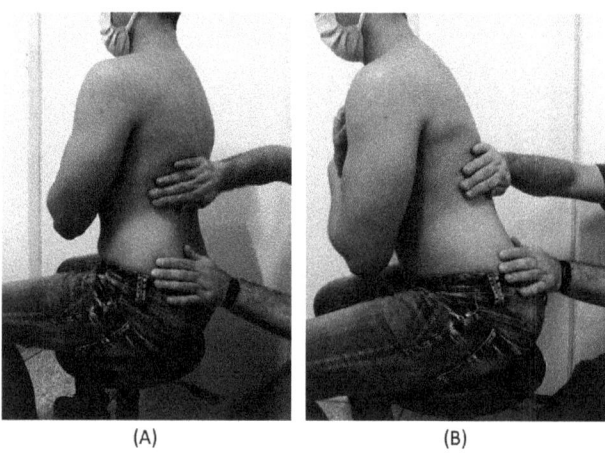

Figure 2. (**A**) Trunk position (90°) and researcher's hands contact at the beginning of the technique. (**B**) 30° trunk flexion and researcher's hands contact at the end of the technique.

2.5.3. Placebo

The subjects were not submitted to the technique of manual thoracolumbar fascia release, but they slowly performed ten repetitions of active trunk flexion-extension (30°) in the same position as the experimental situation. Due to the fact that touch can provide not only well-recognized discriminative input to the brain, but also an affective input, there was no touch from the researcher at this stage [16].

2.6. Statistical Analysis

Data were described as mean (95% confidence interval). The normality and homogeneity of the variables were assessed by the Shapiro-Wilk test and the Levene test, respectively. The effects and interactions in the two moments (pre and post) and three situations (C, Plac, Exp) were evaluated by factorial variance analysis (ANOVA 2 × 3) allowing comparisons between-tests, within-tests, and with interaction. The Tukey test was used as a Post Hoc for multiple comparisons of means. The level of significance adopted for all tests was 5%. Estimates of effect size and power were calculated using the GPower® program version 3.1 (Heinrich-Heine-University Düsseldorf, Germany).

3. Results

There was no statistical differences between-tests, within-tests, nor interaction. The minimal detectable change (MDC: post-pre) for PPT was 3% (−1.14 points) to the control, 8% (+2.45 points) to the placebo, and 13% (+4.28 points) to the experimental. The MDC for NPRS was 0.005% to the control, 0.09% to the placebo, and 0.04% to the experimental, i.e., a change less than 0.3 points in the NPRS. The MDC for ODI was 13% (+2.22 points) to the control, 2% (+0.19 points) to the placebo, and 1% (0.03 points) to the experimental (Table 2).

Table 2. Statistical results between-tests, within-tests and interaction for outcomes.

Outcomes	Control Mean (95% CI)	Placebo Mean (95% CI)	Experimental Mean (95% CI)	Between-Tests				Within-Tests				Interaction			
				p	F	η^2	Power	p	F	η^2	Power	p	F	η^2	Power
PPT (N/cm^2) PT	37.25 (32.63–41.86)	29.37 (23.93–34.81)	30.38 (24.70–36.06)	0.40	0.90	0.47	0.99	0.56	0.34	0.25	0.90	0.06	2.80	0.73	1.00
PPT (N/cm^2) FU	36.11 (30.90–41.31)	31.82 (26.12–37.52)	34.66 (28.01–41.32)												
NPRS (score) PT	3.41 (2.69–4.12)	3.80 (3.06–4.53)	3.00 (2.30–3.69)	0.06	2.79	0.73	1.00	0.80	0.06	0.05	0.25	0.61	0.48	0.32	0.97
NPRS (score) FU	3.43 (2.76–4.09)	3.48 (2.73–4.22)	3.14 (2.38–3.89)												
ODI (%) PT	15.82 (12.91–18.74)	17.51 (14.42–20.59)	19.26 (16.29–22.23)	0.007	5.01	0.83	1.00	0.73	0.11	0.07	0.31	0.97	0.02	0.02	0.11
ODI (%) FU	18.04 (15.00–21.09)	17.70 (14.65–20.76)	19.29 (16.22–22.36)												

CI: confidence interval; PPT: pressure pain threshold (N: Newtons); NPRS: visual numeric pain scale; ODI: Oswestry Disability Index; PT: pre-test; FU: follow-up. η^2: Eta partial. Sample size = 41. Factorial ANOVA (2 × 3).

4. Discussion

The aim of our work was to verify the immediate effect of a single specific thoracolumbar myofascial release technique in individuals with CLBP, concerning pain intensity and disability, in comparison with control and placebo situations. The main findings show that our dosage and specific technique may not have been enough to provide effects on pain intensity and disability in individuals with CLBP. An important aspect that might explain our findings is that the myofascial techniques found in the literature are heterogeneous regarding duration, frequency, and intensity [3,4]. In this sense, a previous study applied four sessions of myofascial treatment, each lasting 40 min, compared to a sham therapy [4]. Ajimsha and colleagues (2014) [3] also used a myofascial technique of 40 min applied in several sites, while in our work the technique lasted five minutes and was applied in only one tissue in addition to a trunk movement.

Our findings demonstrated that although six participants showed a reduction in the NPRS consistent with the MCID [31,40,41], the magnitude of the subjects' pain measured by NPRS was not statistically significant between-test, within-tests, nor interaction. In addition, regarding the PPT measure, no significant difference was observed between-tests, within-tests, nor with interaction according to the MCID of the PPT, which in the literature considered a change of 15% [42]. In addition, the average value found in the present study was around 34 N/cm^2 (3.5 Kgf/cm^2), representing a threshold lower than that reported in the literature [33,43]. According to Fischer (1987) [43], asymptomatic people are expected to report pain or discomfort to PPT test when reaching 55 N/cm^2 (5.6 kgf/cm^2) in men and 37 N/cm^2 (3.8 kgf/cm^2) in women, while Pöntinen (1998) [33] found a pain threshold of 39 N/cm^2 (4.0 kgf/cm^2) in a research with participants with CLBP.

These results probably have suffered interference related to the heterogeneity of the studied population regarding the poor prognosis by SBST, with 56% of the participants classified as low risk, 24.4% medium risk and 19.5% high risk. In addition, four participants of high risk and two of medium risk showed a significant improvement at NPRS in the intervention situation. According to Fritz et al. (2011) [26], there is a relationship between the risk categories and the magnitude of the participants' improvement at the end of the analysis, in which individuals with a higher risk of poor prognosis, presented a greater report of pain attenuation [26].

In terms of the heterogeneity of our sample, some differences related to age and gender must be considered. The reduction in shear strain and increase in thickness of the posterior layer of the TLF in CLBP patients are more significant in the male gender, with a positive correlation between shear strain and low back pain duration [24]. In this sense, range of motion and physical function, body composition, fat distribution pattern, hormonal factors, or structural and/or movement pattern differences between males and females also might need to be considered [24,44]. With aging, biochemical, cellular, and functional changes occur in addition to changes in the structure of the extracellular matrix, and these age-related alterations in fascial tissues lead to densification and fibrosis (thixotropic behavior of hyaluronic acid and collagen synthesis increase thickness) contributing to pain occurrence [17,44].

Concerning functionality outcome, the ODI questionnaire revealed no significant difference between-tests, within-tests, nor with interaction. Lauridsen et al. (2006) [27] evaluated the response capacity of the ODI and MCID of ODI for patients with CLBP and pointed out that a MCID around 12–13 points is clinically important. In addition, in the present study, the interval between applications of the questionnaires was 24 h, which probably influenced the results obtained as it reduced confounding and memory factors, since the objective was to evaluate the effectiveness of the technique. The article on the development of the Brazilian version of the ODI [35] discusses this interference of the retest time in the results and also states that a longer interval improves the chances of reducing the final percentage due to the influence of the natural course of the associated CLBP symptoms.

The time factor calls into question the need to follow-up, because in addition to the natural course of low back pain, it is known that a short-term MT intervention can improve pain and disability but without retention effects after three-months follow-up [1,4]. Nevertheless, habitual loading will result in a high rate of collagen synthesis in a basal state simply as a result of a constant effect of loading from the previous 24–48 h. Magnusson et al. (2010) [45] observed that after cessation of exercise and up to 18–36 h thereafter, there is a negative net balance in collagen levels, whereas the balance is positive for up to 72 h after exercise. However, the connective tissue requires a certain restitution period, since, without sufficient rest, a continuous loss of collagen is likely to occur, which might render the tissue vulnerable. Habitual physical exercises thus results in a higher turnover of collagen, whereas inactivity lowers collagen synthesis and also the turnover [45].

Considering these facts, it is accepted that CLBP has biological, psychological, and social components in several different extensions in addition to the biomechanics involved in its development. It must be considered that each subject has different painful experiences and different outcomes throughout life, where multiple areas of the brain are activated during a pain experience [18,46]. Moreover, these central areas have other primary functions, i.e., movement execution, sensory location, and emotional awareness, which are overloaded in chronic pain, and may explain the emergence of psychosocial problems among other motor and sensory changes that are beyond the scope of this study [46–48].

The multicausality and variety of outcomes presented by chronic pain, in addition to the non-linear interaction arising from the complexity of the interaction of causal factors, may explain the fact that a single session of myofascial mobilization was not enough to modify the threshold and intensity of the pain and functional capacity [49–51]. Additionally, a rehabilitation program focused not only on tissue but also on complementary issues such as exercise, pain education, and behavioral strategies is important [47,49,52–54].

Limitations

The results probably have been influenced by different factors such as the heterogeneity of the studied population regarding the poor prognosis by SBST and the interval between experimental conditions and measurement time points. In addition, other factors, such as the myofascial technique applied compared with other thoracolumbar myofascial approaches, the characteristics of the sample regarding age and gender, or the pain intensity of the sample at baseline (3.7/10), could also have influenced the results. Finally, trunk flexion-extension range of motion and psychological aspects were not evaluated in our work and should be considered.

Another limitation is that there is still no way to quantify the pressure applied by the therapist's hand during manual therapy techniques, making it difficult to reproduce the studied technique. Much of the effects of MT relies on the ability of the physical therapist to sense the changes in the tissue. The biological effects of touch can also change the effectiveness of the treatment, depending on the state of either the physical therapist or the patient. This variability means that interrater reliability is low, and therefore prevents MT from being considered evidence-based [9].

5. Conclusions

This study provides evidence that a single trial of thoracolumbar myofascial release technique was not enough to reduce pain and disability in subjects with CLBP. Further investigations combining other interventions with myofascial mobilization and those with prolonged treatments are required. The mechanisms underlying these responses merit further investigation. We recommend the design of studies that take into account the bio-psychosocial aspects of individuals with CLBP in addition to analyzing the effects of myofascial mobilization at the structural level of the tissue.

Author Contributions: Conceptualization, L.R.P., L.S.V., A.C.R.L. and F.L.M.M.; methodology, A.C.R.L. and L.R.P.; validation, L.R.P., L.S.V., A.C.R.L., C.Q.G. and F.L.M.M.; formal analysis, J.S.C.F.; investigation, L.R.P.; resources, L.R.P., S.d.S.G.B. and P.A.T.; data curation, L.R.P., A.C.R.L. and J.S.C.F.; writing—original draft preparation, L.R.P.; writing—review and editing, L.R.P., A.C.R.L., M.T.S.d.A., D.d.C.d.S.-C., M.X.O., S.F.d.F., R.T., M.B.-F. and V.A.M.; visualization, L.R.P., A.C.R.L., R.T. and F.L.M.M.; supervision, F.L.M.M. and A.C.R.L.; project administration, L.R.P.; funding acquisition, L.R.P. All authors have read and agreed to the published version of the manuscript.

Funding: This research received no external funding.

Institutional Review Board Statement: The study was conducted according to the guidelines of the Declaration of Helsinki, and approved by the Institutional Ethics and Research Committee of Federal University of Jequitinhonha and Mucuri Valleys (protocol code 3.435.537 in 3 July 2019).

Informed Consent Statement: Informed consent was obtained from all subjects involved in the study.

Data Availability Statement: The data presented in this study are available on request from the corresponding author. The data are not publicly available due to the privacy guarantee of the data collected individually.

Acknowledgments: We thank the volunteers, authors, and collaborators. For the loan of equipment and for providing the technique used in the experiment, we thank Leonardo Sette, Cristiano Queiroz, Sílvia Ballesteros, and Patrícia Tavares. Data collections: Federal University of Jequitinhonha and Mucuri Valleys.

Conflicts of Interest: The authors declare no conflict of interest.

References

1. Boff, T.A.; Pasinato, F.; Ben, Â.J.; Bosmans, J.E.; van Tulder, M.; Carregaro, R.L. Effectiveness of Spinal Manipulation and Myofascial Release Compared with Spinal Manipulation Alone on Health-Related Outcomes in Individuals with Non-Specific Low Back Pain: Randomized Controlled Trial. *Physiotherapy* **2020**, *107*, 71–80. [CrossRef] [PubMed]
2. Global Burden of Disease Study 2013 Collaborators. Global, Regional, and National Incidence, Prevalence, and Years Lived with Disability for 301 Acute and Chronic Diseases and Injuries in 188 Countries, 1990–2013: A Systematic Analysis for the Global Burden of Disease Study 2013. *Lancet* **2015**, *386*, 743–800. [CrossRef]
3. Ajimsha, M.S.; Daniel, B.; Chithra, S. Effectiveness of Myofascial Release in the Management of Chronic Low Back Pain in Nursing Professionals. *J. Bodyw. Mov. Ther.* **2014**, *18*, 273–281. [CrossRef]
4. Arguisuelas, M.D.; Lisón, J.F.; Sánchez-Zuriaga, D.; Martínez-Hurtado, I.; Doménech-Fernández, J. Effects of Myofascial Release in Non-Specific Chronic Low Back Pain: A Randomized Clinical Trial. *Spine* **2017**, *42*, 627–634. [CrossRef] [PubMed]
5. Arguisuelas, M.D.; Lisón, J.F.; Coloma, P.S. Clinical Biomechanics Effects of Myofascial Release in Erector Spinae Myoelectric Activity and Lumbar Spine Kinematics in Non-Specific Chronic Low Back Pain: Randomized. *Clin. Biomech.* **2019**, *63*, 27–33. [CrossRef]
6. Casato, G.; Stecco, C.; Busin, R. Role of Fasciae in Nonspecific Low Back Pain. *Eur. J. Transl. Myol.* **2019**, *29*, 159–163. [CrossRef] [PubMed]
7. Mense, S. Innervation of the Thoracolumbar Fascia. *Eur. J. Transl. Myol.* **2019**, *29*, 151–158. [CrossRef]
8. Schilder, A.; Hoheisel, U.; Magerl, W.; Benrath, J.; Klein, T.; Treede, R.D. Sensory Findings after Stimulation of the Thoracolumbar Fascia with Hypertonic Saline Suggest Its Contribution to Low Back Pain. *Pain* **2014**, *155*, 222–231. [CrossRef]
9. Ajimsha, M.S.; Al-Mudahka, N.R.; Al-Madzhar, J.A. Effectiveness of Myofascial Release: Systematic Review of Randomized Controlled Trials. *J. Bodyw. Mov. Ther.* **2015**, *19*, 102–112. [CrossRef]
10. Akhtar, M.W.; Karimi, H.; Gilani, S.A. Effectiveness of Core Stabilization Exercises and Routine Exercise Therapy in Management of Pain in Chronic Nonspecific Low Back Pain: A Randomized Controlled Clinical Trial. *Pak. J. Med. Sci.* **2017**, *33*, 1002–1006. [CrossRef]
11. Searle, A.; Spink, M.; Ho, A.; Chuter, V. Exercise Interventions for the Treatment of Chronic Low Back Pain: A Systematic Review and Meta-Analysis of Randomised Controlled Trials. *Clin. Rehabil.* **2015**, *29*, 1155–1167. [CrossRef] [PubMed]
12. van Middelkoop, M.; Rubinstein, S.M.; Verhagen, A.P.; Ostelo, R.W.; Koes, B.W.; van Tulder, M.W. Exercise Therapy for Chronic Nonspecific Low-Back Pain. *Best Pract. Res. Clin. Rheumatol.* **2010**, *24*, 193–204. [CrossRef] [PubMed]
13. van Middelkoop, M.; Rubinstein, S.M.; Kuijpers, T.; Verhagen, A.P.; Ostelo, R.; Koes, B.W.; van Tulder, M.W. A Systematic Review on the Effectiveness of Physical and Rehabilitation Interventions for Chronic Non-Specific Low Back Pain. *Eur. Spine J.* **2011**, *20*, 19–39. [CrossRef]
14. Wang, X.Q.; Zheng, J.J.; Yu, Z.W.; Bi, X.; Lou, S.J.; Liu, J.; Cai, B.; Hua, Y.H.; Wu, M.; Wei, M.L.; et al. A Meta-Analysis of Core Stability Exercise versus General Exercise for Chronic Low Back Pain. *PLoS ONE* **2012**, *7*, e52082. [CrossRef]
15. Bialosky, J.E.; Bishop, M.D.; Penza, C.W. Placebo Mechanisms of Manual Therapy: A Sheep in Wolf's Clothing? *J. Orthop. Sports Phys. Ther.* **2017**, *47*, 301–304. [CrossRef]

16. McGlone, F.; Wessberg, J.; Olausson, H. Discriminative and Affective Touch: Sensing and Feeling. *Neuron* **2014**, *82*, 737–755. [CrossRef]
17. Wilke, J.; Schleip, R.; Klingler, W.; Stecco, C. The Lumbodorsal Fascia as a Potential Source of Low Back Pain: A Narrative Review. *BioMed Res. Int.* **2017**, *2017*, 5349620. [CrossRef]
18. Bishop, M.D.; Torres-Cueco, R.; Gay, C.W.; Lluch-Girbés, E.; Beneciuk, J.M.; Bialosky, J.E. What Effect Can Manual Therapy Have on a Patient's Pain Experience? *Pain Manag.* **2015**, *5*, 455–464. [CrossRef]
19. De Coninck, K.; Hambly, K.; Dickinson, J.W.; Passfield, L. Measuring the Morphological Characteristics of Thoracolumbar Fascia in Ultrasound Images: An Inter-Rater Reliability Study. *BMC Musculoskelet. Disord.* **2018**, *19*, 180. [CrossRef]
20. Krause, F.; Wilke, J.; Vogt, L.; Banzer, W. Intermuscular Force Transmission along Myofascial Chains: A Systematic Review. *J. Anat.* **2016**, *228*, 910–918. [CrossRef] [PubMed]
21. Wilke, J.; Krause, F.; Vogt, L.; Banzer, W. What Is Evidence-Based about Myofascial Chains: A Systematic Review. *Arch. Phys. Med. Rehabil.* **2016**, *97*, 454–461. [CrossRef]
22. Wilke, J.; Niederer, D.; Vogt, L.; Banzer, W. Remote Effects of Lower Limb Stretching: Preliminary Evidence for Myofascial Connectivity? *J. Sports Sci.* **2016**, *34*, 2145–2148. [CrossRef]
23. Bordoni, B.; Marelli, F.; Morabito, B.; Sacconi, B. The Indeterminable Resilience of the Fascial System. *J. Integr. Med.* **2017**, *15*, 337–343. [CrossRef]
24. Langevin, H.M.; Fox, J.R.; Koptiuch, C.; Badger, G.J.; Greenan-Naumann, A.C.; Bouffard, N.A.; Konofagou, E.E.; Lee, W.N.; Triano, J.J.; Henry, S.M. Reduced Thoracolumbar Fascia Shear Strain in Human Chronic Low Back Pain. *BMC Musculoskelet. Disord.* **2011**, *12*, 203. [CrossRef] [PubMed]
25. Findley, T.; Chaudhry, H.; Stecco, A.; Roman, M. Fascia Research—A Narrative Review. *J. Bodyw. Mov. Ther.* **2012**, *16*, 67–75. [CrossRef] [PubMed]
26. Fritz, J.M.; Beneciuk, J.M.; George, S.Z. Relationship between Categorization with the STarT Back Screening Tool and Prognosis for People Receiving Physical Therapy for Low Back Pain. *Phys. Ther.* **2011**, *91*, 722–732. [CrossRef] [PubMed]
27. Lauridsen, H.H.; Hartvigsen, J.; Manniche, C.; Korsholm, L.; Grunnet-Nilsson, N. Responsiveness and Minimal Clinically Important Difference for Pain and Disability Instruments in Low Back Pain Patients. *BMC Musculoskelet. Disord.* **2006**, *7*, 82. [CrossRef]
28. WHO. *WHO Guidelines on Physical Activity and Sedentary Behaviour*; WHO: Geneva, Switzerland, 2020.
29. Department of Health and Human Services. *Executive Summary Physical Activity Guidelines for Americans*, 2nd ed.; U.S. Department of Health and Human Services: Washington, DC, USA, 2019; pp. 1–7.
30. Bhadauria, E.A.; Gurudut, P. Comparative Effectiveness of Lumbar Stabilization, Dynamic Strengthening, and Pilates on Chronic Low Back Pain: Randomized Clinical Trial. *J. Exerc. Rehabil.* **2017**, *13*, 477–485. [CrossRef] [PubMed]
31. Childs, J.D.; Piva, S.R.; Fritz, J.M. Responsiveness of the Numeric Pain Rating Scale in Patients with Low Back Pain. *Spine* **2005**, *30*, 1331–1334. [CrossRef]
32. Antonaci, F.; Sand, T.; Lucas, G.A. Pressure Algometry in Healthy Subjects: Inter-Examiner Variability. *Scand. J. Rehabil. Med.* **1998**, *30*, 3–8. [CrossRef] [PubMed]
33. Pöntinen, P.J. Reliability, Validity, Reproducibility of Algometry in Diagnosis of Active and Latent Tender Spots and Trigger Points. *J. Musculoskelet. Pain* **1998**, *6*, 61–71. [CrossRef]
34. Frank, L.; McLaughlin, P.; Vaughan, B. The Repeatability of Pressure Algometry in Asymptomatic Individuals over Consecutive Days. *Int. J. Osteopath. Med.* **2013**, *16*, 143–152. [CrossRef]
35. Vigatto, R.; Alexandre, N.M.C.; Filho, H.R.C. Development of a Brazilian Portuguese Version of the Oswestry Disability Index. *Spine* **2007**, *32*, 481–486. [CrossRef] [PubMed]
36. Johnsen, L.G.; Hellum, C.; Nygaard, Ø.P.; Storheim, K.; Brox, J.I.; Rossvoll, I.; Leivseth, G.; Grotle, M. Comparison of the SF6D, the EQ5D, and the Oswestry Disability Index in Patients with Chronic Low Back Pain and Degenerative Disc Disease. *BMC Musculoskelet. Disord.* **2013**, *14*, 148. [CrossRef]
37. Saltychev, M.; Mattie, R.; McCormick, Z.; Bärlund, E.; Laimi, K. Psychometric Properties of the Oswestry Disability Index. *Int. J. Rehabil. Res.* **2017**, *40*, 202–208. [CrossRef]
38. Chaitow, L. What's in a Name: Myofascial Release or Myofascial Induction? *J. Bodyw. Mov. Ther.* **2017**, *21*, 749–751. [CrossRef] [PubMed]
39. Martínez-Jiménez, E.M.; Becerro-de-Bengoa-Vallejo, R.; Losa-Iglesias, M.E.; Rodríguez-Sanz, D.; Díaz-Velázquez, J.I.; Casado-Hernández, I.; Mazoteras-Pardo, V.; López-López, D. Acute Effects of Myofascial Induction Technique in Plantar Fascia Complex in Patients with Myofascial Pain Syndrome on Postural Sway and Plantar Pressures: A Quasi-Experimental Study. *Phys. Ther. Sport* **2020**, *43*, 70–76. [CrossRef] [PubMed]
40. Farrar, J.T.; Young, J.P.; LaMoreaux, L.; Werth, J.L.; Poole, R.M. Clinical Importance of Changes in Chronic Pain Intensity Measured on an 11-Point Numerical Pain Rating Scale. *Pain* **2001**, *94*, 149–158. [CrossRef]
41. Kovacs, F.M.; Abraira, V.; Royuela, A.; Corcoll, J.; Alegre, L.; Cano, A.; Muriel, A.; Zamora, J.; Gil Del Real, M.T.; Gestoso, M.; et al. Minimal Clinically Important Change for Pain Intensity and Disability in Patients with Nonspecific Low Back Pain. *Spine* **2007**, *32*, 2915–2920. [CrossRef] [PubMed]
42. Voogt, L.; de Vries, J.; Meeus, M.; Struyf, F.; Meuffels, D.; Nijs, J. Analgesic Effects of Manual Therapy in Patients with Musculoskeletal Pain: A Systematic Review. *Man. Ther.* **2015**, *20*, 250–256. [CrossRef] [PubMed]

43. Fischer, A.A. Pressure Algometry over Normal Muscles. Standard Values, Validity and Reproducibility of Pressure Threshold. *Pain* **1987**, *30*, 115–126. [CrossRef]
44. Zügel, M.; Maganaris, C.N.; Wilke, J.; Jurkat-Rott, K.; Klingler, W.; Wearing, S.C.; Findley, T.; Barbe, M.F.; Steinacker, J.M.; Vleeming, A.; et al. Fascial Tissue Research in Sports Medicine: From Molecules to Tissue Adaptation, Injury and Diagnostics: Consensus Statement. *Br. J. Sports Med.* **2018**, *52*, 1497. [CrossRef]
45. Magnusson, S.P.; Langberg, H.; Kjaer, M. The Pathogenesis of Tendinopathy: Balancing the Response to Loading. *Nat. Rev. Rheumatol.* **2010**, *6*, 262–268. [CrossRef]
46. Mertens, P.; Blond, S.; David, R.; Rigoard, P. Anatomy, Physiology and Neurobiology of the Nociception: A Focus on Low Back Pain (Part A). *Neurochirurgie* **2015**, *61*, S22–S34. [CrossRef]
47. Puentedura, E.J.; Flynn, T. Combining Manual Therapy with Pain Neuroscience Education in the Treatment of Chronic Low Back Pain: A Narrative Review of the Literature. *Physiother. Theory Pract.* **2016**, *32*, 408–414. [CrossRef] [PubMed]
48. Wallwork, S.B.; Bellan, V.; Catley, M.J.; Moseley, G.L. Neural Representations and the Cortical Body Matrix: Implications for Sports Medicine and Future Directions. *Br. J. Sports Med.* **2016**, *50*, 990–996. [CrossRef]
49. Cholewicki, J.; Breen, A.; Popovich, J.M.; Peter Reeves, N.; Sahrmann, S.A.; Van Dillen, L.R.; Vleeming, A.; Hodges, P.W. Can Biomechanics Research Lead to More Effective Treatment of Low Back Pain? A Point-Counterpoint Debate. *J. Orthop. Sports Phys. Ther.* **2019**, *49*, 425–436. [CrossRef] [PubMed]
50. Bittencourt, N.F.N.; Meeuwisse, W.H.; Mendonça, L.D.; Nettel-Aguirre, A.; Ocarino, J.M.; Fonseca, S.T. Complex Systems Approach for Sports Injuries: Moving from Risk Factor Identification to Injury Pattern Recognition—Narrative Review and New Concept. *Br. J. Sports Med.* **2016**, *50*, 1309–1314. [CrossRef]
51. Huysmans, E.; Ickmans, K.; Van Dyck, D.; Nijs, J.; Gidron, Y.; Roussel, N.; Polli, A.; Moens, M.; Goudman, L.; De Kooning, M. Association Between Symptoms of Central Sensitization and Cognitive Behavioral Factors in People With Chronic Nonspecific Low Back Pain: A Cross-Sectional Study. *J. Manip. Physiol. Ther.* **2018**, *41*, 92–101. [CrossRef] [PubMed]
52. Wiech, K.; Ploner, M.; Tracey, I. Neurocognitive Aspects of Pain Perception. *Trends Cogn. Sci.* **2008**, *12*, 306–313. [CrossRef]
53. Louw, A.; Puentedura, E.J.; Diener, I.; Zimney, K.J.; Cox, T. Pain Neuroscience Education: Which Pain Neuroscience Education Metaphor Worked Best? *South. African J. Physiother.* **2019**, *75*, 1329. [CrossRef] [PubMed]
54. Wood, L.; Hendrick, P.A. A Systematic Review and Meta-Analysis of Pain Neuroscience Education for Chronic Low Back Pain: Short-and Long-Term Outcomes of Pain and Disability. *Eur. J. Pain* **2019**, *23*, 234–249. [CrossRef] [PubMed]

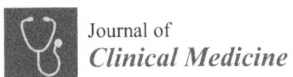

Article

Local Vibration Reduces Muscle Damage after Prolonged Exercise in Men

Anna Piotrowska [1], Wanda Pilch [1], Łukasz Tota [2], Marcin Maciejczyk [2,*], Dariusz Mucha [3], Monika Bigosińska [4], Przemysław Bujas [5], Szczepan Wiecha [6], Ewa Sadowska-Krępa [7] and Tomasz Pałka [2]

1. Institute of Basics Sciences, Faculty of Physiotherapy, University of Physical Education, 31-571 Kraków, Poland; anna.piotrowska@awf.krakow.pl (A.P.); wanda.pilch@awf.krakow.pl (W.P.)
2. Department of Physiology and Biochemistry, Faculty of Physical Education and Sport, University of Physical Education, 31-571 Kraków, Poland; lukasz.tota@awf.krakow.pl (Ł.T.); tomasz.palka@awf.krakow.pl (T.P.)
3. Institute of Biomedical Sciences, Faculty of Physical Education and Sport, University of Physical Education, 31-571 Kraków, Poland; dariusz.mucha@awf.krakow.pl
4. Department of Physical Education, Institute of Physical Culture, State University of Applied Sciences, 33-300 Nowy Sącz, Poland; mbigosin@poczta.onet.pl
5. Institute of Sports, University of Physical Education, 31-571 Kraków, Poland; przemyslaw.bujas@awf.krakow.pl
6. Department of Physical Education and Health, Faculty in Biala Podlaska, Jozef Pilsudski University of Physical Education in Warsaw, 21-500 Biala Podlaska, Poland; szczepan.wiecha@awf-bp.edu.pl
7. Institute of Sport Sciences, The Jerzy Kukuczka Academy of Physical Education, 40-065 Katowice, Poland; e.sadowska-krepa@awf.katowice.pl
* Correspondence: marcin.maciejczyk@awf.krakow.pl

Abstract: Prolonged exercise can lead to muscle damage, with soreness, swelling, and ultimately reduced strength as a consequence. It has been shown that whole-body vibration (WBV) improves recovery by reducing the levels of stress hormones and the activities of creatine kinase (CK) and lactate dehydrogenase (LDH). The aim of the study was to demonstrate the effect of local vibration treatment applied after exercise on the level of selected markers of muscle fiber damage. The study involved 12 untrained men, aged 21.7 ± 1.05 years, with a VO$_2$peak of 46.12 ± 3.67 mL·kg^{-1}·min^{-1}. A maximal intensity test to volitional exhaustion was performed to determine VO$_2$peak and individual exercise loads for prolonged exercise. The subjects were to perform 180 min of physical effort with an intensity of 50 ± 2% VO$_2$peak. After exercise, they underwent a 60 min vibration treatment or placebo therapy using a mattress. Blood samples were taken before, immediately after the recovery procedure, and 24 h after the end of the exercise test. Myoglobin (Mb) levels as well as the activities of CK and LDH were recorded. Immediately after the hour-long recovery procedure (vibration or placebo), the mean concentrations of the determined indices were significantly different from baseline values. In the vibration group, significantly lower values of Mb ($p = 0.005$), CK ($p = 0.030$), and LDH ($p = 0.005$) were seen. Differences were also present 24 h after the end of the exercise test. The results of the vibration group compared to the control group differed in respect to Mb ($p = 0.002$), CK ($p = 0.029$), and LDH ($p = 0.014$). After prolonged physical effort, topical vibration improved post-workout recovery manifested by lower CK and LDH activity and lower Mb concentration compared to a control group.

Keywords: DOMS; vibration; post-exercise muscle damage; physical exercise; recovery

Citation: Piotrowska, A.; Pilch, W.; Tota, Ł.; Maciejczyk, M.; Mucha, D.; Bigosińska, M.; Bujas, P.; Wiecha, S.; Sadowska-Krępa, E.; Pałka, T. Local Vibration Reduces Muscle Damage after Prolonged Exercise in Men. *J. Clin. Med.* **2021**, *10*, 5461. https://doi.org/10.3390/jcm10225461

Academic Editors: Redha Taiar, Mario Bernardo-Filho and Ana Cristina Rodrigues Lacerda

Received: 19 October 2021
Accepted: 18 November 2021
Published: 22 November 2021

Publisher's Note: MDPI stays neutral with regard to jurisdictional claims in published maps and institutional affiliations.

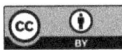

Copyright: © 2021 by the authors. Licensee MDPI, Basel, Switzerland. This article is an open access article distributed under the terms and conditions of the Creative Commons Attribution (CC BY) license (https://creativecommons.org/licenses/by/4.0/).

1. Introduction

Prolonged strenuous exercise can lead to muscle cell damage, with soreness, swelling, and ultimately a decrease in strength as a consequence, especially when the athlete is not used to this type of physical work or performs it after a long absence [1]. The damages take place on the ultrastructure of muscle cells. It has been reported that eccentric contractions [2] and forms of exercise unfamiliar to the body most often contribute to its damage. Clinical symptoms include decreased strength, painful restricted range of movement, stiffness, swelling, and dysfunction of adjacent joints, one of the most common causes of decreased performance in professional athletes. The development of clinical symptoms is usually delayed, occurring between 8 to 20 h after exercise and, as a result of the complex sequences of local and systemic physiological responses, may persist for 24 to 48 h after the injury has occurred [1,3]. This comprehensive picture of subjective and objective symptoms is defined as Delayed Onset Muscle Soreness (DOMS). Among the physiological and biochemical changes, the development of an inflammatory state is followed by an increase in the activity of cellular enzymes and inflammatory metabolites in the blood, a loss of muscle strength, and a decline in endurance [1,4].

Currently, there is growing interest in new methods of biological regeneration, aimed to accelerate the pace of recovery and reduce post-exercise skeletal muscle damage [5]. Scientific reports have mostly evaluated the use of systemic cryotherapy [6] and massage [7]. However, there are also studies evaluating various forms of vibration. Different protocols have incorporated the use of vibration either before, during breaks between efforts, or after the physical performance. Preliminary meta-analyses have shown promising results while also emphasizing the need for further research on this topic [8].

Vibration as a stimulus that positively affects health has been known for a long time, but the exact mechanism and effectiveness are yet to be understood [9]. The largest scientific study used cold whole-body vibration (WBV). The stimulus was applied in a standing position through the feet. WBV has been demonstrated to improve muscle perfusion and improve lymph flow. It significantly affects the supply of oxygen and other components important for the working muscle [10–12]. Recently, WBV has also been evaluated as a post-exercise recovery treatment to reduce muscle pain and loss of muscle strength after exercise [13,14]. Apart from subjective indicators, a decrease in stress hormones [15] and creatine kinase (CK) activity [16] has been observed. Vibration as a mechanical stimulus used in the form of WBV is absorbed mainly by the skeletal system.

The local application of vibration in wellness has been evaluated in a few studies. In addition to WBV, its local use is another form of stimulus propagation that causes smaller changes in the skeletal system. However, the reaction of the soft tissues to this stimulus is strong, as shown in biochemical studies [17] and thermal imaging [18]. Locally applied vibration contributes to the development of neuromuscular adaptations after both single and multiple uses [19]. Vibration applied locally will be absorbed by the soft tissues and will have the greatest impact on them. Therefore, we expect the effect to be equally effective despite the use of a gentler local vibration stimulus.

Changes in the levels of biochemical indicators can assess the degree of damage a muscle cell endures after prolonged physical exertion. Therefore, a research question was posed: will the use of local vibration affect specific indices present immediately after physical exercise and increase the rate of post-exercise recovery by reducing the concentration of post-exercise biochemical indices of muscle cell damage? Our hypothesis assumed that vibration treatment, thanks to increased vascular flow and improved tissue drainage, would reduce the blood markers of muscle damage.

2. Materials and Methods

2.1. Ethics Declaration

The research was carried out in the Laboratory of Vibrotherapy and the Laboratory of Physiological Basis of Adaptation, Central Scientific and Research Laboratory, University of Physical Education in Krakow during September–October 2019. The respondents gave written consent to participate in the research, were explained the purpose and method of the research, and were informed about the possibility of resignation at any stage without giving a reason. The project was approved by the Bioethical Committee of PMWSZ in Opole (No. KB/56/N02/2019) in accordance with the Declaration of Helsinki. The proposed intervention in the form of vibrotherapy met the guidelines for reporting research using whole-body vibration as a treatment regimen in humans [20,21].

2.2. Study Protocol

The protocol included two series of studies: a preliminary one and a main one (Figure 1). In the preliminary study, a basic interview and basic medical examination were performed, and body composition was estimated with the use of an analyzer. At this stage, a graded test until volitional exhaustion was performed during which selected physiological indicators were measured. The obtained values of the graded tests made it possible to estimate the individual exercise load at a level of $50 \pm 2\%$ VO$_2$peak necessary for the implementation of the pivotal test.

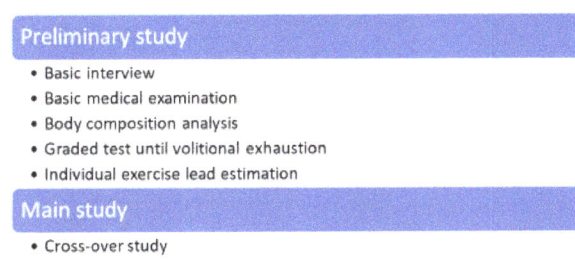
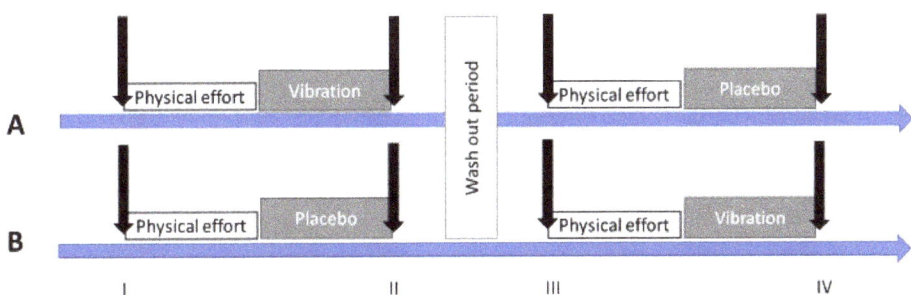

Figure 1. Study protocol with preliminary and main study details. (**A**,**B**) are the names of the groups taking part in the cross-over study. Black arrows represent the instants of time that blood samples were taken. Intervention type: vibration or placebo. I—first blood sampling (before physical effort); II—second blood sampling (1 h after physical effort); III—third blood sampling (before second physical effort); IV—fourth blood sampling (1 h after second physical effort).

Our study included 12 untrained but physically active male students from the University of Physical Education in Krakow who met the inclusion criteria, and in the medical examination, there were no contraindications to the use of vibrotherapy (Table 1).

Table 1. Inclusion and exclusion criteria.

Inclusion Criteria	Exclusion Criteria
- Male gender - Age 19–23 years - BMI within the range of valid values - No additional physical activity, apart from the physical activity covered by the study program - No previous athletic experience	Contraindications to participation in vibrotherapy treatments [22]: • Occurring in the past: tumors, cardiovascular diseases, thrombosis, surgical interventions involving the musculoskeletal system, acute back pain, advanced diabetes; • Currently present: pacemaker, acute inflammation, recovery period after endoprosthesis of the hip or knee joint, infectious diseases; • Occurring during or after the treatment: headache or dizziness, nausea.

In the main study (experimental intermittent study), men were randomly divided into two 6-person groups: A and B. All examined men performed a physical effort with individual estimated load. After exercise, the participants were subjected to vibration treatments or a placebo treatment. In the first part, group A received vibrotherapy treatments after exercise while group B served as the control group by resting on placebo mattresses after exercise. After two weeks, the protocols were changed and the participants from group A received treatment on placebo mattresses, while group B received vibration treatments. Blood was collected before (0), immediately after the renewal procedure (I), and 24 h (II) after the end of the exercise test (Figure 1).

2.3. Study Group

The participants' baseline characteristics (mean ± SD) were an age of 21.7 ± 1.05 years, a body height (BH) of 179.3 ± 4.3 cm, a body mass (BM) of 76.01 ± 3.4 kg, a percentage of body fat (BFP) of $13.72 \pm 2.7\%$, a lean body mass (LBM) of 65.56 ± 2.97 kg, a Body Mass Index (BMI) of 23.64 ± 0.54, and a VO$_2$peak of 46.12 ± 3.67 mL·kg^{-1}·min^{-1}. The values of the physiological indices monitored during the exercise test until exhaustion are presented in Table 2. During the entire research project, the subjects were advised not to change their current diet and refrain from consuming alcohol and taking up additional forms of physical activity.

Table 2. Maximal values of variables measured in graded test.

Variable	Mean	SD	Min	Max
WLmax [W]	273.6	33.2	230	330
VO$_2$peak [L·min^{-1}]	3.28	0.63	2.27	4.22
VO$_2$peak [mL·kg^{-1}·min^{-1}]	43.2	7.8	31.5	58.5
HRmax [bpm]	185.36	8.19	167	195
VEmax [L·min^{-1}]	131.5	36.3	75.4	174.9
FRmax [breaths·min^{-1}]	53.4	9.6	36	67
TVmax [L]	2.60	0.52	1.86	3.49

WLmax—maximal workload; VO$_2$peak—peak oxygen uptake; HRmax—maximal heart rate; VEmax—maximal ventilation; FRmax—maximal breathing frequency; TVmax—maximal tidal volume.

2.4. Data Collection

The body compositions (BH, BM, BMI, BFP, LBM) were estimated with the use of an analyzer (JAWON MEDICAL IOI-353-CE0197-Korea certificate). A graded test until volitional exhaustion [23] was performed on a cycloergometer during which maximal heart rate (HRmax), peak oxygen consumption (VO$_2$peak), maximal pulmonary ventilation (VEmax), maximal breathing frequency (FRmax), maximal tidal volume (TVmax) and the amount of total work performed (TW) were measured. During the test, the levels of cardiopulmonary indices were recorded based on the "breath-by-breath" method using an ergospirometer. Data were averaged every 30 s. The highest registered value of oxygen uptake was considered as peak oxygen uptake. The obtained maximum values of the graded tests made it possible to estimate the individual exercise load at a level of $50 \pm 2\%$ VO$_2$peak necessary for the implementation of the pivotal test.

The following measuring devices were used: cycloergometer (ER 900D, Jaeger, Hoechberg, Germany), ergospirometer (MetaLyzer, Cortex, Leipzig, Germany), and cardiomonitor (RS 400, Polar Elektro, Kempele, Finland). The ergospirometer was calibrated in accordance with the manufacturer's recommendations (gas and volume calibration). All physiological tests at this stage were carried out in the morning in the air-conditioned Laboratory of Physiological Basis of Adaptation of the University of Physical Education in Krakow (PN-EN ISO 9001: 2015).

2.5. Biochemical Analysis

Blood was collected from the antecubital vein in a volume of 15 mL in accordance with the applicable standards of the laboratory diagnostician before (0), immediately after the renewal procedure (I), and 24 h (II) after the end of the exercise test.

Myoglobin (Mb), CK, and LDH determinations were performed using the enzyme immunoassay technique—ELISA, using the E-LizaMat3000 apparatus (DRG Instruments Gmbh, Marburg, Germany) with use of kits: Mb: EIA-3955 (DRG GmbH, Marburg, Germany), sensitivity (the lowest detectable level: 5 ng/mL); CK: EIA-4361 (DRG GmbH, Marburg, Germany), sensitivity (the lowest detectable level: 0.5 ng/mL); LDH: MAK066 (Sigma-Aldrich Co., St. Louis, MO, USA). To determine changes in plasma volumes of the blood samples, the following was determined: hemoglobin concentrations using the Drabkin method and hematocrit levels using the micro-hematocrit method. Changes in plasma volume (%ΔPV) were calculated using the formula of Dill and Costila [24] modified by Harisson et al. [25] The concentrations of biochemical markers in the blood samples collected after exercise were corrected for %ΔPV.

2.6. Intervention

All examined men performed 180 min of physical effort on cycloergometer at a relative intensity of $50 \pm 2\%$ VO$_2$peak. A 10 min warm-up using the same intensity was performed prior to beginning the test. Immediately after exercise, the body was dried and BM was re-measured followed by a four-minute shower (water temperature: 21 ± 2 °C).

The participants in the vibration group then underwent a 60 min lower body vibration massage in a reclining position using a RAM Vitberg+ Massage Device (Vitberg, Nowy Sącz, Poland) (Figure 2. The duration of the treatment was determined according to the manufacturer's information and consisted of two 30 min cycles. The therapeutic stimulus generated by the device was cycloidal vibrations directed in three perpendicular directions, with a small amplitude, a low to medium frequency, and a variable sequence of impulses (f = 20–52 Hz, A = 0.1–0.5 mm, a = 6.9–13.5 m/s^2). During the 60 min treatment, the vibrations were interrupted at different values of frequency, amplitude, and acceleration (Figure 3). The device has a TUV Rheinland certificate (No. 0197) and a quality certificate for class IIa medical devices (No. HD60118119001).

Placebo treatments were carried out on specially designed Vitberg+ placebo devices, which in terms of shape, appearance, and equipment were identical to the active ones. They generated the same sound signals during individual phases of the placebo treatment but did not produce the vibrations tested in the experimental group.

2.7. Statistical Analysis

The test results for groups A and B using the vibrating devices and placebo devices were blinded, and the following groups were identified as vibrated (V) and placebo (C). All results were presented as arithmetic means with standard deviations. In order to assess the significance of differences between groups, and time changes, analysis of variance (ANOVA) with repeated measurements was used. Afterwards, post hoc analysis was carried out using Tukey's test. Data distribution was checked using the Shapiro–Wilk test. Homogeneity of variance within the groups was tested via Levene's test (variance of the analyzed parameters was similar in both groups). The effect size (partial eta squared (η^2)) was calculated and interpreted as small (0.01), medium (0.06), or large (0.14) [26]. Additionally, in post hoc analysis, the effect size (d-Cohen) between groups was calculated and interpreted as small (0.20), medium (0.50), or large (0.80) [26]. Observed statistical power (post hoc power) is also reported. Statistically significant results were defined as a p-value of <0.05. The following software was used to perform the calculations: STATISTICA 13.1 (StatSoft, Tulsa, OK, USA).

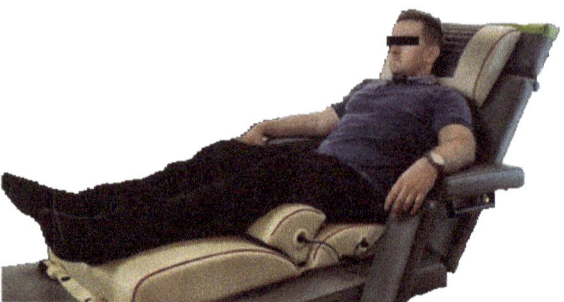

Figure 2. The position of the body on the device generating the vibration stimulus (illustrative photo).

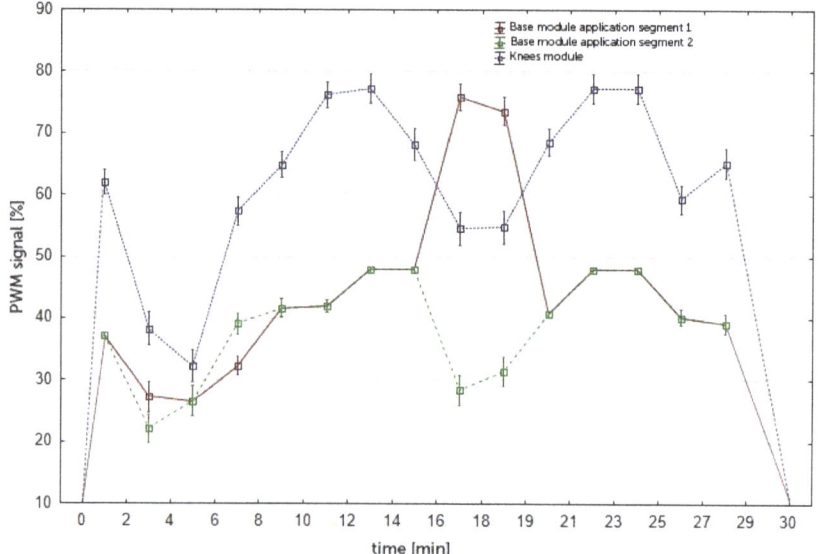

Figure 3. Voltage-current characteristics of the Knees program with the Knees S module (PWM: Pulse Width Modulation).

3. Results

In the study, significant time changes were noted for LDH (f = 156.7, $p < 0.001$, $\eta^2 = 0.87$, observed power: 1.0), CK (f = 3427.7, $p < 0.001$, $\eta^2 = 0.99$, observed power: 1.0), and Mb (f = 20.46, $p < 0.001$, $\eta^2 = 0.48$, observed power: 0.99). The studied groups differ with regard to the examined indices (LDH: f = 4.5, $p = 0.04$, $\eta^2 = 0.17$, observed power: 0.47; CK: f = 4.56, $p = 0.049$, $\eta^2 = 0.17$, observed power: 0.47; Mb: f = 4.61, $p = 0.04$, $\eta^2 = 0.18$, observed power: 0.26). Moreover, there were significant interactions between the analyzed factors (group × time): (LDH: f = 15.02, $p < 0.001$, $\eta^2 = 0.41$, observed power: 0.99; CK: f = 8.06, $p = 0.001$, $\eta^2 = 0.27$, observed power: 0.94; Mb: f = 4.56, $p = 0.04$, $\eta^2 = 0.25$, observed power 0.48).

Post-hoc analysis indicated that the concentrations of Mb and activities of CK and LDH in the C and V groups taken before exercise (0) did not differ significantly. Immediately after an hour-long recovery procedure (vibration or placebo) (I), the mean concentrations of the indices increased significantly in relation to the baseline in both groups. All values differed between C and V groups. Similar differences were seen in the results obtained 24 h after the end of the exercise test (II). Thus, the average values of Mb concentrations and activities of CK and LDH in the V group were significantly lower than in the C group. After 24 h from the end of the exercise test, a significant decrease in Mb concentrations and

LDH activity was observed in group V while the CK activity was still increasing but was significantly lower than in the control group. Twenty-four hours after the exercise, the Mb concentration in the vibration group was similar to baseline measurement (Table 3).

Table 3. The concentration of myoglobin (Mb), activity of creatine kinase (CK), and lactate dehydrogenase (LDH) before (0), immediately after the renewal procedure (I), and 24 h (II) after the end of the exercise test in the group subjected to post-exercise therapy (V) and in the control group (C).

Variable	Group/p-Value	0	I	II
Mb (μg/L)	C	14.84 ± 4.21	32.32 ± 19.21 **	21.67 ± 8.48 **
	V	15.22 ± 4.31	23.82 ± 14.88 **	14.28 ± 5.51
	p (d)	0.506	0.005 * (0.44)	0.002 * (1.06)
CK (IU/L)	C	213.53 ± 34.49	306.04 ± 37.28 **	611.11 ± 55.27 **
	V	205.06 ± 25.52	270.89 ± 37.17 **	564.95 ± 41.08 **
	p (d)	0.501	0.030 * (0.94)	0.029 * (0.96)
LDH (IU/L)	C	172.23 ± 14.31	214.94 ± 13.92 **	210.48 ± 14.82 **
	V	174.64 ± 13.09	197.66 ± 13.80 **	194.14 ± 14.02
	p (d)	0.691	0.005 * (1.25)	0.014 * (1.13)

* significant differences ($p < 0.05$) between groups: C and V (post hoc); ** significant group difference to baseline (post hoc); d—effect size (d-Cohen).

The effectiveness of the vibration treatments in accelerating recovery after prolonged physical exercise was assessed by analyzing the dynamic changes in concentrations of biochemical indicators (Δ) recorded immediately after the renewal procedure (I) and after 24 h of restitution (II). The average value of the increases/decreases of the analyzed variables (ΔMb, ΔLDH, and ΔCK) in men subjected to vibrations differed significantly compared to the control group (Table 4).

Table 4. Differences in the concentration of myoglobin (Mb), activity of creatine kinase (CK), and lactate dehydrogenase (LDH) in the blood 1 h and 24 h after exercise in the group subjected to post-exercise therapy (V) and in the control group (C).

Variable	Group	ΔI—0	ΔII—0	ΔII—I
ΔMb	C	17.48 ± 15.61	6.83 ± 5.51 **	−10.65 ± 11.16 **
	V	8.59 ± 11.71	−0.94 ± 2.73 **	−9.53 ± 10.71 **
	p	0.003 *	0.000 *	0.729
ΔCK	C	92.51 ± 18.34	397.57 ± 21.33 **	305.06 ± 21.33 **
	V	65.80 ± 19.76	356.89 ± 24.61 **	294.09 ± 23.67 **
	p	0.002 *	0.003 *	0.245
ΔLDH	C	42.70 ± 12.00	38.24 ± 12.87 **	−4.46 ± 2.90 **
	V	23.01 ± 8.85	19.50 ± 11.76 **	−3.51 ± 7.51 **
	p	0.000 *	0.001 *	0.707

* significant differences ($p < 0.05$) between groups: C and V; ** significant group differences at three time points.

4. Discussion

In our study, we indicated that the use of vibration treatments after prolonged exercise may reduce the increase in indicators of post-exercise muscle damage. The observed lower concentrations and activities of markers reflecting the degree of muscle fiber damage after exercise in subjects receiving vibrotherapy compared to placebo procedures constitutes important evidence of the effectiveness of post-exercise vibration treatments in recovery after prolonged exercise. In our opinion, this effect may translate into a reduction in DOMS symptoms.

The cycloidal vibrations with variable parameters of intensity, amplitude, and frequency (Figure 2) produced significant reductions in CK and LDH activities and Mb concentrations compared to the control group. The comparison of results obtained in the control group made it possible to identify differences in the values of the tested parameters.

The selected time points (after 1 h of recovery and after 24 h from the end of exercise) illustrated that the selected physical effort caused an increase in the examined parameters (I). After 24 h, Mb and LDH had already decreased in both groups. For CK, the time of 24 h was too short, and the activity of this enzyme continued to increase. Such changes are characteristic of strain injuries, as previously observed [27,28]. However, the proposed protocol using vibratory therapy allowed the capturing of significant differences.

As indicated in the introduction, the effectiveness of vibration in sports has not been fully established. The available data indicate that vibration therapy can be used preventively as well as therapeutically after physical effort [29]. Vibrations increase neuromuscular activity by modulating proprioceptive function and increase muscle strength [8,29]. Vibrotherapy has effects on hormone levels and lymphatic drainage, leading to a reduction in pain and improvement in mood [30]. The mechanism for pain relief, one of the primary symptoms of DOMS, involves the activation of large diameter fibers while suppressing the transfer activity of small diameter fibers [31,32]. The mechanism of action in relieving other symptoms of DOMS can be drawn from the work published by Weerakkody et al. [33] The authors concluded that vibration results in the stimulation of large diameter afferent nerve fibers within a muscle which block the neurological "gate" in the spinal cord, preventing the symptoms of DOMS from being transmitted to the brain. In addition, they carried out tests at various frequencies which allowed for the selection of the optimal parameter (80 Hz).

In additional studies, the role of vibratory stimuli in reducing the symptoms of DOMS has been expanded upon. Koeda et al. [34] demonstrated the effectiveness of vibrations applied to the elbow flexor muscles. In addition to the beneficial but subjective effects observed by the authors of this work, vibration resulted in an increase in range of motion and blood flow. The latter effect is illustrated by an increase in skin temperature after applying a vibratory stimulus [18]. However, this relationship is not so obvious. In the study of Moreira-Marconi et al. [35], when using a 60 s exposure to WBV, the skin temperature of the posterior lower limbs decreased. The authors associated this finding with a redistribution of blood to working muscles. This is another difference between the action of local vibrations, as in our study, and WBV.

Vibration has been shown to significantly reduce the amount of interleukin-6 released and the influx of morphotic blood components involved in the inflammatory response [36,37]. All these mechanisms allow one to control the severity and extent of inflammation caused by prolonged exercise.

A study concerning the effect of vibrotherapy on muscle soreness and CK activity after eccentric exercise was conducted by Bakhitiary et al. [38]. The main difference between the protocols used by Bakhitiary et al. and us was in the timing of when the vibration was applied. In our work, it was used post-workout. Bakhitiary et al. randomized 50 untrained volunteers into two equal groups: one received vibrotherapy and one received no therapy. Vibratory stimuli (50 Hz) were applied locally to the left and right quadriceps, thigh, and calf muscles for 1 min. Then, both groups performed physical exercise with a predominance of eccentric contractions on the treadmill at a speed of 4 km/h. After 24 h, serum CK activity and the level of subjective pain directly related to the DOMS were measured. The results showed a significantly increased mean value of DOMS symptoms and CK activity in the non-vibration group as compared to the vibrated group. The authors of the study indicated that this proves that vibration applied before exercise can prevent and control DOMS. Similarly, in the paper by Imtiyaz et al. [39], the authors tried to determine how vibration and massage affect not the alleviation of DOMS-related ailments but also its prevention. Two experimental groups received vibration therapy (50 Hz vibration for five minutes) or manual massage (15 min) just before exercise with a predominance of eccentric contractions. The control group did not receive any treatment. The following characteristics were assessed to document changes in the muscle's condition: muscle soreness (pain sensation), range of motion, maximum isometric force (MIF), one-repetition maximum, and the selected biochemical indices, LDH and CK. The results of the study showed that muscle pain was significantly less in the experimental groups (vibration and massage) compared to the control group at 24, 48, and 72 h after exercise. The experimental and control group showed no significant differences in MIF. The use of vibration therapy resulted in significantly lower LDH and CK activities at 48 h after exercise compared to the control group. According to the authors of the cited study, vibration therapy and massage are equally useful in preventing DOMS. In our research, vibration therapy was performed during the rest period after prolonged exercise, in contrast to the therapies being performed before exercise in the above-cited study. Despite this difference, it also observed lower Mb concentrations and lower CK and LDH activity compared to the group without vibration treatment.

Vibration applied after exercise, like in our study, was the subject of individual works [13,36]. In our previous research [36], using cycloidal vibrations with variable parameters of intensity, amplitude, and frequency after intense physical exertion in men produced a significant reduction in the concentration of Mb measured at 1 h and 24 h after exercise compared to the control group. These studies also assessed the level of metalloproteinase-2, an enzyme involved in the remodeling of the extracellular matrix, in which the concentration decreased in the vibrated group after exercise.

Currently, many devices use vibratory stimuli, most often with constant parameters describing the generated vibrations. Their impact on the body is multifaceted. Vasodilation is observed, resulting in improved blood and lymph circulation [11], reduced pain after intense exercise, and lowered levels of biochemical markers indicating damage to muscle cells [8,27]. A systematic review, published in 2019, included 10 studies with a total of 258 participants [8]. The authors of the meta-analysis reported that vibration significantly improved not only the subjective symptoms of DOMS as assessed by the VAS scale at several time points after exercise (24, 48, and 72) but also significantly improved CK levels after 24 and 48 h, but not 72 h. Our study also indicated significantly lower CK levels in the groups subjected to vibrotherapy after 24 h, which is in line with the previously observed results.

The studies cited above have confirmed vibration to reduce muscle soreness after exercise and improve the status of markers indicating the severity of inflammation and ultrastructural muscle damage. However, comparing studies involving vibrotherapy can be difficult due to the different vibratory parameters used in pre-exercise or post-exercise protocols. These parameters have a huge impact on the biological effects of treatments. The influence of vibration using both high and low frequencies on the autonomic functions of the cardiovascular system was investigated by Liu et al. [40]. The impact of vibrations on post-exercise changes in heart rate variability and peripheral arterial tension was assessed. The subjects received vibration treatments (0, 5, and 15 Hz) in random order for 10 min. The study confirmed that low-frequency vibration applied after exercise can reduce peripheral vascular tone and accelerate the recovery of the pre-paroxysmal heart rhythm. This effect was more pronounced at 15 Hz than at 5 Hz. The authors indicated these effects are a result of a decrease in the activity of the sympathetic nerves to the heart. Vibration stimuli lead to the taking over of the heart's activity by the parasympathetic nervous system. These results encourage the use of vibration therapy after exercise, as done in our study, thanks to its ability to amplify the effects of cardiovascular influence and acceleration of post-workout recovery.

This study shows the effect of local vibration applied after prolonged physical exertion in young, healthy men. The analysis of the literature shows the complex relationship between the sex of the study participants and the use of the vibration stimulus. In the study of Shibata et al. [41], the gender differences in subjective response to whole-body vibration (WBV) under standing posture was measured. Males and females rated the discomfort of the test stimuli including fore-and-aft, lateral, and vertical vibration. Subjective scale for discomfort caused by WBV exposure was obtained. The authors concluded that there are gender differences in subjective discomfort, and that females are subjectively more sensitive for fore-and-aft and lateral WBV exposure, especially at higher vibration magnitude. The gender differences were also reported by Sañudo et al. in knee stability in response to WBV [42]. On the other hand, this stimulus may affect men and women differently, but the effect may be directly related to differences in body composition. Investigating whether WBV's effect on force-time characteristics is dependent on time and sex was the aim of Merrigan et al.'s study [43]. Participants performed a static quarter squat with WBV (30 Hz; 2–4 mm) and then performed the isometric mid-thigh pull. In women, the rate of force development (RFD) was moderately affected immediately post-WBV. In men, however, the effect of WBV on RFD existed 15 min after exposure. Men produced more peak force (PF) than women. All RFD bands were greater in men than in women, but relative to fat-free mass, PF, and RFD, there were no differences between women and men. This indicates that the results obtained in this study concern only males, and confirmation of such an effect in females requires additional studies with female participants.

5. Limitation of the Study

The use of the cross-over model allowed for obtaining interesting results, but still, the basic limitation of the project is the small number of respondents. Despite the small sample size, we observed large effect size and significance of intergroup differences. We did not calculate the sample size a-priori, and therefore, we suggest that future research on this topic should include a larger sample with high statistical power.

Another limitation is the lack of blood samples after 48 and 72 h, which may provide a more complete insight into the removal rate of the biochemical markers tested. The research presented in this paper concerned the effects of local vibration in young, physically active men, and the conclusions drawn from it also apply only to this group.

6. Conclusions

In summary, local cycloidal-oscillating vibration reduces the activity of CK, LDH, and concentration of Mb compared to the control group, immediately and 24 h after performing 180 min moderate intensity exercise on a cycloergometer in young, physically active men.

The introduction of treatments using local vibration after exercise can reduce post-exercise muscle damage and shorten recovery time. Such action may allow for the development of an effective, not overburdening recovery protocol in young, physically active men.

Author Contributions: Conceptualization, T.P., E.S.-K., W.P. and A.P.; methodology, T.P., M.B. and M.M.; software, A.P.; validation, D.M., Ł.T. and S.W.; formal analysis, M.B., M.M.; investigation, T.P.; resources, A.P.; data curation, M.B.; writing—original draft preparation A.P.; writing—review and editing, W.P., Ł.T., T.P. and M.M.; visualization A.P.; supervision, T.P. and W.P.; project administration, P.B.; funding acquisition T.P. and M.M. All authors have read and agreed to the published version of the manuscript.

Funding: This research was funded by Narodowe Centrum Badań i Rozwoju (Poland), Grant Number: POIR.01.01.01-00-1208. The APC was funded within the framework of the program of the Ministry of Science and Higher Education (Poland) under the name "Regional Initiative for Perfection" within the years 2019–2022, project No. 022/RID/2018/19 in the total of 11,919,908 PLN.

Institutional Review Board Statement: The study was conducted according to the guidelines of the Declaration of Helsinki and approved by the Ethics Committee of Opole Medical School (Poland) (KB/56/N02/2019).

Informed Consent Statement: Informed consent was obtained from all subjects involved in the study.

Data Availability Statement: The data presented in this study are available on request from the corresponding author.

Conflicts of Interest: The authors declare no conflict of interest.

References

1. Hotfiel, T.; Freiwald, J.; Hoppe, M.W.; Lutter, C.; Forst, R.; Grim, C.; Bloch, W.; Hüttel, M.; Heiss, R. Advances in Delayed-Onset Muscle Soreness (DOMS): Part I: Pathogenesis and Diagnostics. *Sportverletz.-Sportschaden* **2018**, *32*, 243–250. [CrossRef] [PubMed]
2. Hody, S.; Croisier, J.L.; Bury, T.; Rogister, B.; Leprince, P. Eccentric Muscle Contractions: Risks and Benefits. *Front. Physiol.* **2019**, *10*, 536. [CrossRef] [PubMed]
3. Yu, J.Y.; Jeong, J.G.; Lee, B.H. Evaluation of Muscle Damage Using Ultrasound Imaging. *J. Phys. Ther. Sci.* **2015**, *27*, 531–534. [CrossRef] [PubMed]
4. Banfi, G.; Colombini, A.; Lombardi, G.; Lubkowska, A. *Metabolic Markers in Sports Medicine*, 1st ed.; Elsevier Inc.: Amsterdam, The Netherlands, 2012; Volume 56. [CrossRef]
5. Kunysz-Rozborska, M. Wellness in Contemporary Sport. *Qual. Sport* **2017**, *3*, 48. [CrossRef]
6. Rose, C.; Edwards, K.M.; Siegler, J.; Graham, K.; Caillaud, C. Whole-Body Cryotherapy as a Recovery Technique after Exercise: A Review of the Literature. *Int. J. Sports Med.* **2017**, *38*, 1049–1060. [CrossRef] [PubMed]
7. Guo, J.; Li, L.; Gong, Y.; Zhu, R.; Xu, J.; Zou, J.; Chen, X. Massage Alleviates Delayed Onset Muscle Soreness after Strenuous Exercise: A Systematic Review and Meta-Analysis. *Front. Physiol.* **2017**, *8*, 747. [CrossRef] [PubMed]
8. Lu, X.; Wang, Y.; Lu, J.; You, Y.; Zhang, L.; Zhu, D.; Yao, F. Does Vibration Benefit Delayed-Onset Muscle Soreness?: A Meta-Analysis and Systematic Review. *J. Int. Med. Res.* **2019**, *47*, 3–18. [CrossRef]
9. Bernardo-Filho, M.; Bemben, D.; Stark, C.; Taiar, R. Biological Consequences of Exposure to Mechanical Vibration. *Dose-Response* **2018**, *16*, 1–2. [CrossRef]
10. Fuller, J.T.; Thomson, R.L.; Howe, P.R.C.; Buckley, J.D. Effect of Vibration on Muscle Perfusion: A Systematic Review. *Clin. Physiol. Funct. Imag.* **2013**, *33*, 1–10. [CrossRef]
11. Manimmanakorn, N.; Manimmanakorn, A.; Phuttharak, W.; Hamlin, M.J. Effects of Whole Body Vibration on Glycemic Indices and Peripheral Blood Flow in Type II Diabetic Patients. *Malays. J. Med. Sci.* **2017**, *24*, 55–63. [CrossRef]
12. Morel, D.S.; da Fontoura Dionello, C.; Moreira-Marconi, E.; Brandao-Sobrinho-Neto, S.; Paineiras-Domingos, L.L.; Souza, P.L.; da Cunha de Sá-Caputo, D.; Dias, G.; Figueiredo, C.; Carmo, R.C.R.; et al. Relevance of Whole Body Vibration Exercise in Sport: A Short Review With Soccer, Diver and Combat Sport. *Afr. J. Tradit. Complement. Altern. Med.* **2017**, *14*, 19–27. [CrossRef]
13. Aminian-Far, A.; Hadian, M.R.; Olyaei, G.; Talebian, S.; Bakhtiary, A.H. Whole-Body Vibration and the Prevention and Treatment of Delayed-Onset Muscle Soreness. *J. Athl. Train.* **2011**, *46*, 43–49. [CrossRef] [PubMed]
14. Manimmanakorn, N.; Ross, J.J.; Manimmanakorn, A.; Lucas, S.J.E.; Hamlin, M.J. Effect of Whole-Body Vibration Therapy on Performance Recovery. *Int. J. Sports Physiol. Perform.* **2015**, *10*, 388–395. [CrossRef]
15. Kim, S.S.; Ju, S.B.; Park, G.D. Changes in Stress Hormone Levels with the Application of Vibrations before Resistance Exercises at Different Intensities. *J. Phys. Ther. Sci.* **2015**, *27*, 2845–2847. [CrossRef]
16. Timon, R.; Tejero, J.; Brazo-Sayavera, J.; Crespo, C.; Olcina, G. Effects of Whole-Body Vibration after Eccentric Exercise on Muscle Soreness and Muscle Strength Recovery. *J. Phys. Ther. Sci.* **2016**, *28*, 1781–1785. [CrossRef] [PubMed]
17. Couto, B.P.; Silva, H.R.; Filho, A.G.; Da Silveira Neves, S.R.; Ramos, M.G.; Szmuchrowski, L.A.; Barbosa, M.P. Acute Effects of Resistance Training with Local Vibration. *Int. J. Sports Med.* **2013**, *34*, 814–819. [CrossRef]
18. Pilch, W.; Czerwińska Ledwig, O.; Chitryniewicz-Rostek, J.; Nastałek, M.; Krężałek, P.; Jędrychowska, D.; Totko-Borkusewicz, N.; Uher, I.; Kaško, D.; Tota, L.; et al. The Impact of Vibration Therapy Interventions on Skin Condition and Skin Temperature Changes in Young Women with Lipodystrophy: A Pilot Study. *Evid.-Based Complement. Altern. Med.* **2019**, *2019*, 8436325. [CrossRef]
19. Souron, R.; Besson, T.; Millet, G.Y.; Lapole, T. Acute and Chronic Neuromuscular Adaptations to Local Vibration Training. *Eur. J. Appl. Physiol.* **2017**, *117*, 1939–1964. [CrossRef] [PubMed]
20. Van Heuvelen, M.J.G.; Rittweger, J.; Judex, S.; Sañudo, B.; Seixas, A.; Fuermaier, A.; Tucha, O.; Nyakas, C.; Marín, P.J.; Taiar, R.; et al. Reporting Guidelines for Whole-Body Vibration Studies in Humans, Animals and Cell Cultures: A Consensus Statement from an International Group of Experts. *Biology* **2021**, *10*, 965. [CrossRef] [PubMed]
21. Wuestefeld, A.; Fuermaier, A.; Bernardo-Filho, M.; da Cunha de Sá-Caputo, D.; Rittweger, J.; Schoenau, E.; Stark, C.; Marin, P.J.; Seixas, A.; Judex, S.; et al. Towards reporting guidelines of research using whole-body vibration as training or treatment regimen in human subjects—A Delphi consensus study. *PLoS ONE* **2020**, *15*, e0235905. [CrossRef] [PubMed]
22. Piotrowska, A.; Czerwińska-Ledwig, O. Effect of local vibrotherapy in sitting or lying position in two time protocols on the cellulite grade and change of body circumferences in women with cellulite. *J. Cosmet. Dermatol.* **2021**, 1–10. [CrossRef]
23. Żuchowicz, A.; Kubica, R.; Tyka, A. Exercise Thermoregulation after Physical Training in Warm and Temperate Environments. *J. Hum. Kinet.* **1999**, *1*, 1999.
24. Dill, D.B.; Costill, D.L. Calculation of Percentage Changes in Volumes of Blood, Plasma, and Red Cells in Dehydration. *J. Appl. Physiol.* **1974**, *37*, 247–248. [CrossRef]
25. Harrison, M.; Graveney, M.; Cochrane, L. Some Sources of Error in the Calculation of Relative Change in Plasma Volume. *Eur. J. Appl. Physiol. Occup. Physiol.* **1982**, *50*, 13–21. [CrossRef]
26. Cohen, J. *Statistical Power Analysis for the Behavioral Sciences*; Routledge Academic: New York, NY, USA, 1988. [CrossRef]
27. Ziemann, E.; Kasprowicz, K.; Kasperska, A.; Zembro, A. Do High Blood Hepcidin Concentrations Contribute to Low Ferritin Levels in Young Tennis Players at the End of Tournament Season? *J. Sports Sci. Med.* **2013**, *12*, 249–258.

28. Freire, L.A.; de Brito, M.A.; Esteves, N.S.; Tannure, M.; Slimani, M.; Znazen, H.; Bragazzi, N.L.; Brito, C.J.; Soto, D.A.S.; Gonçalves, D.; et al. Running Performance of High-Level Soccer Player Positions Induces Significant Muscle Damage and Fatigue Up to 24 h Postgame. *Front. Psychol.* **2021**, *12*, 708725. [CrossRef]
29. Veqar, Z.; Imtiyaz, S. Vibration Therapy in Management of Delayed Onset Muscle Soreness. *J. Clin. Diagn. Res.* **2014**, *8*, 1–5. [CrossRef]
30. Uher, I. Vibration Therapy and Its Influence on Health. *Biomed. J. Sci. Tech. Res.* **2018**, *6*, 3–7. [CrossRef]
31. Lundeberg, T.; Nordemar, R.; Ottoson, D. Pain Alleviation by Vibratory Stimulation. *Pain* **1984**, *20*, 25–44. [CrossRef]
32. Rittweger, J. Vibration as an Exercise Modality: How It May Work, and What Its Potential Might Be. *Eur. J. Appl. Physiol.* **2010**, *108*, 877–904. [CrossRef]
33. Weerakkody, N.S.; Percival, P.; Hickey, M.W.; Morgan, D.L.; Gregory, J.E.; Canny, B.J.; Proske, U. Effects of Local Pressure and Vibration on Muscle Pain from Eccentric Exercise and Hypertonic Saline. *Pain* **2003**, *105*, 425–435. [CrossRef]
34. Koeda, T.; Ando, T.; Inoue, T.; Kamisaka, K.; Tsukamoto, S.; Torikawa, T.; Hirasawa, J.; Yamazaki, M.; Ida, K.; Mizumura, K. A Trial to Evaluate Experimentally Induced Delayed Onset Muscle Soreness and Its Modulation by Vibration. *Environ. Med.* **2003**, *47*, 26–30. [CrossRef]
35. Moreira-Marconi, E.; Moura-Fernandes, M.C.; Lopes-Souza, P.; Teixeira-Silva, Y.; Reis-Silva, A.; Marchon, R.M.; De Oliveira Guedes-Aguiar, E.; Paineiras-Domingos, L.L.; Da Cunha De Sá-Caputo, D.; Morel, D.S.; et al. Evaluation of the Temperature of Posterior Lower Limbs Skin during the Whole Body Vibration Measured by Infrared Thermography: Cross-Sectional Study Analysis Using Linear Mixed Effect Model. *PLoS ONE* **2019**, *14*, e0212512. [CrossRef]
36. Tyka, A.K.; Pałka, T.; Piotrowska, A.; Żiżka, D.; Pilch, W.; Cebula, A.; Tyka, A. The Effect of Vibro-Massage on the Level of Selected Marker of Muscle Damageand Connective Tissues after Long-Term Physical Exercise in Males. *J. Kinesiol. Exerc. Sci. Antropomotoryka* **2018**, *82*, 21–27. [CrossRef]
37. Broadbent, S.; Rousseau, J.J.; Thorp, R.M.; Choate, S.L.; Jackson, F.S.; Rowlands, D.S. Vibration Therapy Reduces Plasma IL6 and Muscle Soreness after Downhill Running. *Br. J. Sports Med.* **2010**, *44*, 888–894. [CrossRef]
38. Bakhtiary, A.H.; Safavi-Farokhi, Z.; Aminian-Far, A. Influence of Vibration on Delayed Onset of Muscle Soreness Following Eccentric Exercise. *Br. J. Sports Med.* **2007**, *41*, 145–148. [CrossRef] [PubMed]
39. Imtiyaz, S.; Veqar, Z.; Shareef, M.Y. To Compare the Effect of Vibration Therapy and Massage in Prevention of Delayed Onset Muscle Soreness (DOMS). *J. Clin. Diagn. Res.* **2014**, *8*, 133–136. [CrossRef] [PubMed]
40. Liu, K.; Wang, J.; Hsu, C.; Liu, C.; Chen, C.P.C. Low-Frequency Vibration Facilitates Post-Exercise Cardiovascular Autonomic Recovery. *J. Sports Sci. Med.* **2021**, *20*, 431–437. [CrossRef] [PubMed]
41. Shibata, N.; Ishimatsu, K. Gender difference in subjective response to whole-body vibration under standing posture. *Int. Arch. Occup. Environ. Health* **2012**, *85*, 171–179. [CrossRef] [PubMed]
42. Sanudo, B.; Feria, A.; Carrasco, L.; de Hoyo, M.; Santos, R. Gender differences in knee stability in response to whole-body vibration. *J. Strength Cond. Res.* **2012**, *26*, 2156–2165. [CrossRef]
43. Merrigan, J.; Dabbs, N.; Jones, M. Isometric Mid-thigh Pull Kinetics: Sex Differences and Response to Whole-Body Vibration. *J. Strength Cond. Res.* **2020**, *34*, 2407–2411. [CrossRef] [PubMed]

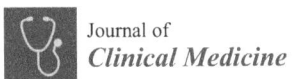

Article

Focus on the Scapular Region in the Rehabilitation of Chronic Neck Pain Is Effective in Improving the Symptoms: A Randomized Controlled Trial

Norollah Javdaneh [1], Tadeusz Ambroży [2,*], Amir Hossein Barati [3], Esmaeil Mozafaripour [4] and Łukasz Rydzik [2,*]

1. Department of Biomechanics and Sports Injuries, Kharazmi University, Tehran 14911-15719, Iran; njavdaneh68@gmail.com
2. Institute of Sports Sciences, University of Physical Education, 31-571 Krakow, Poland
3. Department of Health and Exercise Rehabilitation, Shahid Beheshti University of Tehran, Tehran 19839-69411, Iran; ahbarati20@gmail.com
4. Department of Health and Sports Medicine, University of Tehran, Tehran 14179-35840, Iran; e.mozafaripour@yahoo.com
* Correspondence: tadek@ambrozy.pl (T.A.); lukasz.gne@op.pl (Ł.R.)

Abstract: Chronic neck pain is a common human health problem. Changes in scapular posture and alteration of muscle activation patterns of scapulothoracic muscles are cited as potential risk factors for neck pain. The purpose of this study was to compare the effects of neck exercise training (NET) with and without scapular stabilization training (SST) on pain intensity, the scapula downward rotation index (SDRI), forward head angle (FHA) and neck range of motion (ROM) in patients with chronic neck pain and scapular dyskinesia. A total of sixty-six subjects with chronic neck pain and scapular dyskinesia were randomly divided into three groups: neck exercise training, n = 24, combined training (NET + SST), n = 24 and a control group, n = 24. Pain intensity, SDRI, FHA and ROM were measured by the numerical rating scale, caliper, photogrammetry and IMU sensor, respectively. When the combined intervention group consisting of NET and SST was compared with NET alone at six weeks, there was a statistically significant difference in pain intensity, SDRI, FHA and cervical ROM for flexion and extension ($p \leq 0.05$). Adding scapular exercises to neck exercises had a more significant effect in decreasing pain intensity, SDRI, FHA and increased cervical ROM than neck exercises alone in patients with chronic neck pain. These findings indicate that focus on the scapular posture in the rehabilitation of chronic neck pain effectively improves the symptoms.

Keywords: therapeutic exercises; chronic neck pain; scapular dyskinesia

1. Introduction

Neck pain that lasts for three months or more is determined as chronic neck pain. The mechanism of nonspecific neck pain is still not clearly understood. While neck pain as etiology is multifactorial and includes working conditions, sedentary lifestyle, postural abnormalities, previous trauma to the neck region and altered neuromuscular control of cervical muscles are the main risk factors for nonspecific neck pain stated in the literature [1]. Changes in scapular posture and muscle activation patterns are cited as potential risk factors for chronic neck pain (CNP) [1]. Subjects with chronic neck pain tend to have more protracted shoulders compared with asymptomatic issues [2]. An altered kinematic of the scapula may be present in subjects with chronic neck pain, which can play a substantial role in the maintaining or intensifying of symptoms in these patients [3,4]. The underlying mechanisms in the relationship between altered scapular kinematics and CNP may be due to changes in the length–tension relationships of muscles that connect the scapula, head, cervical spine and chest. Altered behaviors of muscles, such as the trapeziuses, levator

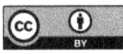

scapula and rhomboid minor, which are directly connected to the cervical spine, may cause compression and shear forces on the neck area and cause pain in this region [4].

Scapular downward rotation syndrome (SDRS) is a common scapular alignment impairment. It is reported that, most often, SDRS typically leads to shortened levator scapula (LS), and lengthened upper trapezius (UT) and serratus anterior (SA) muscles [5]. Furthermore, the lower trapezius (LT) weakness can play a substantial role in insufficient scapular upward rotation [5]. The scapulothoracic muscles play an essential role in transferring the load between the upper limb and the spine [6]. Studies have shown a change in the recruitment of muscle patterns in subjects with neck pain compared to healthy subjects. Individuals with chronic neck pain have different muscle activation patterns and kinematics than individuals without a disorder [1,7]. Subjects with neck pain have less muscle strength and activity than healthy people [8,9]. Pain sensitivity and axioscapular muscle activity have altered in neck pain patients compared with healthy controls [10]. Researchers have shown a relationship between decreased muscle strength and endurance with chronic nonspecific neck pain [11]. Neck stabilization exercises have been popular for managing and preventing spinal dysfunction by recruiting local muscles and regulating the over-activity of surface muscles [12,13]. A systematic literature review on the influence of exercise intervention for chronic neck disorders showed that exercise training has an essential role in the cure of neck pain but stated that more studies are needed to examine the effect of each type of exercise [14].

Even though many studies have been done on chronic neck pain, little is known about the potential benefits of scapular exercise on chronic neck pain [6,15]. According to a systematic review, scapular exercise may improve symptoms of neck pain, but the effects of scapular exercise on pain and dysfunction in the neck region remain unclear because the number of studies was small and recommended that further high quality research is needed [16].

Some studies have used these exercises in combination to treat people with chronic neck pain [15,17–19]. Most of the above assignments have not considered the role of scapula condition in treating neck pain, and postural variables have been less studied. Furthermore, due to the lack of comparison between these training interventions, the effect size of this exercise in each region is not known. Scapular dyskinesia also needs to be considered during the management of chronic neck pain. Rehabilitation exercises that aim to return functionality of the scapular muscles are deemed necessary to render a successful result. Therefore, the purpose of this study is to evaluate the effectiveness of adding the scapular stabilization training to the neck exercise training on pain, the scapula downward rotation index, forward head angle and neck ROM in the patient's chronic neck pain with scapular dyskinesia. We hypothesized that adding scapular stabilization training to neck exercise training will increase treatment efficacy on these variables.

2. Materials and Methods

2.1. Study Design

This study was a three-arm randomized control trial, with two intervention groups and a control group, and was conducted according to the Consolidated Standards of Reporting Trials (CONSORT) guidelines [15] and registered at UMIN-CTR Clinical Trial (ID: UMIN000043938). A total of 72 patients were recruited from two rehabilitation and physiotherapy centers between May 2020 and October 2020 in Tehran city. All expected outcomes were collected at the Noor Health Center. The study was conducted following the Helsinki Convention and approved by the Ethics Committee of the Sports Science Research Center (ID: IR.KHU.REC.1398.011). Written informed consent was obtained from each patient to be included in this study. Participants were assessed before the study and after 6 weeks of intervention (end of the exercise intervention) by a physiotherapist blinded to the participants' groups. An external assistant physiotherapist, blinded to the participants' allocation groups, was responsible for collecting patient data. The independent variables were neck exercise, combined exercise (neck exercise + scapular stabilization exercise), control group and time (pre-intervention, post-intervention). The dependent variables were pain intensity, scapula downward rotation index and forward head angle.

2.2. Participants

Patients with chronic neck pain were recruited through a text message on social networks and via flyers displayed at the hospitals. They were selected based on the eligibility criteria listed below. A total of 72 patients with ongoing chronic neck pain volunteered for this study. In this study, chronic neck pain was identified as neck pain with no specific cause, such as inflammation, disease and infection, but was stimulated by palpation, and neck movement [20].

Inclusion criteria involved people between 20 and 50 years of age who had a history of ongoing bilateral neck pain for three months or more. Furthermore, moderate pain intensity (between 3 and 7 based on VAS) and having bilateral scapula downward rotation (participants had to score 5 mm or above on the base scapula downward rotation index) were among the inclusion criteria. Exclusion criteria were any previous shoulder or neck surgery, fibromyalgia and pathology and having a poor general health status that would interfere with the exercises during the study. The inclusion/exclusion criteria were confirmed by a physician and three physiotherapists, by history and physical examination.

Sample size calculations using G*Power software (v3.1.9.2, Heinrich-Heine-University, Dusseldorf, Germany) as in the previous studies [21,22] resulted in 66 patients (22 patients per group). Considering an effect size of 0.23, a statistical power of 0.8%, and an alpha of 0.05 (two-tailed test), a total sample size of 66 was required (22 patients per group). An allowance was made for a 10% dropout rate, increasing the sample size to 72 patients (24 per group). Patients were randomized by the slot-drawing method into one of three groups: group (1) neck exercise training; group (2) combined (neck exercise training plus scapular stabilization training); group (3) control group (Figure 1). The allocation was by sealed opaque envelopes, and patients were assigned to each group by a sealed envelope containing one of the three groups. For the allocation of participants, computerized random numbers were used. In this study, the assessor was blinded; however, patients were aware of what treatment they were participating in. The inclusion/exclusion criteria and outcome measurements were assessed by an orthopedic surgeon and physiotherapist, blinded to the study's procedures. The outcome assessors and data analysts were kept blinded to the group allocation to intervention or control group.

2.3. Outcome Measure(s)

Pain intensity was measured with the Visual Analogue Scale (VAS). Patients were instructed to assess the severity of neck pain experienced last week on a 0–10 cm horizontal line (0 = painless and 10 = worst pain imaginable) [23]. The VAS has been shown to have excellent test–retest reliability (ICC = 0.97) and high validity (r with a 5-point verbal descriptive scale = 0.71–0.78) to evaluate pain perception. An alteration of two points or more was identified as the minimal clinically important difference in patients with chronic neck pain [23].

The scapula downward rotation index (SDRI) and forward head angle were measured by caliper and photogrammetry, respectively. The modified Kibbler method was used to measure the SDRI and was conducted on the dominant hand side using a caliper. The SDRI was calculated using the following equation: the distance between the second thoracic vertebra and spine of the scapula minus the distance between the seventh thoracic vertebra and the inferior angle of the scapula. Positive values demonstrated downward rotation scapula [21,24]. The interclass correlation coefficient (ICC) of the inter-rater reliability was 0.85 and the ICCs of the intra-rater reliabilities were 0.88–0.96 [21,24].

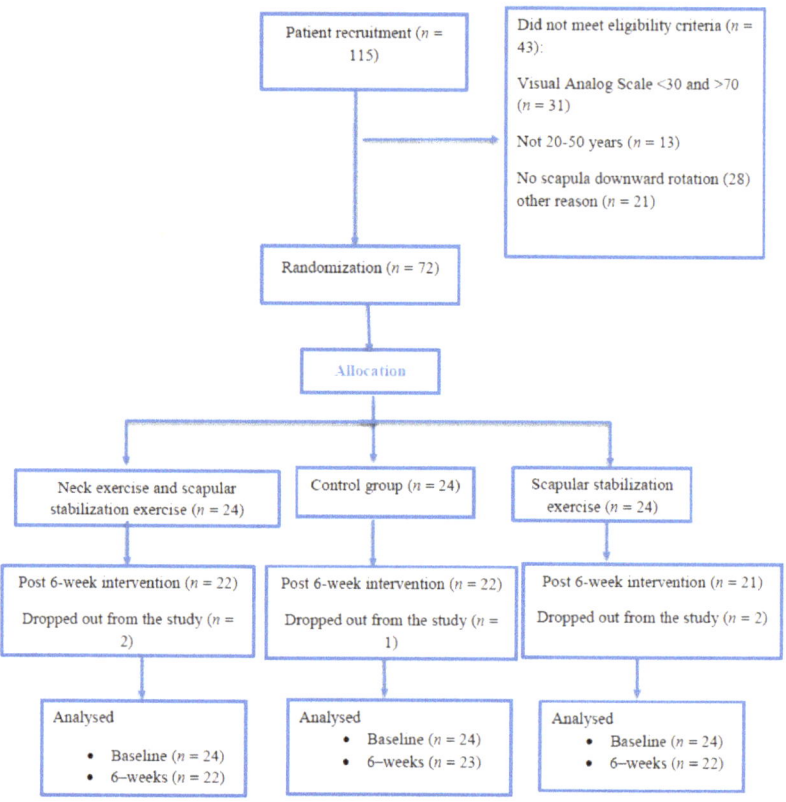

Figure 1. CONSORT flow diagram of the study.

Forward head posture was measured using photogrammetry (Canon PowerShot, SX130IS). This is the angle composed at the intersection of a horizontal line through the seventh cervical vertebra and a line to the tragus of the ear. The craniovertebral angle (CVA) was analyzed using postural assessment software (Sony Cyber-shot DSC-P93, Sony, San Jose, CA, USA). A craniovertebral angle less than 48°–50° is defined as forward head posture [25]. Craniovertebral angles have been proven to be valid measures of posture when compared with similar angles measured on radiographs [25].

The MyoMotion (Noraxon Inc., Scottsdale, AZ, USA) 3D motion analysis system was used to investigate the cervical ROM. A small inertial measurement unit (IMU) sensor placed on a body segment tracked 3D angular orientation. The IMU 3D motion analysis is acceptable in its validity and reliability for the cervical ROM [26]. The MyoMotion IMU sensors include a 3D accelerometer, gyroscope and magnetometer, and when placed on a body segment, can be used to determine the segment's three-dimensional orientation. The IMU 3D motion analysis is completely wireless and does not require calibration. For the cervical ROM assessment, an IMU sensor was pasted to the head (middle of the front of the head) using a flexible and adjustable strap. The cervical ROM changes were recorded with the sampling frequency at 200 Hz [26]. The calibration posture was sitting straight with neutral head positioning and the arms next to the body with the elbows bent at 90° to determine the value of the 0° angle in the cervical joint [26]. Data were analyzed using the Noraxon MyoResearch 3.14.32 Windows software (Noraxon Inc., Scottsdale, AZ, USA). The patient performed flexion and extension movements in the sagittal plane. The ICC of each movement was over 0.8.

2.4. Rehabilitation Interventions

Neck exercise training (NET): The composition and progress of the exercises were designed according to the exercises presented in previous studies [22,27–29]. The exercises included craniocervical flexion using the stabilizer pressure biofeedback unit, neck isometric exercises using Thera-band and neck stability exercises in supine, prone, quadrupedal and bipedal positions. Further details on the exercise protocol are reported in the study by Javdaneh et al. [22]. NET was implemented once a day (three days per week, for six weeks). More details on the interventions and exercise are reported in Table A1.

Scapular stabilization training (SST): Scapular stabilization exercise training covered exercises for the muscles influencing scapular alignment related to chronic neck pain [21]. The composition of the SST was planned based on prior research [21]. The progressive SST training was designed based on sports medicine principles [30]. Exercises included: non- resistive SUR exercise [31], wall facing arm lift, prone arm lift, backward rocking arm lift [32], elevation of the arm in line with the lower trapezius muscle fibers, elevation of the arm in the plane of the scapula [33], shoulder shrug, [34] and stretching of levator scapular and the pectoralis minor muscle [35]. The exercises were performed three days per week, for six weeks (18 sessions in total). More details on the interventions and exercise are reported in Table A2.

The exercise training was implemented under the surveillance of three physiotherapists and an athletic trainer, who had more than five years of experience in the treatment of the musculoskeletal system. Each training session took 40–60 min. It was composed of 10 min of warm-up exercises, 30 min of scapular exercises and a 5 min cool-down.

The control group participated in a session in which they were taught a home exercise program that mainly focused on the posture of the body during daily work and demonstrations of lifting, pressing, pulling tasks and office ergonomics. After the end of the interventions, the control group received a comprehensive rehabilitation program.

2.5. Statistical Analysis

The Statistical Package for the Social Sciences (SPSS, IBM Corporation, Armonk, NY, USA) version 19.0 was used for statistical analysis. A Shapiro–Wilk test was performed to test the normality of the data. The variance of repeated measures (RM-ANOVA) was used to examine the differences between groups. Effect sizes were calculated and were interpreted according to Cohen d (trivial < 0.2, small = 0.2–0.5, medium = 0.5–0.8 or large > 0.8). Mathematically, Cohen's effect size is denoted by; $d = M_1 - M_2/S$. A level of 0.05 was identified as being of statistical significance.

3. Results

One hundred fifteen subjects were screened and 72 were selected and randomized after consideration of the inclusion and exclusion criteria. Five patients withdrew from the study due to personal reasons before completing the interventions (two from the neck exercise group, two from the combined group and one person from the control group). There was a high degree of adherence to the two interventions (18 sessions for both intervention groups). No adverse events were reported. The baseline and demographic characteristics of the 72 patients included in the study are reported in Table 1. At the baseline, there were no significant differences between groups in any of the demographic characteristics and clinical variables. Finally, the data of 67 subjects were analyzed after the intervention.

Table 1. Demographic characteristics of the participants for all groups at baseline. All values are expressed as mean ± SD.

Variables		Groups (No.)			p	Gender Differences
		NET (n = 24)	Combined (n = 24)	Control (n = 24)		p
Age (year)		32.58 ± 6.37	34.25 ± 8.01	35.41 ± 7.77	0.77	0.84
Weight (kg)		75.65 ± 4.10	78.5 ± 5.00	76.23 ± 4.05	0.73	0.078
Height (cm)		178 ± 5.20	179 ± 5.28	177 ± 5.68	0.74	0.001
BMI (kg/m^2)		24.20 ± 2.17	24.33 ± 2.07	24.08 ± 2.05	0.83	0.017
Duration of symptoms (year)		3.18 ± 1.54	4.25 ± 1.85	3.40 ± 1.104	0.57	0.69
VAS at baseline (0–100)		57.15 ± 6.33	59.70 ± 6.15	58.65 ± 6.44	0.83	0.91
SDRI at baseline		1.5 ± 0.13	1.59 ± 0.17	1.59 ± 0.14	0.91	0.80
FHA at baseline		40.50 ± 2.88	39.87 ± 2.90	39.79 ± 2.85	0.87	0.76
Neck flexion ROM at baseline		46.37 ± 4.76	46.33 ± 4.97	45.62 ± 5.40	0.80	0.71
Neck extension ROM at baseline		37.83 ± 4.76	37.58 ± 5.35	37.58 ± 5.35	0.85	0.68
Gender (n)	Female	13	14	14	0.67	
	Male	11	10	10		

NET: neck exercises training; Combined: neck exercises + scapular stabilization training; BMI: body mass index; VAS: visual analogous scale; SDRI: scapula downward rotation index; FHA: forward head angle; ROM: range of motion.

The results showed a significant effect of time ($p < 0.001$), group ($p < 0.001$) and time by group interaction ($p < 0.001$) for VAS, ROM, SDRI and FHP. Significant differences between groups were found for VAS after the intervention. Reduction in the severity of pain (VAS) was significantly higher in the combined group (neck exercise and scapular stabilization exercise) than the neck exercise alone and control groups. For VAS, between neck exercise intervention vs. combined intervention (effect size (ES) = -2.71, $p = 0.001$), neck exercise vs. control (ES = 4.16; $p = 0.001$) and combined group vs. control (ES = 5.45; $p = 0.001$) significant differences were observed (Table 2).

Significant differences between groups were found for the scapular downward rotation index and forward head angle after the interventions. For the scapular downward rotation index, differences between the neck exercise training group vs. combined group (ES = -3.56, $p = 0.001$), and combined intervention vs. control (ES = -4.55; $p = 0.001$) were observed as significant, and in neck exercise vs. control (ES = 0.74; $p = 0.43$) no significant difference was observed. For forward head angle, differences between the neck exercise training group vs. combined group (ES = -1.86, $p = 0.001$), neck exercise vs. control (ES = -1.23; $p = 0.001$) and combined intervention vs. control (ES = -3.09; $p = 0.001$) were observed to be significant (Table 2).

Significant differences between groups were found for neck flexion and extension ROM at six weeks. For neck flexion ROM, differences between the neck exercise training group vs. combined training (ES = 1.54, $p = 0.024$), combined training vs. control (ES = 3.47; $p = 0.001$) and also combined training vs. control (ES = 1.90.; $p = 0.01$) were observed to be significant. For neck extension ROM, differences between neck exercise training vs. combined training (ES = 1.57, $p = 0.025$), neck exercise training vs. control (ES = 3.07; $p = 0.001$) and also combined training vs. control (ES = 4.06; $p = 0.001$) were observed as significant (Table 2).

Table 2. VAS, SDRI, FHA and ROM scores differences between groups.

Variables	Group	Pre-Training [a]	Post-Training [a]	NET vs. Combined Mean Difference (%95 CI)	NET vs. Combined ES (p-Value)	NET vs. Control Mean Difference (%95 CI)	NET vs. Control ES (p-Value)	Combined vs. Control Mean Difference (%95 CI)	Combined vs. Control ES (p-Value)
Pain, 0–100 (mL)	NET	57.15 ± 6.33	31.55 ± 5.15	8.32 (5.32, 12.45)	2.71 (0.001) *	−13.77 (−17.25, −9.25)	4.16 (0.001) *	−22.10 (−27.1, −17.2)	6.66 (0.001) *
	Combined	59.70 ± 6.15	12.35 ± 4.74						
	Control	58.65 ± 6.44	57.60 ± 6.54						
SDRI	NET	1.5 ± 0.13	1.40 ± 0.14	0.257 (0.12, 0.39)	3.56 (0.001) *	−0.084 (−0.22, 0.05)	0.74 (0.430)	−0.342 (−0.47, −0.20)	4.55 (0.001) *
	Combined	1.59 ± 0.17	0.87 ± 0.21						
	Control	1.59 ± 0.14	1.56 ± 0.13						
FHA	NET	40.50 ± 2.88	44.54 ± 3.12	−2.12 (−3.93, −0.31)	1.86 (0.001) *	2.85 (1.04, 4.66)	1.23 (0.001) *	4.97 (3.17, 6.67)	3.09 (0.001) *
	Combined	39.87 ± 2.90	49.41 ± 3.06						
	Control	39.79 ± 2.85	39.54 ± 3.24						
Neck flexion ROM	NET	46.37 ± 4.76	59.16 ± 5.32	−3.83 (−7.25, −0.40)	1.54 (0.024) *	5.66 (2.24, 9.09)	1.90 (0.001) *	9.50 (6.07, 12.9)	3.47 (0.001) *
	Combined	46.33 ± 4.97	66.87 ± 4.27						
	Control	45.62 ± 5.40	48.58 ± 6.04						
Neck extension ROM	NET	37.83 ± 4.76	52.83 ± 6.10	−3.92 (−7.53, −0.43)	1.57 (0.025) *	7.64 (4.08, 11.20)	3.07 (0.001) *	11.62 (8.06, 15.18)	4.06 (0.001) *
	Combined	37.58 ± 5.35	61.04 ± 7.18						
	Control	37.58 ± 5.35	37.45 ± 5.15						

NET: neck exercises training; Combined: neck exercises + scapular stabilization training; ES: effect size; SDRI: scapula downward rotation index; FHA: forward head angle; ROM: range of motion; [a] mean ± standard deviation, * statistically significant difference ($p < 0.05$).

4. Discussion

The results of this study indicated that VAS, SDRI and FHA decreased in neck exercises training alone (except SDRI) and in combined intervention in subjects with CNP and scapular dyskinesia. The results also showed a significant increase in the cervical ROM after the intervention. This study revealed that a combined intervention group including neck exercise training and scapular stabilization exercise training was superior to neck exercise training alone in improving the variables of subjects with CNP.

The results of this study are relative to improvements in VAS compliance with prior studies investigating the effects of neck exercise training [22,28]. The mechanism through which neck exercise training reduces chronic neck pain may be based on the notion that exercise training increments activity in the motor pathways, thereby exerting an inhibitory effect on pain receptors in the central nervous system [36]. Furthermore, it may be that the development in neuromuscular control from neck exercise training decreases the compression placed on the joints. The afferent input induced by exercise applications may stimulate neural inhibitory systems at various levels in the spinal cord and activate descending inhibitory pathways from the midbrain and decrease pain [37].

The results of this study are consistent with the results of previous studies. Thompson et al. showed a positive impact of a progressive neck exercise program, including isometric strengthening exercises of the cervical flexors, extensors and side flexors, upper limb strengthening exercises and cervical stretching exercises on people with chronic neck pain [18]. Ylinen et al. showed that both strength and endurance training, including dynamic neck exercises of the neck, shoulders and upper extremities, were effective methods for decreasing pain and disability in women with chronic, nonspecific neck pain [19].

Correcting the scapula position passively or actively has been shown to decrease chronic neck pain [38,39]. Combination therapies are recommended due to better pain intensity than manual therapy or exercise alone [40]. It was demonstrated that the correction of the scapular position may decrease the tension in the axioscapular muscles and abnormal cervical loads, and therefore the pain decreases [6]. Another reason for reduced pain is the reduction of downward pulling tension due to special exercises for upward rotation muscles of the scapula. The downward pulling tension due to sustained scapular downward rotation defects arose in participants. The sustained compressive force of posterior neck spine can induce pain by a downward pull on the neck spine or facets via the levator scapula and upper trapezius muscles. The exercise training may have altered the tension–length relationship of the tightened scapular downward rotator muscles, causing the reduction in downward pulling tension, and consequently decreasing the force on the neck facet joints [41]. The main action of the levator scapulae muscle is to elevate and downwardly rotate the scapulae. With its connection to the upper four neck vertebrae and vertically oriented muscle fibers position, this condition puts undesirable pressure on the upper part and a potential compressive force on the lower part of the cervical vertebrae. Therefore, decreased levator scapulae muscle activity may help to reduce shear force and compressive load on the neck region during active neck movements [2] and thus reduce pain intensity.

The scapula exercise in the current study focused on increasing activation of the upward rotation muscles of the scapula. The serratus anterior, upper trapezius and lower trapezius muscles are considered as scapular upward rotator muscles. These exercises may have caused a decrease in the imbalance between these muscles. Improving the function and strength of the weak muscles and the balance between the scapular upward and downward rotator muscles can improve scapular alignment. By increasing hyperextension and cervical lordosis, the upper trapezius could generate forward head posture. The intervention should manage the extreme activity of the upper trapezius muscle to correct forward head posture and decrease neck pain [42]. Therefore, scapula exercises combined with other interventions may reduce the activity of the upper trapezius, improving scapular alignment and proper scapular rhythm, and ultimately affecting the head-forward angle.

In both programs of the present study, training also significantly increased the neck flexion and extension ROM; however, this increase was substantially higher in the combined group. Altered scapular posture has been detected in subjects with NP, which may be an effective mechanism for intensification of symptoms in these patients [1,43]. Scapular downward rotation syndrome can participate in long comparative loading of the neck region via the transition of the weight of the upper extremities to the cervical spine [3,4]. As observed, exercise therapy reduced pain and it is likely that this reduction in pain will release the muscles from tension and allow the joint to move more.

This study also has several limitations. First, we did not evaluate the long-term effect of the six-week neck exercise with scapular exercise intervention. Even though the six-week neck exercise with scapular exercise intervention is effective on symptoms in the patients with neck pain and scapular dyskinesia, the results may not be generalized for the longer term. Second, in this study, we used patients with scapular downward rotation defects, so other forms of scapular dyskinesia or healthy subjects may have different results. Therefore, this limitation makes it difficult to generalize the results. Finally, we recruited the patients for six weeks; therefore, a longitudinal study of the long-term effects with follow-up is necessary.

5. Conclusions

The results suggest that neck exercise training combined with the scapular stabilization exercise was more effective for reducing pain, forward head angle, scapula upward rotation and increasing cervical ROM in patients' chronic neck pain with scapular downward rotation defects. These findings indicate that focus on the scapular posture in the rehabilitation of chronic neck pain effectively improves the symptoms.

Author Contributions: Conceptualization, N.J., and E.M.; methodology, N.J., and E.M.; software, N.J. and E.M.; validation, N.J., E.M. and A.H.B.; formal analysis, N.J., E.M. and A.H.B.; investigation, N.J. and E.M.; resources, N.J.; data curation, N.J. and E.M.; writing—original draft preparation, N.J. and N.J., Ł.R., T.A.; writing—review and editing, N.J. and A.H.B., Ł.R., T.A.; visualization, N.J. and E.M.; supervision, N.J., Ł.R., T.A.; project administration, N.J., and E.M.; funding acquisition, Ł.R., T.A. All authors have read and agreed to the published version of the manuscript.

Funding: Open Access financed by the programme of the Minister of Science and Higher Education entitled 'Regional Initiative for Perfection' within the years 2019–2022, project No. 022/RID/2018/19, in the total of 11919908 PLN.

Institutional Review Board Statement: The study was conducted according to the guidelines of the Declaration of Helsinki and approved by the Ethics Committee of the Sports Science Research Center (ID: IR.KHU.REC.1398.011).

Informed Consent Statement: Informed consent was obtained from all subjects involved in the study.

Data Availability Statement: The datasets analyzed during the current study are available from the corresponding author on reasonable request.

Acknowledgments: The authors would like to thank all the participants who took part in this study.

Conflicts of Interest: The authors declare no conflict of interest.

Appendix A

Table A1. Details of the neck exercise training.

Exercise	Week	Dosage	Description
Craniocervical flexion exercise	1–6	5–10 reps × 5–10 s	In the first phase of training, the subjects were requested to do a slow and controlled craniocervical flexion task in the supine status. The patient concentrated on feeling the back of the head slide in the cephalad and caudad directions on the supporting surface. Then, the patient performed craniocervical flexion to sequentially reach 5 pressure targets, in 2 mmHg increments, from a baseline of 20 mmHg to the final level of 30 mmHg. For each target level, the contraction duration was increased to 10 s, and the patient was trained to perform 10 repetitions, with 5 s rest periods between each contraction. After completing one step, the exercise then progressed to training at the next target level, up to the final target of 30 mmHg.
cervical bracing exercise	1 2 3 4 5 6	8 reps × 8 s 8 reps × 10 s 10 reps × 12 s 10 reps × 15 s 12 reps × 15 s 12 reps × 18 s	The patients were asked to maintain the positions and contractions during the exercises. Participants held the contraction for 10 s at each position, with 8 repetitions. All exercise repetitions were increased progressively from 8 to 12.
cervical isometric exercises	1 2 3 4 5 6	5 reps × 8 s 5 reps × 10 s 7 reps × 12 s 7 reps × 15 s 8 reps × 15 s 8 reps × 18 s	In this phase, the patient exerted force in the opposite direction of the applied resistance.

Table A2. Details of the scapular stabilization exercise.

Exercise	Week	1 Repetition Maximum (%)	Resistance Type	Targeted Repetitions	Description
Scapular upward rotation	1, 2 3 4 5 6	- Yellow Red Green Blue	body weight resistive elastic band	10–15 reps × 3 sets 10 reps × 3 sets	The subjects stood with their backs against the wall, with wall contact from head to buttock, and feet shoulder width apart. In the starting position, the shoulder was abducted 90° with the elbow flexed 90°. The subjects were instructed to slide their arms up the wall. The sliding movement ended when the shoulder reached 180° of abduction. The subject was then instructed to maintain the arm position for 3 s.
Wall facing arm lift	1, 2 3 4 5 6	- 30 40 50 60	body weight Dumbbell	10–15 reps × 3 sets 10 reps × 3 sets	The subject stood facing the wall and contacted it from nose to knees with feet shoulder width apart. In the starting position, shoulder abducted 90° with elbow flexed 90°. The subjects were instructed to slide their arms up the wall when the shoulder reached 145° of abduction. The subject was then instructed to lift both hands with elbows extended until they were in the full abduction position.
Backward rocking arm lift	1, 2 3 4 5 6	- 30 40 50 60	body weight Dumbbell	10–15 reps × 3 sets 10 reps × 3 sets	Initially, the subjects were placed in the quadruped position and instructed to rock backward slowly until the buttocks touched both heels. The subject was then instructed to lift the arm.
Arm raise overhead in line with the lower trapezius muscle fibers	1, 2 3 4 5 6	- 30 40 50 60	body weight Dumbbell	10–15 reps × 3 sets 10 reps × 3 sets	The subjects performed shoulder abduction in the plane of the scapula above 120° in the standing position.
Shoulder abduction in the plane of the scapula above 120°	1, 2 3 4 5 6	- 30 40 50 60	body weight Dumbbell	10–15 reps × 3 sets 10 reps × 3 sets	The subjects performed shoulder abduction in the plane of the scapula above 120° in the standing position.
Shoulder shrug	1, 2 3 4 5 6	- 30 40 50 60	body weight Dumbbell	10–15 reps × 3 sets 10 reps × 3 sets	The subjects stood with their feet positioned shoulder-width apart. The subjects were instructed to move both of their shoulders until high as possible, and then lowers them, while not bending the elbows or moving the body at all.
Levator scapula and pectoralis minor muscle stretched	1 2 3 4 5 6			10 s × 3 sets 15 s × 3 sets 20 s × 3 sets 25 s × 3 sets 30 s × 3 sets 30 s × 3 sets	Levator scapula stretching; Subject sat, hand positioned in the interscapular region and performed cervical lateral flexion. Corner/wall stretch done for pectoralis minor.

References

1. Yildiz, T.I.; Cools, A.; Duzgun, I. Alterations in the 3-dimensional scapular orientation in patients with non-specific neck pain. *Clin. Biomech.* **2019**, *70*, 97–106. [CrossRef]
2. Szeto, G.P.; Straker, L.; Raine, S. A field comparison of neck and shoulder postures in symptomatic and asymptomatic office workers. *Appl. Ergon.* **2002**, *33*, 75–84. [CrossRef]
3. Cagnie, B.; Struyf, F.; Cools, A.; Castelein, B.; Danneels, L.; O'Leary, S. The Relevance of Scapular Dysfunction in Neck Pain: A Brief Commentary. *J. Orthop. Sports Phys. Ther.* **2014**, *44*, 435–439. [CrossRef]
4. Helgado, T.H.; Kristjansson, E.; Mottram, S.; Karduna, A.; Jonsson, H., Jr. Altered scapular orientation during arm elevation in patients with insidious onset neck pain and whiplash-associated disorder. *J. Orthop. Sports Phys. Ther.* **2010**, *40*, 784–791. [CrossRef]
5. Sahrmann, S. *Diagnosis and Treatment of Movement Impairment Syndromes*; Elsevier Health Sciences: Amsterdam, The Netherlands, 2001.
6. Van Dillen, L.R.; McDonnell, M.K.; Susco, T.M.; Sahrmann, S.A. The Immediate Effect of Passive Scapular Elevation on Symptoms With Active Neck Rotation in Patients With Neck Pain. *Clin. J. Pain* **2007**, *23*, 641–647. [CrossRef] [PubMed]
7. Szeto, G.P.Y.; Straker, L.M.; O'Sullivan, P.B. EMG median frequency changes in the Neck—Shoulder stabilizers of symptomatic office workers when challenged by different physical stressors. *J. Electromyogr. Kinesiol.* **2005**, *15*, 544–555. [CrossRef] [PubMed]
8. Miranda, I.F.; Neto, E.S.W.; Dhein, W.; Brodt, G.A.; Loss, J.F. Individuals With Chronic Neck Pain Have Lower Neck Strength Than Healthy Controls: A Systematic Review With Meta-Analysis. *J. Manip. Physiol. Ther.* **2019**, *42*, 608–622. [CrossRef] [PubMed]
9. Castelein, B.; Cools, A.; Parlevliet, T.; Cagnie, B. Are chronic neck pain, scapular dyskinesis and altered scapulothoracic muscle activity interrelated?: A Case–Control study with surface and Fine—Wire EMG. *J. Electromyogr. Kinesiol.* **2016**, *31*, 136–143. [CrossRef]
10. Christensen, S.W.; Hirata, R.P.; Graven-Nielsen, T. Altered pain sensitivity and axioscapular muscle activity in neck pain patients compared with healthy controls. *Eur. J. Pain* **2017**, *21*, 1763–1771. [CrossRef]
11. Barton, P.M.; Hayes, K.C. Neck flexor muscle strength, efficiency, and relaxation times in normal subjects and subjects with unilateral neck pain and headache. *Arch. Phys. Med. Rehabil.* **1996**, *77*, 680–687. [CrossRef]
12. Jull, G.A.; Richardson, C.A. Motor control problems in patients with spinal pain: A new direction for therapeutic exercise. *J. Manip. Physiol. Ther.* **2000**, *23*, 115–117. [CrossRef]
13. Tsiringakis, G.; Dimitriadis, Z.; Triantafylloy, E.; McLean, S. Motor control training of deep neck flexors with pressure biofeedback improves pain and disability in patients with neck pain: A systematic review and meta-analysis. *Musculoskelet. Sci. Pract.* **2020**, 102220. [CrossRef] [PubMed]
14. Gross, A.; Kay, T.M.; Paquin, J.P.; Blanchette, S.; Lalonde, P.; Christie, T.; Dupont, G.; Graham, N.; Burnie, S.J.; Gelley, G. Exercises for mechanical neck disorders. *Cochrane Database Syst. Rev.* **2015**. Available online: https://www.cochranelibrary.com/cdsr/doi/10.1002/14651858.CD004250.pub5/abstract (accessed on 28 June 2015). [CrossRef] [PubMed]
15. Celenay, S.T.; Kaya, D.O.; Akbayrak, T. Cervical and scapulothoracic stabilization exercises with and without connective tissue massage for chronic mechanical neck pain: A prospective, randomised controlled trial. *Man. Ther.* **2016**, *21*, 144–150. [CrossRef] [PubMed]
16. Seo, Y.G.; Park, W.H.; Lee, C.S.; Kang, K.C.; Min, K.B.; Lee, S.M.; Yoo, J.C. Is Scapular Stabilization Exercise Effective for Managing Nonspecific Chronic Neck Pain?: A Systematic Review. *Asian Spine J.* **2020**, *14*, 122. [CrossRef]
17. Yildiz, T.I.; Turgut, E.; Duzgun, I. Neck and Scapula-Focused Exercise Training on Patients With Nonspecific Neck Pain: A Randomized Controlled Trial. *J. Sport Rehabil.* **2018**, *27*, 403–412. [CrossRef]
18. Thompson, D.; Oldham, J.; Woby, S. Does adding cognitive-behavioural physiotherapy to exercise improve outcome in patients with chronic neck pain? A randomised controlled trial. *Physiotherapy* **2016**, *102*, 170–177. [CrossRef]
19. Ylinen, J.; Takala, E.-P.; Nykänen, M.; Häkkinen, A.; Mälkiä, E.; Pohjolainen, T.; Karppi, S.-L.; Kautiainen, H.; Airaksinen, O. Active neck muscle training in the treatment of chronic neck pain in women: A randomized controlled trial. *JAMA* **2003**, *289*, 2509–2516. [CrossRef]
20. Bovim, G.; Schrader, H.; Sand, T. Neck pain in the general population. *Spine* **1994**, *19*, 1307–1309. [CrossRef]
21. Javdaneh, N.; Letafatkar, A.; Shojaedin, S.; Hadadnezhad, M. Scapular exercise combined with cognitive functional therapy is more effective at reducing chronic neck pain and kinesiophobia than scapular exercise alone: A randomized controlled trial. *Clin. Rehabil.* **2020**, *34*, 1485–1496. [CrossRef]
22. Javdaneh, N.; Molayei, F.; Kamranifraz, N. Effect of adding motor imagery training to neck stabilization exercises on pain, disability and kinesiophobia in patients with chronic neck pain. *Complement. Ther. Clin. Pr.* **2021**, *42*, 101263. [CrossRef] [PubMed]
23. Pool, J.J.; Ostelo, R.W.; Hoving, J.L.; Bouter, L.M.; De Vet, H.C. Minimal clinically important change of the Neck Disability Index and the Numerical Rating Scale for patients with neck pain. *Spine* **2007**, *32*, 3047–3051. [CrossRef]
24. Lee, J.-H.; Cynn, H.-S.; Choi, W.-J.; Jeong, H.-J.; Yoon, T.-L. Various shrug exercises can change scapular kinematics and scapular rotator muscle activities in subjects with scapular downward rotation syndrome. *Hum. Mov. Sci.* **2016**, *45*, 119–129. [CrossRef]
25. Singla, D.; Veqar, Z.; Hussain, M.E. Photogrammetric assessment of upper body posture using postural angles: A literature review. *J. Chiropr. Med.* **2017**, *16*, 131–138. [CrossRef] [PubMed]

26. Yoon, T.-L.; Kim, H.-N.; Min, J.-H. Validity and reliability of an inertial measurement Unit—Based 3-dimensional angular measurement of cervical range of motion. *J. Manip. Physiol. Ther.* **2019**, *42*, 75–81. [CrossRef]
27. Celenay, S.T.; Akbayrak, T.; Kaya, D.O. A comparison of the effects of stabilization exercises plus manual therapy to those of stabilization exercises alone in patients with nonspecific mechanical neck pain: A randomized clinical trial. *J. Orthop. Sports Phys. Ther.* **2016**, *46*, 44–55. [CrossRef] [PubMed]
28. Dusunceli, Y.; Ozturk, C.; Atamaz, F.; Hepguler, S.; Durmaz, B. Efficacy of neck stabilization exercises for neck pain: A randomized controlled study. *J. Rehabil. Med.* **2009**, *41*, 626–631. [CrossRef] [PubMed]
29. Chung, S.; Jeong, Y.-G. Effects of the craniocervical flexion and isometric neck exercise compared in patients with chronic neck pain: A randomized controlled trial. *Physiother. Theory Pract.* **2018**, *34*, 916–925. [CrossRef]
30. Medicine, A. *ACSM's Guidelines for Exercise Testing and Prescription*; Lippincott Williams & Wilkins: Philadelphia, PA, USA, 2013.
31. Ha, S.-M.; Kwon, O.-Y.; Yi, C.-H.; Cynn, H.-S.; Weon, J.-H.; Kim, T.-H. Effects of scapular upward rotation exercises on alignment of scapula and clavicle and strength of scapular upward rotators in subjects with scapular downward rotation syndrome. *J. Electromyogr. Kinesiol.* **2016**, *26*, 130–136. [CrossRef] [PubMed]
32. Ha, S.-M.; Kwon, O.-Y.; Cynn, H.-S.; Lee, W.-H.; Park, K.-N.; Kim, S.-H.; Jung, D.-Y. Comparison of electromyographic activity of the lower trapezius and serratus anterior muscle in different arm-lifting scapular posterior tilt exercises. *Phys. Ther. Sport* **2012**, *13*, 227–232. [CrossRef]
33. Ekstrom, R.A.; Donatelli, R.A.; Soderberg, G.L. Surface electromyographic analysis of exercises for the trapezius and serratus anterior muscles. *J. Orthop. Sports Phys. Ther.* **2003**, *33*, 247–258. [CrossRef]
34. Choi, W.-J.; Cynn, H.-S.; Lee, C.-H.; Jeon, H.-S.; Lee, J.-H.; Jeong, H.-J.; Yoon, T.-L. Shrug exercises combined with shoulder abduction improve scapular upward rotator activity and scapular alignment in subjects with scapular downward rotation impairment. *J. Electromyogr. Kinesiol.* **2015**, *25*, 363–370. [CrossRef]
35. Lynch, S.S.; Thigpen, C.A.; Mihalik, J.P.; Prentice, W.E.; Padua, D. The effects of an exercise intervention on forward head and rounded shoulder postures in elite swimmers. *Br. J. Sports Med.* **2010**, *44*, 376–381. [CrossRef] [PubMed]
36. Kaka, B.; Ogwumike, O.O. Effect of neck stabilization and dynamic exercises on pain, disability and fear avoidance beliefs in patients with non-specific neck pain. *Physiotherapy* **2015**, *101*, e704. [CrossRef]
37. Christian, G.F.; Stanton, G.J.; Sissons, D.; How, H.Y.; Jamison, J.; Alder, B.; Fullerton, M.; Funder, J.W. Immunoreactive ACTH, beta-endorphin, and cortisol levels in plasma following spinal manipulative therapy. *Spine* **1988**, *13*, 1411–1417. [CrossRef] [PubMed]
38. Ha, S.-M.; Kwon, O.-Y.; Yi, C.; Jeon, H.-S.; Lee, W.-H. Effects of passive correction of scapular position on pain, proprioception, and range of motion in neck-pain patients with bilateral scapular downward-rotation syndrome. *Man. Ther.* **2011**, *16*, 585–589. [CrossRef] [PubMed]
39. Lluch, E.; Arguisuelas, M.D.; Quesada, O.C.; Noguera, E.M.; Puchades, M.P.; Rodríguez, J.A.P.; Falla, D. Immediate effects of active versus passive scapular correction on pain and pressure pain threshold in patients with chronic neck pain. *J. Manip. Physiol. Ther.* **2014**, *37*, 660–666. [CrossRef] [PubMed]
40. Miller, J.; Gross, A.; D'Sylva, J.; Burnie, S.J.; Goldsmith, C.H.; Graham, N.; Haines, T.; Brønfort, G.; Hoving, J.L. Manual therapy and exercise for neck pain: A systematic review. *Man. Ther.* **2010**, *15*, 334–354. [CrossRef]
41. Ha, S.-M.; Kwon, O.-Y.; Park, K.-N. Effects of 6-week self-scapular upward rotation exercise on downward pulling tension in subjects with scapular downward rotation syndrome. *Phys. Ther. Korea* **2012**, *19*, 32–37. [CrossRef]
42. Struyf, F.; Nijs, J.; Mollekens, S.; Jeurissen, I.; Truijen, S.; Mottram, S.; Meeusen, R. Scapular-focused treatment in patients with shoulder impingement syndrome: A randomized clinical trial. *Clin. Rheumatol.* **2013**, *32*, 73–85. [CrossRef] [PubMed]
43. Helgadottir, H.; Kristjansson, E.; Mottram, S.; Karduna, A.; Jonsson, H., Jr. Altered alignment of the shoulder girdle and cervical spine in patients with insidious onset neck pain and Whiplash—Associated disorder. *J. Appl. Biomech.* **2011**, *27*, 181–191. [CrossRef] [PubMed]

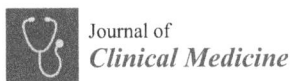

Article

Adiponectin Is a Contributing Factor of Low Appendicular Lean Mass in Older Community-Dwelling Women: A Cross-Sectional Study

Leonardo Augusto Costa Teixeira [1,2,3], Jousielle Marcia dos Santos [1,3,4], Adriana Netto Parentoni [1,3], Liliana Pereira Lima [1,3,4], Tamiris Campos Duarte [1,2], Franciane Pereira Brant [1,2], Camila Danielle Cunha Neves [1,4], Fabiana Souza Máximo Pereira [2,3,5], Núbia Carelli Pereira Avelar [6], Ana Lucia Danielewicz [6], Amanda Aparecida Oliveira Leopoldino [7], Sabrina Paula Costa [1,3], Arthur Nascimento Arrieiro [1,2], Luana Aparecida Soares [1,3], Ana Caroline Negreiros Prates [1,3], Juliana Nogueira Pontes Nobre [4], Alessandra de Carvalho Bastone [1,3], Vinicius Cunha de Oliveira [1,2,3], Murilo Xavier Oliveira [1,2,3], Pedro Henrique Scheidt Figueiredo [1,3], Henrique Silveira Costa [1,3], Vanessa Amaral Mendonça [1,2,3,4], Redha Taiar [8,*] and Ana Cristina Rodrigues Lacerda [1,2,3,4,*]

1. Physiotherapy Department, Federal University of Jequitinhonha and Mucuri Valleys, Diamantina 39803-371, Brazil
2. Postgraduate Program in Health Sciences (PPGCS), Federal University of Jequitinhonha and Mucuri Valleys (UFVJM), Diamantina 39803-371, Brazil
3. Postgraduate Program in Rehabilitation and Functional Performance (PPGReab), Federal University of Jequitinhonha and Mucuri Valleys, Diamantina 39803-371, Brazil
4. Postgraduate Multicenter Program in Physiological Sciences (PPGCF), Federal University of Jequitinhonha and Mucuri Valleys (UFVJM), Diamantina 39803-371, Brazil
5. Medicine School, University of Jequitinhonha and Mucuri Valleys (UFVJM), Diamantina 39803-371, Brazil
6. Department of Health Sciences, University of Santa Catarina (UFSC), Araranguá 88040-900, Brazil
7. Postgraduate Program in Health Sciences, Faculty of Medical Science of Minas (FCMMG), Belo Horizonte 30130-110, Brazil
8. MATériaux et Ingénierie Mécanique (MATIM), Université de Reims Champagne-Ardenne, 51100 Reims, France
* Correspondence: redha.taiar@univ-reims.fr (R.T.); lacerda.acr@ufvjm.edu.br (A.C.R.L.)

Abstract: Inflammaging is a chronic, sterile, low-grade inflammation that develops with advanced age in the absence of overt infection and may contribute to the pathophysiology of sarcopenia, a progressive and generalized skeletal muscle disorder. Furthermore, a series of biomarkers linked to sarcopenia occurrence have emerged. To aid diagnostic and treatment strategies for low muscle mass in sarcopenia and other related conditions, the objective of this work was to investigate potential biomarkers associated with appendicular lean mass in community-dwelling older women. This is a cross-sectional study with 71 older women (75 ± 7 years). Dual-energy X-ray absorptiometry was used to assess body composition. Plasmatic blood levels of adipokines (i.e., adiponectin, leptin, and resistin), tumor necrosis factor (TNF) and soluble receptors (sTNFr1 and sTNFr2), interferon (INF), brain-derived neurotrophic factor (BDNF), and interleukins (IL-2, IL-4, IL-5, IL-6, IL-8, and IL-10) were determined by enzyme-linked immunosorbent assay. Older women with low muscle mass showed higher plasma levels of adiponectin, sTNFr1, and IL-8 compared to the regular muscle mass group. In addition, higher adiponectin plasma levels explained 14% of the lower appendicular lean mass. High adiponectin plasmatic blood levels can contribute to lower appendicular lean mass in older, community-dwelling women.

Keywords: aging; appendicular muscle mass; inflammaging; biomarkers; adiponectin; sarcopenia

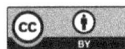

1. Introduction

According to the International Classification of Diseases (ICD-10-MC), sarcopenia is a gradual and generalized muscle disease that consists of the progressive loss of muscle mass, muscle strength, and/or physical function [1]. Older people with loss of muscle mass experience a marked decline in strength, and physical function [2]. Low muscle mass and function may result in a reduced quality of life, a loss of independence, a need for long-term care, an increased risk of falls and fractures, and mortality [1,2]. Cognitive impairment, fear of falling, depressive symptoms, a poor or fair self-perception of health, and inflammation are a few of the characteristics that might predispose a person to sarcopenia [3].

A continuous, sterile, low-grade inflammation known as "inflammaging" may contribute to the clinical symptoms of chronic diseases [4–6]. Thus, inflammaging can contribute to the etiology of sarcopenia and to the dysfunction of skeletal muscle tissue, establishing a vicious cycle of inflammation and muscle wasting [5]. High levels of interleukin-6 (IL-6), interleukin-8 (IL-8), tumor necrosis factor (TNF), interferon (IFN), granulocyte stimulating factor, high-temperature monocytes, and serine protease are frequently associated with deteriorated physical function, reduced muscle mass, and decreased muscular strength in older individuals [7].

Moreover, previous research has demonstrated a negative correlation between inflammatory biomarkers and chronic conditions [6]. In older people with sarcopenia, high levels of IL-6 and soluble tumor necrosis factor receptor 2 (sTNFr2) were reported [4]. Additionally, sarcopenia can affect the signaling pathway for adiponectin activation [8] to prevent muscle atrophy and inflammation while fostering muscle regeneration [8–10]. Despite the current literature indicating a link between biomarkers and sarcopenia, especially in women [8], few studies have used DXA to assess appendicular lean mass (ALM). With this regard, current literature often estimates lean mass indirectly or infers muscle mass using a muscular performance test. Since muscle and adipose tissue are related to the release of adipocytokines, it is imperative to assess them using the most recommended method [7–10]. Furthermore, few studies provide information on the association between muscle mass and a large panel of biomarkers analyzed simultaneously.

It is challenging to identify a single biomarker that can characterize sarcopenia due to the complex pathophysiology and the multiple pathways that cause muscle wasting and sarcopenia [4,8]. Therefore, the aims of the present study were: (1) To classify older community-dwelling women according to the ALM using dual-energy X-ray absorptiometry (DXA), one of the most recommended methods to assess the body composition, as with normal or low ALM. (2) To compare anthropometric parameters, muscle strength, and a broad panel of biomarkers (IL-2, IL-4, IL-5, IL-6, IL-8, IL-10, TNF, sTNFr1, sTNFr2, adiponectin, leptin, resistin, and BDNF) between older community-dwelling women groups stratified according to the ALM. (3) To investigate contributing factors to low ALM in older community-dwelling women. (4) To contribute to the development of strategies for early diagnosis and/or treatment of low muscle mass in sarcopenia and other conditions affected by muscle mass in older women.

2. Materials and Methods

2.1. Design

This cross-sectional study was approved by the Ethics Committee of the Universidade Federal dos Vales do Jequitinhonha e Mucuri (UFVJM) with number 1.461.306. All participants signed an informed consent form. The assessments were performed in the Laboratório de Fisiologia do Exercício (LAFIEX) and Laboratório de Inflamação e Metabolismo (LIM) of the UFVJM between June 2016 and June 2017.

2.2. Sample

To identify older women compatible with the assessment procedures, community-dwelling older women were recruited based on their registration at the Basic Health Units (BHU) in Diamantina, Minas Gerais, Brazil. All participants were visited at home and answered a questionnaire with information about their medical history, life habits, and comorbidities. The exclusion criteria were age (<65), cognitive decline evaluated by the Mini Mental State Examination [3], subjects unable to walk independently, hospitalized or had suffered fractures in the last three months, presence of neoplasm in the last five years, in palliative care, subjects that performed physical activity on a regular basis (more than three times a week), and subjects with severe visual and auditory impairment and with acute cardiorespiratory diseases.

2.3. Procedures

Three planned sessions included assessments. At first, they completed the clinical health interviews after signing the permission form, and the eligibility criteria were checked. On the newly scheduled day, the participants had examinations of their body composition in the morning while abstaining from food, liquids, and medicine. After a 15-min pause for rest and a standard meal, all participants started the handgrip strength test. To describe the inflammatory profile, blood samples were taken from the participants twenty-four hours after body composition [11].

2.4. Biomarker Assessment

Blood was drawn from the patient's upper limb through antecubital venipuncture and preserved in 10-mL heparin tubes. After collecting blood, the samples were centrifuged at 3000 rpm in a centrifuge for 10 min. Plasma samples were stored in the freezer $-80\ °C$ until the analysis. After six months of storage, the inflammatory blood profile was evaluated by measuring the plasma levels of biomarkers IL-2, IL-4, IL-5, IL-6, IL-8, IL-10, IFN, TNF, adiponectin, leptin, resistin, BDNF, and soluble receptors sTNFR1 and sTNFr2 by an immunoenzymatic technique (ELISA sandwich) (DuoSet, R&D Systems, Minneapolis, MN, USA) according to the manufacturer's instructions [11].

2.5. Muscle Stregth

Handgrip strength (HGS) was evaluated using a Jamar dynamometer®. The participants were instructed to stay seated, with a neutral fist, an elbow flexed 90 degrees, and a neutral shoulder. The HGS measure, i.e., an isometric contraction of the dominant hand applied on the handles of the dynamometer, was expressed in kilogram force (kgf). The mean of three measurements was used for analysis [2,12].

2.6. Body Composition

Body composition was measured using DXA with Encore Software 2005 (Lunar Radiation Corporation, Madison, WI, USA, model DPX). The same assessor performed all body composition evaluations in the morning. After screening by DXA at the ALM, total fat mass and total trunk mass were obtained.

2.7. Dependent Variable—Appendicular Muscle Mass

From the sum of the lean muscle masses of the arms and legs obtained by DXA, it was possible to determine the ALM [2,13]. According to the Foundation for the National Institutes of Health Sarcopenia Project (FNIH) [13] and European Working Group on Sarcopenia in Older People (EWGSOP 2018) [2] the criteria for the low appendicular muscle mass was less than 15.00 kg. The participants were classified into two groups: one with normal ALM and the other with low ALM.

2.8. Independent Variables

The following sixteen independent variables (total fat mass, trunk fat mass and biomarkers IL-2, IL-4, IL-5, IL-6, IL-8, IL-10, IFN, TNF, adiponectin, leptin, resistin, BDNF, sTNFR1, and sTNFr2) were included as possible independent factors associated with ALM.

2.9. Analyses

GPower software version 3.1.9.2, was used to calculate the sample size. We estimated the sample size from previous work, which found a correlation between adiponectin and sarcopenia of 0.24 and an effect size of 0.31 [14]. In addition, considering an alpha error of 5% and a power of 80%, a sample size of 71 old people was determined.

The Statistical Package for the Social Sciences, version 22.0 (SPSS Statistics; IBM, Armonk, NY, USA), and MedCalc Statistical Software, version 13.1 (MedCalc Software, Ostend, Belgium), were used to conduct statistical analyses. Data normality was verified by the Kolmogorov–Smirnov test. Continuous variables were expressed as the mean and standard deviation ($\pm$ SD). The *t*-test for parametric variables or Mann–Whitney-test for nonparametric variables were used to compare the mean differences of continuous variables among subjects with and without low ALM. Pearson or Spearman correlations analysis was used to investigate the relationship between ALM and anthropometric variables and biomarkers.

Univariate and stepwise multivariate linear regression were used to confirm the determinants of ALM. In each multivariate model adjusted for age, variables related to ALM in the univariate analysis ($p < 0.1$) were included. Four assumptions were used in the linear regression analysis: linearity, residual distribution, homoscedasticity, and the absence of multicollinearity. Scatter plots were used to assess the linearity of the independent variables and residuals, and a histogram was used to look at the distribution of residuals. The scatter plot confirmed the homoscedasticity, which was defined by the evenly distributed residuals in the regression line. The variance inflation factor (VIF) values below 10.0 were used to define the absence of multicollinearity. Additionally, the autocorrelation of the variables was verified by the Durbin–Watson test, and the values between 1.5 and 2.5 showed that there was no autocorrelation in the data. Statistical significance was set at 5%.

3. Results

Characteristics of Subjects

Four hundred and eleven elderly women were recruited based on their registration at the BHU. Of these, one hundred and ten addresses were not located, and thirty-one were not age-appropriate. Two hundred and seventy elderly women were interviewed in their homes, and one hundred and fourteen did not meet the inclusion criteria. One hundred and fifty-six older community-dwelling women were eligible for the evaluation procedures. Eighty-five elderly women did not complete all assessments, while seventy-one completed all procedures (Figure 1).

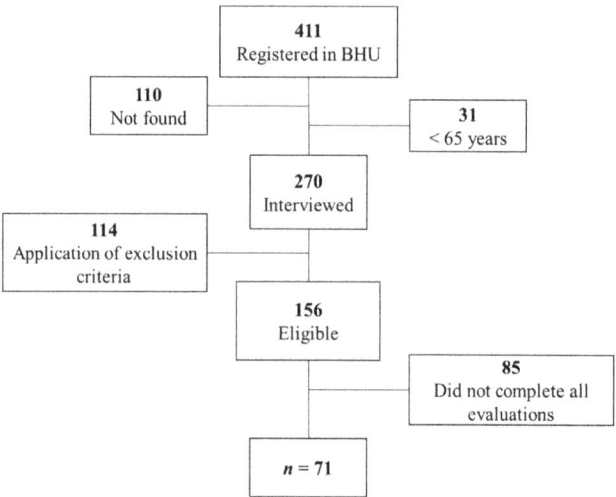

Figure 1. Sample recruitment flowchart. Abbreviations: BHU: basic health units.

Seventy-one older community-dwelling women (75 ± 7 years old) participated in the study. The characteristics of body composition, muscle strength, and biomarker plasma levels are presented in Table 1.

Table 1. Characteristics of older community-dwelling women. (n = 71).

	Mean (± SD)
Age (years)	75 (7)
Appendicular lean mass (kg)	14.38 (2.63)
Trunk fat mass (kg)	12.44 (4.29)
Total fat mass (kg)	23.01 (6.82)
HGS (kgf)	19.9 (6.38)
Adiponectin (µg/mL)	49.34 (6.94)
BDNF (µg/mL)	2.51 (0.93)
IFN (ng/mL)	1.56 (1.52)
IL 2 (ng/mL)	5.13 (8.51)
IL 4 (ng/mL)	2.39 (3.10)
IL 5 (ng/mL)	1.05 (1.21)
IL 6 (ng/mL)	17.45 (4.23)
IL 8 (ng/mL)	23.73 (9.03)
IL10 (ng/mL)	2.13 (3.40)
Leptin (µg/mL)	1.84 (0.27)
Resistin (µg/mL)	1.62 (0.35)
sTNFr1 (µg/mL)	3.93 (3.29)
sTNFr2 (µg/mL)	2.11 (0.48)
TNF (ng/mL)	1.31 (1.87)

Data presented as mean ± standard deviation (SD). Abbreviations: BDNF: brain-derived neurotrophic factor; HGS: handgrip strength; sTNFr1: soluble tumor necrosis factor receptor 1; sTNFr2: soluble tumor necrosis factor receptor 2; IFN: interferon; TNF: tumor necrosis factor; IL-10: interleukin-10; IL-5: interleukin-5; IL-4: interleukin-4; IL-2: interleukin-2. IL-6: interleukin-6; IL-8: interleukin-8.

The low ALM group presented lower values of trunk fat mass, total fat mass, and HGS. Furthermore, plasma levels of adiponectin, IL-8, and sTNFr1 were higher in the low ALM group compared to the normal ALM group ($p < 0.05$) (Table 2).

Table 2. Anthropometric variables, muscle strength, and biomarker blood levels stratified according to the appendicular lean mass in older community-dwelling women. (n = 71).

	Normal ALM (n = 22)	Low ALM (n = 49)	p-Value
Age (years)	73 (7)	75 (7)	0.19
ALM (kg)	17.49 (1.41)	12.98 (1.66)	<0.01 *
Trunk fat mass (kg)	16.73 (2.67)	10.52 (3.40)	<0.01 *
Total fat mass (kg)	29.87 (5.08)	19.92 (5.02)	<0.01 *
HGS (kgf)	25.38 (5.74)	17.47 (5.02)	<0.01 *
Adiponectin (µg/mL)	46.11 (9.61)	50.79 (4.78)	0.01 *
BDNF (µg/mL)	2.27 (0.83)	2.62 (0.97)	0.12
IFN (ng/mL)	1.46 (0.34)	1.61 (1.82)	0.25
IL-2 (ng/mL)	4.12 (0.39)	5.58 (10.25)	0.89
IL-4 (ng/mL)	1.98 (0.17)	2.57 (3.73)	0.21

Table 2. *Cont.*

	Normal ALM (n = 22)	Low ALM (n = 49)	p-Value
IL-5 (ng/mL)	0.74 (0.16)	1.20 (1.44)	0.17
IL-6 (ng/mL)	16.58 (2.81)	17.84 (4.70)	0.32
IL-8 (ng/mL)	20.71 (4.75)	25.08 (10.15)	0.01 *
IL-10 (ng/mL)	1.59 (0.30)	2.37 (4.08)	0.46
Leptin (μg/mL)	1.90 (0.20)	1.81 (0.29)	0.47
Resistin (μg/mL)	1.59 (0.34)	1.64 (0.36)	0.55
sTNFr1 (μg/mL)	2.74 (2.62)	4.46 (3.45)	0.03 *
sTNFr2 (μg/mL)	1.98 (0.41)	2.17 (0.51)	0.23
TNF (ng/mL)	1.06 (0.17)	1.43 (2.25)	0.14

Data presented as mean ± standard deviation (SD). Abbreviations: ALM = appendicular lean mass; BDNF = brain-derived neurotrophic factor; HGS: handgrip strength; Stnfr1 = soluble tumor necrosis factor receptor 1; STNFr2 = soluble tumor necrosis factor receptor 2; IFN = interferon; TNF = tumor necrosis factor; IL-10 = interleukin-10; IL-5 = interleukin-5; IL-4 = interleukin-4; IL-2 = interleukin-2. IL-6 = interleukin-6; IL-8 = interleukin-8. Note: * p-value < 0.05.

There was a significant positive correlation between ALM and trunk fat mass (r = 0.78; $p < 0.01$) and a significant negative correlation between ALM and adiponectin (r = −0.26; p = 0.03), IL-8 (r = −0.26; p = 0.03), and sTNFr-1 (r = −0.25; p = 0.04) (Table 3). In univariate regression analyses, having ALM as a dependent variable revealed that the blood adiponectin, sTNFr1, and IL-8 levels were negatively associated with ALM in older women. In multivariate analyses, including trunk fat mass and biomarkers as independent variables, the trunk fat mass and adiponectin composed the model that better explained the ALM. Therefore, in clinical terms, total trunk fat and adiponectin predicted ALM in community-dwelling older women. Overall, these outcomes explained 65% (β = 0.76; adjusted R^2 = 0.65; p = 0.001) of the ALM, and adiponectin explained 14% of the ALM variability (β = −0.39; R^2 = −0.14; p < 0.01) of community-dwelling older women (Table 3).

Table 3. Independent contributors to appendicular lean mass in community-dwelling older women (n = 71).

Independent Variables	r	Univariate			Multivariate		p-Value
		R^2 Adjusted	β	p-Value	R^2 Adjusted	β	
Trunk fat mass	0.78 ± 0.01	0.58	0.76	<0.01 *	0.65	0.76	0.001 *
Adiponectin	−0.26 ± 0.03	0.14	−0.39	0.001 *			
IL-8	−0.26 ± 0.03	0.03	−0.22	0.06			NS
sTNFr-1	−0.25 ± 0.04	0.05	−0.26	0.03 *			NS

B: beta coefficient; r: coefficient of Spearman correlation; R2 adjusted: adjusted coefficient of determination. BDNF: brain-derived neurotrophic factor; STNFR1: soluble tumor necrosis factor receptor 1; IL-8: interleukin-8. NS: non significance. Note: * p-value < 0.05.

4. Discussion

To our knowledge, this is the first study to assess the association between appendicular muscle mass using DXA and a broad panel of blood biomarkers related to sarcopenia. In our screening, low appendicular muscle mass or the risk of sarcopenia was present in 69% of the community-dwelling older women. Handgrip strength (HGS), total fat mass, and trunk fat mass were significantly lower in the low ALM group. Regarding biomarkers, plasma levels of adiponectin, sTNFr1, and IL-8 were higher in the low ALM group and demonstrated an association with adiponectin, sTNFr1, and IL-8 with ALM. In clinical terms, community-dwelling older women with less muscle mass had higher blood levels of these biomarkers (Table 2). Of note, our post-hoc analysis from linear multiple regression (correlation coefficient of 0.26 between ALM and adiponectin) revealed a large effect size of 0.35 and a power of 0.85 [14].

Noteworthy, older women with low ALM also presented low HGS, as in cases of confirmed sarcopenia [1,2,14,15]. There is still debate concerning the relationship between biomarkers and sarcopenia [4,5,7,8,10,16,17]. This is because once a skeletal muscle has become a secretory organ, inflammatory and muscle cells can work together to produce the myokines that induce sarcopenia [5,18,19].

There is growing evidence suggesting that chronic low-grade inflammation, or inflammation, could play a key role in the development of sarcopenia [4,5,7,10,15–18]. Thus, high blood level of proinflammatory biomarkers, including IL-6, IL-8, and IL-15, can affect skeletal muscle mass and are suggestive of inflammation, whereas high blood level of anti-inflammatory biomarkers, i.e., IL-4, IL-10, and IL-15 can counteract the generation and activity of proinflammatory cytokines and consequently the muscle atrophy and sarcopenia [5,10,17–22].

Among all evaluated biomarkers, adiponectin, IL-8, and sTNFr1 correlated negatively with ALM (Table 3). It is unclear whether IL-8, a chemotactic factor that leads to inflammation, contributes to sarcopenia [10,23]. As seen in cachexia and frailty, higher levels of IL-8 indicate a more prepared and active innate immune response [24]. The findings of the present study reinforce a previous work, including older people from the United Kingdom, which demonstrated the effect between higher levels of IL-8, and lower ALM, i.e., subjects with higher risk of sarcopenia [25].

Thus, the findings of the study are consistent with studies that found an increase in sTNFr1 blood levels to be negatively linked to muscle mass parameters [26]. Furthermore, over a five-year period, computed tomography as well as the Jamar dynamometer revealed a significant link between increased sTNFr1 blood levels and loss of muscle mass and strength [26]. However, Lustosa et al. (2017) found greater sTNFr1 blood levels in older individuals who were not sarcopenic [27]. In this sense, as the connection between sTNFr1 and sarcopenia or low muscle mass remains unclear, further research is needed.

Sarcopenia is linked to the adipokines, i.e., leptin and adiponectin [16], which are secreted by adipose and musculoskeletal tissues [10]. Currently, it is unclear whether leptin and muscle mass or sarcopenia interact [5,10,28]. As far as we know, leptin blood levels have proinflammatory effects [29]. The study by Li et al. (2019), which included older sarcopenic and nonsarcopenic individuals, showed that sarcopenic individuals had considerably higher leptin blood levels, which were linked to the severity and risk of sarcopenia [30]. In accordance, Kohara et al. (2011) observed that high leptin blood levels are greater in individuals with sarcopenia and visceral obesity than in individuals with only one condition, suggesting that leptin blood levels are associated with sarcopenia, independent of visceral fat [31]. Although leptin blood levels were lower in the low ALM group in our sample, this difference was not statistically significant.

A biomarker with antidiabetic, anti-inflammatory, and antiatherogenic properties is adiponectin [8,16,32]. It is produced by skeletal muscle and adipose tissue, has metabolic effects primarily in the liver and skeletal muscle, and modulates inflammatory processes by preventing the production of proinflammatory markers, including IL-6, IL-18, and TNF- [16,32,33]. A positive muscle function regulator also directly produces injured fibers and triggers the metabolism of muscle cells [8,9,31–33].

According to a meta-analysis, including seven studies, those with sarcopenia ($n = 557$) were more likely to have higher levels of adiponectin [8]. In addition, the prevalence of sarcopenia was reported to differ between men and women, and meta-regression analysis revealed an important role for females in explaining the association between sarcopenia and adiponectin, suggesting that women have higher levels of adiponectin than men, as they seem to express more plasma adiponectin than men, regardless of fat mass and BMI, due to the influence of sex hormones [8]. However, adiponectin blood levels in studies using DXA did not differ significantly between subgroups in analysis [8]. In another line, our findings are consistent with the results of Rossi et al. (2019), who compared the inflammatory profile of the Brazilian seniors and observed that the sarcopenic group had a higher concentration of adiponectin [16]. Although increased adiponectin levels in sarcopenia are still being studied [4,5,8,10,16], some possible mechanisms have been proposed to explain the peculiarity: down-regulation of adiponectin receptor signaling [8,32], deposition of adipose tissue in muscles that may influence adiponectin expression [8,34], and activation of catabolism related to the presence of other comorbidities [8,33]. Of note, adiponectin blood level was significantly higher in the low ALM group in our sample and was inversely associated with ALM ($r = -0.259$; $p = 0.02$) explaining 14% of the ALM variability ($\beta = -0.39$; $R^2 = -0.14$; $p < 0.00$), occurring independently of the total fat mass or trunk fat mass.

Therapeutic targets for the treatment of sarcopenia might include anti-inflammatory cytokines [5,33]. It is generally agreed upon that regulating IL-6 levels may be a therapeutic approach to keep skeletal muscle healthy [5,33,35]. Considering the evidence of adiponectin's anti-inflammatory and regenerative role, our findings point to it as a potential biomarker linked to muscle damage brought on by low ALM and encourage more study into diagnostics and therapy.

The development of chronic inflammation and sarcopenia may be influenced by adipose tissue, which can also lead to sarcopenia and sarcopenic obesity [10,16,35]. As a result, obese people who have more visceral subcutaneous adipose tissue are more likely to have greater levels of adiponectin, indicating that the distribution of adipose tissue also influences the release of adipokines [10,34]. Thus, understanding that body fat, especially trunk fat, is metabolically active and secretes inflammatory biomarkers, including adiponectin [34], it is important to highlight that the best model that explained the low appendicular muscle mass was adiponectin and the trunk fat mass (Table 3) in older community-dwelling women. In addition, to clarify the relationship between ALM, fat mass, and adiponectin, we evaluated additional models using adiponectin as a dependent variable, including total fat mass, total lean mass, and ALM as independent variables. Therefore, we found that ALM was the only significant predictor [$F (1, 69) = 12.79$; $p < 0.01$; $R^2 = 0.14$; $\beta = -0.39$], explaining 14% of adiponectin, reinforcing the association between muscle mass and adiponectin independently of body fat.

When the model of the analysis was adjusted for age, the results remained the same ($R = 0.80$; adjusted $R^2 = 0.63$; $p < 0.001$), suggesting that trunk fat mass and adiponectin are possible predictors of appendicular muscle mass in older community-dwelling women. Thus, our findings together allow us to speculate on the involvement of adiponectin in the modulation of inflammatory control and ALM, influencing positively the balance between the anti-inflammatory (IFN, IL-4, IL-5, and IL-10) and proinflammatory biomarkers (IL-2, IL-6, sTNFr2, and TNF) in community-dwelling older women. However, the biomarkers were dosed systemically in our group, but possibly future research that measures the biomarkers directly in the muscle would provide more illuminating results. More research advances are needed to explore whether there is a cause-effect relationship in the interaction between muscle and biomarkers.

Notably, there was no difference in the clinical, sociodemographic, cultural, or functional variables between the older, normal, and low ALM groups, showing there was no data interpretation bias. The present study's stronger points were its methodological rigor, use of one of the most recommended methods to measure body composition, participants fasting prior to body composition and blood level assessments, the blinding of the evaluators to the DXA and strength test, as well as the rigor in the exclusion criteria used.

The contribution of the present study is to show that high levels of adiponectin are associated with lower appendicular muscle mass in community-dwelling elderly women. The practical implications of this study are as follows: (1) Older women with lower ALM assessed by DXA also have lower HGS. Low levels of these clinical features are directly associated with sarcopenia in older women; (2) higher adiponectin levels were associated with lower appendicular muscle mass among community-dwelling older women; (3) contribution to clinical or public health strategies aimed at early assessment and diagnosis of sarcopenia and other diseases related to low muscle mass in old women. The limitation of this study was the short observation time (cross-sectional study); only older community-dwelling women were investigated; our findings should not be extrapolated to the population of clinical settings, long-term care facilities, or hospital environments; and we did not assess a cutoff point for adiponectin to predict ALM. Future studies that determine a cutoff point for adiponectin based on ALM in both sexes may further enhance our understanding of the association of these variables with sarcopenia.

5. Conclusions

High adiponectin levels in the blood contribute to lower ALM in community-dwelling older women. Therefore, initiatives for the diagnosis and treatment of sarcopenia in community-dwelling older women may focus on this adipokine as a possible biomarker of sarcopenia.

Author Contributions: Conceptualization, L.A.C.T., A.N.P., T.C.D., F.P.B. and A.C.R.L.; methodology, L.A.C.T., A.N.P., T.C.D., F.P.B., C.D.C.N., V.A.M. and A.C.R.L.; software, L.A.C.T. and P.H.S.F.; validation, L.A.C.T. and L.P.L.; formal analysis, L.A.C.T., J.M.d.S., L.P.L., V.A.M. and A.C.R.L.; investigation, L.A.C.T., J.M.d.S., A.N.P., L.P.L., T.C.D., F.P.B., C.D.C.N., V.A.M. and A.C.R.L.; resources, A.N.P., V.A.M. and A.C.R.L.; data curation, L.A.C.T., J.M.d.S., A.N.P., L.P.L., T.C.D., F.P.B., C.D.C.N., N.C.P.A., V.A.M. and A.C.R.L.; writing—original draft preparation, L.A.C.T., J.M.d.S., A.N.P., L.P.L., F.P.B., L.A.S., V.A.M. and A.C.R.L.; writing—review and editing, A.N.P., N.C.P.A., A.A.O.L., S.P.C., V.A.M. and A.C.R.L.; visualization, J.M.d.S., A.N.P., L.P.L., F.P.B., F.S.M.P., N.C.P.A., A.L.D., A.A.O.L., S.P.C., A.N.A., L.A.S., A.C.N.P., R.T., J.N.P.N., A.d.C.B., V.C.d.O., M.X.O., P.H.S.F., H.S.C., V.A.M. and A.C.R.L.; supervision, A.N.P., V.A.M. and A.C.R.L.; project administration, A.N.P., V.A.M. and A.C.R.L.; funding acquisition, A.N.P., R.T., A.d.C.B., V.C.d.O., M.X.O., V.A.M. and A.C.R.L. All authors have read and agreed to the published version of the manuscript.

Funding: This study was supported by the Fundação de Amparo a Pesquisa do Estado de Minas Gerais (FAPEMIG), the Conselho Nacional de Desenvolvimento Científico e Tecnológico (Universal CNPq-402574/2021-4), and the Coordenação de Aperfeiçoamento de Pessoal de Nível Superior (CAPES).

Institutional Review Board Statement: The study was conducted according to the guidelines of the Declaration of Helsinki and was approved by the Institutional Ethics and Research Committee of Federal University of Jequitinhonha and Mucuri Valleys (protocol code 1.461.306 on 22 March 2016).

Informed Consent Statement: Informed consent was obtained from all subjects involved in the study.

Data Availability Statement: The data presented in this study are available upon request from the corresponding author. The data are not publicly available due to the privacy guarantee of the data collected individually.

Acknowledgments: The authors are grateful to the old women participants as study volunteers, and the professionals from the Health Department and the Basic Health Units of the municipality of Diamantina, Minas Gerais, for assisting in the conduct of recruitment and facilitating contact with the elderly population of the sample.

Conflicts of Interest: The authors declare no conflict of interest.

References

1. Baumgartner, R.N.; Koehler, K.M.; Gallagher, D.; Romero, L.; Heymsfield, S.B.; Ross, R.R.; Garry, P.J.; Lindeman, R.D. Epidemiology of Sarcopenia among the Elderly in New Mexico. *Am. J. Epidemiol.* **1998**, *147*, 755–763. [CrossRef] [PubMed]
2. Cruz-Jentoft, A.J.; Bahat, G.; Bauer, J.; Boirie, Y.; Bruyère, O.; Cederholm, T.; Cooper, C.; Landi, F.; Rolland, Y.; Sayer, A.A.; et al. Sarcopenia: Revised European consensus on definition and diagnosis. *Age Ageing* **2019**, *48*, 16–31. [CrossRef] [PubMed]
3. de Souza, L.F.; Fontanela, L.C.; Gonçalves, C.; Mendrano, A.L.; Freitas, M.A.; Danielewicz, A.L.; de Avelar, N.C.P. Cognitive and behavioral factors associated to probable sarcopenia in community-dwelling older adults. *Exp. Aging Res.* **2021**, *48*, 150–163. [CrossRef] [PubMed]
4. Curcio, F.; Ferro, G.; Basile, C.; Liguori, I.; Parrella, P.; Pirozzi, F.; Della-Morte, D.; Gargiulo, G.; Testa, G.; Tocchetti, C.G.; et al. Biomarkers in sarcopenia: A multifactorial approach. *Exp. Gerontol.* **2016**, *85*, 1–8. [CrossRef] [PubMed]
5. Pan, L.; Xie, W.; Fu, X.; Lu, W.; Jin, H.; Lai, J.; Zhang, A.; Yu, Y.; Li, Y.; Xiao, W. Inflammation and sarcopenia: A focus on circulating inflammatory cytokines. *Exp. Gerontol.* **2021**, *154*, 111544. [CrossRef] [PubMed]

6. Arrieiro, A.N.; Soares, L.A.; Prates, A.C.N.; Figueiredo, P.H.S.; Costa, H.S.; Simão, A.P.; Neves, C.D.C.; dos Santos, J.M.; Santos, L.M.D.M.; Avelar, N.C.P.; et al. Inflammation Biomarkers Are Independent Contributors to Functional Performance in Chronic Conditions: An Exploratory Study. *Int. J. Med. Sci. Health Res.* **2021**, *5*, 30–37. [CrossRef]
7. Argilés, J.M.; Campos, N.; Lopez-Pedrosa, J.M.; Rueda, R.; Rodriguez-Mañas, L. Skeletal Muscle Regulates Metabolism via Interorgan Crosstalk: Roles in Health and Disease. *J. Am. Med. Dir. Assoc.* **2016**, *17*, 789–796. [CrossRef]
8. Komici, K.; Iacono, A.D.; De Luca, A.; Perrotta, F.; Bencivenga, L.; Rengo, G.; Rocca, A.; Guerra, G. Adiponectin and Sarcopenia: A Systematic Review with Meta-Analysis. *Front. Endocrinol.* **2021**, *12*, 576619. [CrossRef]
9. Fiaschi, T.; Tedesco, F.S.; Giannoni, E.; Diaz-Manera, J.; Parri, M.; Cossu, G.; Chiarugi, P. Globular Adiponectin as a Complete Mesoangioblast Regulator: Role in Proliferation, Survival, Motility, and Skeletal Muscle Differentiation. *Mol. Biol. Cell* **2010**, *21*, 848–859. [CrossRef]
10. Wang, T. Searching for the link between inflammaging and sarcopenia. *Ageing Res. Rev.* **2022**, *77*, 101611. [CrossRef]
11. Neves, C.D.; Lage, V.K.; Lima, L.P.; Matos, M.A.; Vieira, L.; Teixeira, A.L.; Figueiredo, P.H.; Costa, H.S.; Lacerda, A.C.R.; Mendonça, V.A. Inflammatory and oxidative biomarkers as determinants of functional capacity in patients with COPD assessed by 6-min walk test-derived outcomes. *Exp. Gerontol.* **2021**, *152*, 111456. [CrossRef] [PubMed]
12. Dias, J.A.; Ovando, A.C.; Külkamp, W.; Junior, N.G.B. Hand grip strength: Evaluation methods and factors influencing this measure. *Rev. Bras. De Cineantropometria E Desempenho Hum.* **2010**, *12*, 209–216.
13. Studenski, S.A.; Peters, K.W.; Alley, D.E.; Cawthon, P.M.; McLean, R.R.; Harris, T.B.; Ferrucci, L.; Guralnik, J.M.; Fragala, M.S.; Kenny, A.M.; et al. The FNIH Sarcopenia Project: Rationale, Study Description, Conference Recommendations, and Final Estimates. *J. Gerontol. A Biol. Sci. Med. Sci.* **2014**, *69*, 547–558. [CrossRef] [PubMed]
14. Can, B.; Kara, O.; Kizilarslanoglu, M.C.; Arik, G.; Aycicek, G.S.; Sumer, F.; Civelek, R.; Demirtas, C.; Ulger, Z. Serum markers of inflammation and oxidative stress in sarcopenia. *Aging Clin. Exp. Res.* **2016**, *29*, 745–752. [CrossRef]
15. Rossi, F.E.; Lira, F.S.; Silva, B.S.A.; Freire, A.P.C.F.; Ramos, E.M.C.; Gobbo, L.A. Influence of skeletal muscle mass and fat mass on the metabolic and inflammatory profile in sarcopenic and non-sarcopenic overfat elderly. *Aging* **2018**, *31*, 629–635. [CrossRef]
16. Parentoni, A.N.; Lustosa, L.P.; Dos Santos, K.D.; Sá, L.F.; Ferreira, F.O.; Mendonça, V.A. Comparação da força muscular respiratória entre os subgrupos de fragilidade em idosas da comunidade. *Fisioter. E Pesqui.* **2013**, *20*, 361–366. [CrossRef]
17. Peake, J.M.; Della Gatta, P.; Suzuki, K.; Nieman, D.C. Cytokine expression and secretion by skeletal muscle cells: Regulatory mechanisms and exercise effects. *Exerc. Immunol. Rev.* **2015**, *21*, 8–25.
18. Pedersen, B.K.; Febbraio, M.A. Muscle as an Endocrine Organ: Focus on Muscle-Derived Interleukin-6. *Physiol. Rev.* **2008**, *88*, 1379–1406. [CrossRef]
19. Pedersen, B.K.; Fischer, C. Physiological roles of muscle-derived interleukin-6 in response to exercise. *Curr. Opin. Clin. Nutr. Metab. Care* **2007**, *10*, 265–271. [CrossRef]
20. Hofmann, S.; Rösen-Wolff, A.; Tsokos, G.; Hedrich, C. Biological properties and regulation of IL-10 related cytokines and their contribution to autoimmune disease and tissue injury. *Clin. Immunol.* **2012**, *143*, 116–127. [CrossRef]
21. Heredia, J.E.; Mukundan, L.; Chen, F.M.; Mueller, A.A.; Deo, R.C.; Locksley, R.M.; Rando, T.A.; Chawla, A. Type 2 Innate Signals Stimulate Fibro/Adipogenic Progenitors to Facilitate Muscle Regeneration. *Cell* **2013**, *153*, 376–388. [CrossRef]
22. Harada, A.; Sekido, N.; Akahoshi, T.; Wada, T.; Mukaida, N.; Matsushima, K. Essential involvement of interleukin-8 (IL-8) in acute inflammation. *J. Leukoc. Biol.* **1994**, *56*, 559–564. [CrossRef]
23. Wilson, D.; Jackson, T.; Sapey, E.; Lord, J.M. Frailty and sarcopenia: The potential role of an aged immune system. *Ageing Res. Rev.* **2017**, *36*, 1–10. [CrossRef] [PubMed]
24. Westbury, L.D.; Fuggle, N.R.; Syddall, H.E.; Duggal, N.A.; Shaw, S.C.; Maslin, K.; Dennison, E.M.; Lord, J.M.; Cooper, C. Relationships Between Markers of Inflammation and Muscle Mass, Strength and Function: Findings from the Hertfordshire Cohort Study. *Calcif. Tissue Res.* **2017**, *102*, 287–295. [CrossRef] [PubMed]
25. Singh, T.; Newman, A.B. Inflammatory markers in population studies of aging. *Ageing Res. Rev.* **2011**, *10*, 319–329. [CrossRef] [PubMed]
26. Schaap, L.A.; Pluijm, S.M.F.; Deeg, D.J.H.; Harris, T.B.; Kritchevsky, S.; Newman, A.B.; Colbert, L.H.; Pahor, M.; Rubin, S.M.; Tylavsky, F.A.; et al. Higher Inflammatory Marker Levels in Older Persons: Associations With 5-Year Change in Muscle Mass and Muscle Strength. *J. Gerontol. Ser. A* **2009**, *64*, 1183–1189. [CrossRef]
27. Lustosa, L.P.; Batista, P.P.; Pereira, D.S.; Pereira, L.S.M.; Scianni, A.; Ribeiro-Samora, G.A. Comparison between parameters of muscle performance and inflammatory biomarkers of non-sarcopenic and sarcopenic elderly women. *Clin. Interv. Aging* **2017**, *12*, 1183–1191. [CrossRef]
28. Abella, V.; Scotece, M.; Conde, J.; Pino, J.; Gonzalez-Gay, M.A.; Gómez-Reino, J.J.; Mera, A.; Lago, F.; Gómez, R.; Gualillo, O. Leptin in the interplay of inflammation, metabolism and immune system disorders. *Nat. Rev. Rheumatol.* **2017**, *13*, 100–109. [CrossRef]
29. Li, C.-W.; Yu, K.; Shyh-Chang, N.; Li, G.-X.; Jiang, L.-J.; Yu, S.-L.; Xu, L.-Y.; Liu, R.-J.; Guo, Z.-J.; Xie, H.-Y.; et al. Circulating factors associated with sarcopenia during ageing and after intensive lifestyle intervention. *J. Cachexia-Sarcopenia Muscle* **2019**, *10*, 586–600. [CrossRef]
30. Kohara, K.; Ochi, M.; Tabara, Y.; Nagai, T.; Igase, M.; Miki, T. Leptin in Sarcopenic Visceral Obesity: Possible Link between Adipocytes and Myocytes. *PLoS ONE* **2011**, *6*, e24531. [CrossRef]

31. Fiaschi, T.; Cirelli, D.; Comito, G.; Gelmini, S.; Ramponi, G.; Serio, M.; Chiarugi, P. Globular adiponectin induces differentiation and fusion of skeletal muscle cells. *Cell Res.* **2009**, *19*, 584–597. [CrossRef] [PubMed]
32. Wolf, A.M.; Wolf, D.; Rumpold, H.; Enrich, B.; Tilg, H. Adiponectin induces the anti-inflammatory cytokines IL-10 and IL-1RA in human leukocytes. *Biochem. Biophys. Res. Commun.* **2004**, *323*, 630–635. [CrossRef] [PubMed]
33. Belizário, J.E.; Fontes-Oliveira, C.C.; Borges, J.P.; Kashiabara, J.A.; Vannier, E. Skeletal muscle wasting and renewal: A pivotal role of myokine IL-6. *SpringerPlus* **2016**, *5*, 619. [CrossRef]
34. Guenther, M.; James, R.; Marks, J.; Zhao, S.; Szabo, A.; Kidambi, S. Adiposity distribution influences circulating adiponectin levels. *Transl. Res.* **2014**, *164*, 270–277. [CrossRef] [PubMed]
35. Sell, H.; Habich, C.; Eckel, J. Adaptive immunity in obesity and insulin resistance. *Nat. Rev. Endocrinol.* **2012**, *8*, 709–716. [CrossRef] [PubMed]

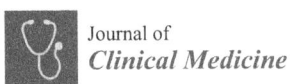

Review

The Effect of Pressotherapy on Performance and Recovery in the Management of Delayed Onset Muscle Soreness: A Systematic Review and Meta-Analysis

Paweł Wiśniowski [1], Maciej Cieśliński [1], Martyna Jarocka [1], Przemysław Seweryn Kasiak [2], Bartłomiej Makaruk [1], Wojciech Pawliczek [1] and Szczepan Wiecha [1,*]

[1] Department of Physical Education and Health in Biala Podlaska, Faculty in Biala Podlaska, Jozef Pilsudski University of Physical Education in Warsaw, 21-500 Biala Podlaska, Poland; pawel.wisniowski@awf.edu.pl (P.W.); maciej.cieslinski@awf.edu.pl (M.C.); martyna.jarocka@awf.edu.pl (M.J.); bartlomiej.makaruk@awf.edu.pl (B.M.); wojciech.pawliczek@awf.edu.pl (W.P.)
[2] Students' Scientific Group of Lifestyle Medicine, 3rd Department of Internal Medicine Cardiology, Medical University of Warsaw, 02-091 Warsaw, Poland; przemyslaw.kasiak1@gmail.com
* Correspondence: szczepan.wiecha@awf.edu.pl; Tel.: +48-833-428-823

Abstract: Background: It has been demonstrated that pressotherapy used post-exercise (Po-E) can influence training performance, recovery, and physiological properties. This study examined the effectiveness of pressotherapy on the following parameters. Methods: The systematic review and meta-analysis were performed according to PRISMA guidelines. A literature search of MEDLINE, PubMed, EBSCO, Web of Science, SPORTDiscus, and ClinicalTrials has been completed up to March 2021. Inclusion criteria were: randomized control trials (RCTs) or cross-over studies, mean participant age between 18 and 65 years, ≥1 exercise mechanical pressotherapy intervention. The risk of bias was assessed by the Cochrane risk-of-bias tool for RCT (RoB 2.0). Results: 12 studies comprised of 322 participants were selected. The mean sample size was $n = 25$. Pressotherapy significantly reduced muscle soreness (Standard Mean Difference; SMD = -0.33; CI = -0.49, -0.18; $p < 0.0001$; $I^2 = 7\%$). Pressotherapy did not significantly affect jump height (SMD = -0.04; CI = -0.36, -0.29; $p = 0.82$). Pressotherapy did not significantly affect creatine kinase level 24–96 h after DOMS induction (SMD = 0.41; CI = -0.07, 0.89; $p = 0.09$; $I^2 = 63\%$). Conclusions: Only moderate benefits of using pressotherapy as a recovery intervention were observed (mostly for reduced muscle soreness), although, pressotherapy did not significantly influence exercise performance. Results differed between the type of exercise, study population, and applied treatment protocol. Pressotherapy should only be incorporated as an additional component of a more comprehensive recovery strategy. Study PROSPERO registration number—CRD42020189382.

Keywords: pressotherapy; compression; regeneration; DOMS

Citation: Wiśniowski, P.; Cieśliński, M.; Jarocka, M.; Kasiak, P.S.; Makaruk, B.; Pawliczek, W.; Wiecha, S. The Effect of Pressotherapy on Performance and Recovery in the Management of Delayed Onset Muscle Soreness: A Systematic Review and Meta-Analysis. *J. Clin. Med.* **2022**, *11*, 2077. https://doi.org/10.3390/jcm11082077

Academic Editor: Antonio Frizziero

Received: 20 February 2022
Accepted: 28 March 2022
Published: 7 April 2022

Publisher's Note: MDPI stays neutral with regard to jurisdictional claims in published maps and institutional affiliations.

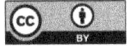

Copyright: © 2022 by the authors. Licensee MDPI, Basel, Switzerland. This article is an open access article distributed under the terms and conditions of the Creative Commons Attribution (CC BY) license (https://creativecommons.org/licenses/by/4.0/).

1. Introduction

Physical activity, especially at the competitive level, causes a lot of negative changes in the human body [1,2]. Inflammation occurs as a result of damage to muscle cells [3] from which creatine kinase (CK), lactate dehydrogenase, and metabolites are released [1,2]. In such cases, we observe decreased efficiency, faster muscle fatigue, a decrease in the range of motion (ROM), and the appearance of pain in places where they are overloaded [4,5]. This phenomenon is exacerbated especially with eccentric exercises (ECC) [6], in which intense exercise may cause Delayed Onset Muscle Soreness (DOMS) [7].

To increase exercise capacity as well as reduce the risk of injury, the key element is the use of training measures related to biological recovery to reduce metabolites to minimum values and to ensure the right amount of energy substrates, including ATP and phosphocreatine [8].

The most commonly used methods of biological recovery include treatments in the field of physical therapy (cold therapy, heat therapy, electrotherapy, compression therapy), manual therapy, massage (myofascial release and self-myofascial release), and pharmacology [9,10]. Of the above methods, in recent years much attention has been paid to compression therapy [11], in which the most frequent mention is External Pneumatic Compression (EPC) [12] as well as Intermittent Pneumatic Compression (IPC) [12]. This is especially seen in football, where over half of the players declared that the use of pressotherapy potentially accelerated regeneration [13].

Among the studies that used EPCs, a positive effect was found to increase flexibility and reduce muscle soreness (MS) [14,15], as well as reducing lymphoedema [16] and lactate [17]. The research conducted by Martin et al. (2015) showed that EPC did not statistically significantly affect the reduction of lactate after the 30-s Wingate test compared to the control group [17]. Similar relationships were found by Haun et al. (2017), in which they did not notice a statistical difference in muscle strength between the control group and the experimental group after resistance training in the form of back squats [11].

Using IPC has been reported to be effective in regeneration with short-term ECC efforts, reduction of fatigue [18], reduction of edema [19], improvement of local blood supply [20], and improvement in the ROM [12]. In subsequent studies, IPC was more effective at reducing high lactate levels than passive rest after exercise [21], and also statistically significantly reduced soft tissue stiffness after ECC training [19] and slightly reduced delayed post-exercise (Po-E) pain after short-term intense exercise [22].

Other studies have shown mitigating the effects of reducing muscle strength immediately after training [18] and improving the speed of a 400-m run [12].

This systematic review and meta-analysis aimed to examine the effectiveness of the pressotherapy to reduce DOMS after exercise. The primary endpoint was to assess pressotherapy the changes in MS and sports performance. The secondary endpoint is to establish the specific benefits on the selected outcomes of muscle functional capacities (e.g., strength, power), muscle damage markers (e.g., serum CK levels), joint ROM, and pain sensation.

2. Materials and Methods

The present review and meta-analysis were reported according to the Preferred Reporting Items for Systematic Reviews and Meta-Analyses (PRISMA) and follow the recommendations of the Cochrane Handbook for Systematic Reviews of Interventions [23]. The PRISMA 2020 statement: an updated guideline for reporting systematic reviews. Systematic Reviews [24].

2.1. Search Strategy and Screening Procedures

Searches were carried out on the following electronic databases: MEDLINE (PubMed and EBSCO), Web of Science, SPORT Discus. We did not have any limits and we searched all articles to March 2021 for studies aimed at determining the effect of pressotherapy on the magnitude and time course of Po-E muscle soreness and sports performance and recovery following exercise-induced muscle damage. We also searched current information about registers and reports in ClinicalTrials.gov. Additionally, we carried out a manual search of the bibliography of the included works and tracked their citations in the Scholar database. We head the same keywords as in databases. There were no associated publications, reports, or registers.

The search algorithm was conducted using PICO's strategy [23] (type of studies, participants, interventions, comparators, and outcome assessment) and combined Medical Subject Headings, free-terms, and matching synonyms of the following related words: (1) population: healthy adults, "middle-aged", "young adults"; (2) intervention: external assisted mechanical therapy, "external counterpulsation", "lymphatic drainage", "pressotherapy", "intermittent pneumatic compression", "pneumatic compression", "pneumatic therapy", "intermittent compression", "compression therapy", "compression massage", "pneumatic massage"); (3) outcome: "Soreness", "DOMS", "inflammation", "muscle fatigue", "recovery", "Delayed Onset Muscle Soreness", "EIMD", "hyperalgesia", "allodynia", "myalgia"; and (4) comparator: control conditions; RCT's studies and cross-over. In addition, we searched the citations included in the identified publications deemed eligible for our study.

2.2. Inclusion Criteria

Those studies in which the title and abstract were related to the aim of the present review were included for full-text request. We included studies that (1) were conducted as randomized control trials (RCT) and cross-over designs; (2) included a mean participant age between 18 and 65 years old. (3) Healthy adults with exercise-induced muscle damage regardless of their level of sports activity and performance (4) were based on at least one exercise intervention described as "External assisted mechanical therapy" (machines).

2.3. Exclusion Criteria

Studies were excluded if (1) outcome measurements were not reported as DOMS max values, or (2) they were not written in English. A third reviewer (SW) resolved cases of initial reviewer disagreement. Nonrandomized experiments, observational studies, secondary studies (any types of evidence syntheses), and opinion pieces (e.g., narrative reviews, editorials) were excluded too.

2.4. Selection Process, Data Collection, Data Extraction, and Management

Two initial reviewers (MJ and MC) independently examined the titles and abstracts of retrieved articles to identify suitable studies and extracted the following information from the included studies: First author's name and year of publication; study design; characteristics of the participants included; mean age; sample size and percentage of female subjects; weekly frequency, period and modality of External assisted mechanical therapy intervention; the reported measurement of Muscle functional capacities (e.g., strength, power), Muscle damage markers (e.g. serum CK levels), Joint ROM, and pain sensation. A third reviewer (SW) resolved cases of author disagreement.

2.5. Risk of Bias Assessment

The risk of bias of RCTs was assessed using the Cochrane risk-of-bias tool for randomized trials (RoB 2.0) [25], in which five domains were evaluated: Randomization process, deviations from intended interventions, missing outcome data, measurement of the outcome, and selection of the reported result. Each domain was assessed for risk of bias. Studies were graded as (1) "low risk of bias" when a low risk of bias was determined for all domains; (2) "some concerns" if at least one domain was assessed as raising some concerns but not at a high risk of bias for any single domain; or (3) "high risk of bias" when a high risk of bias was reached for at least one domain or the studied judgment included some concerns in multiple domains [24]. Assessment for individual randomized, parallel-group trials is presented in Figure 1. For pre-post studies and non-RCTs we used the Quality Assessment Tool for Quantitative Studies [25], in which seven domains were evaluated: Selection bias, study design, confounders, blinding, data collection methods, withdrawals, and dropouts. Each domain was considered strong, moderate, or weak. Studies were classified as "low risk of bias" if they presented no weak ratings; "moderate risk of bias" when there was at least one weak rating; or "high risk of bias" if there were two or more weak ratings [25]. Assessment for individually randomized, cross-over trials is presented in Figure 2. The risk of bias was independently assessed by two reviewers (MJ and PW). A third reviewer (SW) was consulted in case of disagreement.

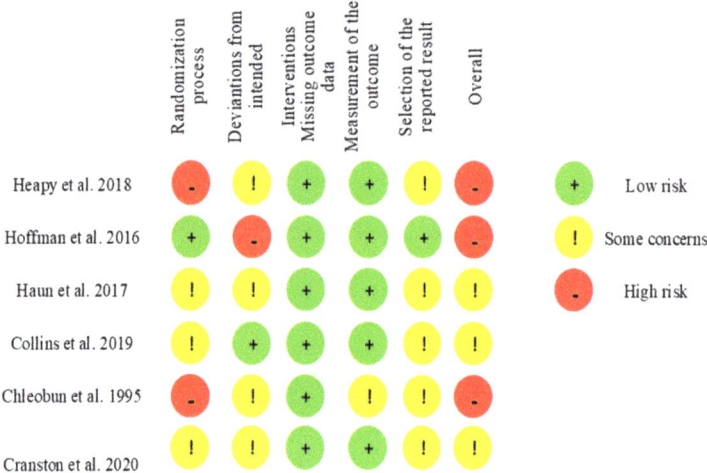

Figure 1. Risk of bias 2 tool. Assessment for individual randomized, parallel-group trials [25].

Author	Randomization process	Deviations from intended interventions	Missing outcome data	Measurement of the outcome	Selection of the reported result	Overall bias
Cochrane et al. 2013	High	Some concerns	Low	Low	Some concerns	Some concerns
Draper et al. 2020	High	Some concerns	Low	Low	Some concerns	High
Northey et al. 2016	High	Some concerns	Low	Some concerns	Some concerns	Some concerns
Velanzuela et al. 2018	High	Some concerns	Low	Low	Some concerns	High
Oliver et al. 2021	High	High	Low	Low	Some concerns	High

Figure 2. Risk of bias 2 tool. Assessment for individually randomized, cross-over trials [25].

2.6. Outcome Measures

Objective results of interest for meta-analyses from included baseline to last available follow-up. Data were typically collected immediately and 24 h, 48 h, 72 h, up to 96 h after the intervention.

2.7. Primary Outcomes

The primary endpoint was to assess the effect changes in MS and sports performance.

2.8. Secondary Outcomes

The secondary endpoint was to assess muscle functional capacities (e.g., strength, power), muscle damage markers (e.g., serum CK levels), and joint ROM and pain sensation.

2.9. Statistical Considerations

Random-effects meta-analyses were performed using the Revman5.4.1 software [26]. Data was represented by Standardized Mean Difference and 95% Confidence Interval (CI). tau-squared Tau^2, chi-squared Chi^2 and I^2 were used to investigate the presence of heterogeneity in meta-analysis. A p value < 0.05 was considered statistically significant.

3. Results

3.1. Results of the Search

A total of 693 articles related to the topic were retrieved through a comprehensive database and other sources search, of which, 169 articles were duplicates. After removing all ineligible articles, a total of 12 RCTs were included in the analysis. The detailed screening process is shown in Figure 3.

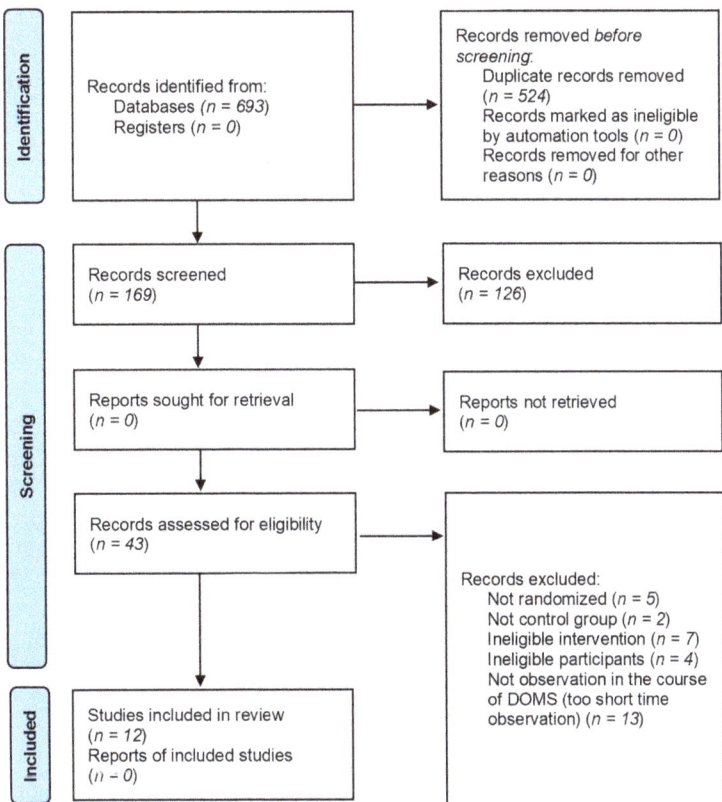

Figure 3. PRISMA flow diagram of included/excluded studies.

3.2. Details of the Intervention Groups in the Included Studies

Characteristics of the included studies are summarized in Table 1.

There were five randomized controlled trials [18,29,30,32,33] and seven randomized crossover trials [11,12,19,27,28,31,34]. Overall, studies included patients from five countries: USA (n = 5), New Zealand (n = 3), Ireland (n = 1), Australia (n = 2), and Spain (n = 1).

The total study population of all selected articles comprised of 322 healthy volunteers with an unequal distribution of sex (n_{male} = 274; n_{female} = 48). Throughout all the studies, mean sample size ranged from 10 to 72 volunteers.

The average sample size of the pressotherapy group was 14.33 and the control group 13.25. The mean age of the study population was 28.1 years. In two studies the mean age was above 40 years. [1,2].

Two studies involved well-trained volunteers [11,33]. Three studies included runners [12,29,31]. One study included strength-trained males [30]. Two studies included physically active volunteers [18,27] and athletes [28,34], another two studies chose healthy participants [19,32]. Detailed information about the training status is presented in the Table 1.

Table 1. The key characteristic of selected studies ($n = 12$).

Author/Country	Design/Publication Year	Participant Cohort (Training Status, Sex, Age)	Sample Size (n)	Experimental vs. Control Condition	DOMS Induction Intervention	Outcome Variables and Time of Measurement Post-Exercise (hrs)	Main Effects [* $p < 0.05$: Pre-Post ($\times$ Time)]	Total Exposition Time	Therapy Parameters
Hoffman et al. [12]/USA	RCT/2016	participants in the 2015 161-km Western States Endurance Run, men (IPC:43 ± 8 years, Massage:46 ± 10 years, con.:45 ± 9 years)	$n = 72$ $n = 24$ exp. (IPC) $n = 25$ exp. (Massage), $n = 23$ con.	45 min post exercises IPC (20 min), 45 min post-exercise Massage (20 min) vs. Placebo therapy (20 min)	161 km ultra-marathon race	400-m run times, Muscle Pain and Soreness, Overall Fatigue (prerace, postrace, post-treatment, 24-168 h post-race day)	400-m run times (pre↔, post 72 h↑, 120 h↓) Lower-Body Muscle Pain and Soreness (pre↔, postrace↑*, posttreatment↑*#, post 24–96 h↑*, post-120–168 h↑) Time and interaction effect* (no group effect) Muscular Fatigue (pre↔, postrace↑, post-treatment↑*#, postrace 24-168 h↑) Time and interaction effect* (no group effect)	20 min ISPC 20 min Massage 20 min Con.	ISPC—80 mmHg Massage—(the 30 s—calf and hamstring, 1 min—quadriceps), compression (2 min—calf and quadriceps, 3 min hamstring, tapotement (30 s leg and quadriceps)
Haun et al. [27]/USA	RCT/2017	endurance-trained male, participating in ≥72 h per week of endurance exercise for at least 3 months. (EPC:21 ± 0.4 years, con:21.1 ± 0.6 years)	$n = 18$ $n = 9$ exp. (EPC) $n = 9$ con.	24 h, 48 h, 72 h post-exercises EPC (1 h) vs. Placebo therapy (1 h) 96 h, 120 h treatments only EPC (1 h) vs. placebo therapy (1 h)	6 km run on the treadmill at an incline of 1% (pre and 16 h)	CK, Muscle Pain, and Soreness (pre-exercises, 72 h to 168 h), Flexibility (pre-exercises, 72 h to 168 h), 6-km run times (pre-exercises, 168 h)	CK (pre, 72 h↑, 96 h↑*, 120 h↑, 144 h↑, 168 h↔) Time effect* (No group or group × interaction effect) Muscle Soreness (pre, 72 h↓*, 96 h↓, 120 h↓*, 144 h↓, 168 h↔) Time effect* (No group or —group effect) Flexibility (pre, 72 h↑, 96 h↔, 120 h↔, 144 h↔, 168 h↓) 6 km run time (pre, 168 h↓)	300 min EPC 300 min EPC Con	EPC—70 mmHg (inflation—30 s/ deflation—30 s)

158

Table 1. Cont.

Study	Design/Year	Participants	Sample	Protocol	Measurements	Results	Intervention	Pressure
Cochrane et al. [18]/NZ	RCO/2013	10 healthy males, involved in physical activity (21.0 ± 1.7 years)	n = 10 n = 10 exp (IPC) n = 10 con.	Immediately post-exercises, 24 h post-exercise, 48 h post-IPC (30 min) vs. Placebo therapy (30 min)	3 sets × 100 rep. strenuous bout of eccentric exercise on BIODEX	CK, VJ, Muscle Dynamometry ISO 75° - CON 30°/s; 180°/s; - ECC 30°/s; 180°/s) (Pre, 24 h, 48 h, post 72 h)	CK (pre, 24 h↑, 48 h↑*, 72 h↑) VJ height (pre, 24 h↓, 48 h↑, 72 h↑) VJ peak power (pre, 24 h↓, 48 h↓, 72 h↓) Peak ISO (pre, 24 h↓*, 48 h↑*, 72 h↑*) Peak CON 30° (pre, 24 h↑*, 48 h↓, 72 h↓) Peak CON 180° (pre, 24 h↓, 48 h↓, 72 h↑) Peak ECC 30° (pre, 24 h↓, 48 h↓, 72 h↑) Peak ECC 180° (pre, 24 h↓, 48 h↑, 72 h↑) Ave ISO 75° (pre, 24 h↓, 48 h↑, 72 h↑) Ave CON 30° (pre, 24 h↓*, 48 h↓, 72 h↓) Ave CON 180° (pre, 24 h↓, 48 h↓, 72 h↓) Ave ECC 30° (pre, 24 h↓, 48 h↓, 72 h↑) Ave ECC 180° (pre, 24 h↑, 72 h↑)	90 min IPC 90 min Con	IPC—cell 1 (distal)—70 mmHg, cells 2–4 80 mmHg, cell 5 (proximal) 60 mmHg/deflation—30 s.
Collins et al. [28]/IE	RCT/2019	21 male team sport athletes (21.6 ± 3.4 years)	n = 21 n = 11 exp. n = 10 con.	Pre-, post-, 24 h post- exercises ECP (20 min) vs. Placebo therapy (20 min)	Max CMJ, 2 × 20 sprint, and second max CMJ	CK, C, T, IgA, sAA, VAS, CMJ height (Pre, post, 24 h post)	CK (pre, post↑*, 24 h↑*) Main effect for time* Cortisol (pre, post↑, 24 h↓) Testosterone (pre, post↑*, 24 h↓*) Main effect for time Alpha-Amylase (pre, post↓*#, 24 h↑*#) Main effect for time, and group Immunoglobulin—A (pre, post↑, 24 h↓) VAS (pre, post↑, 24 h↑*) Main effect for time CMJ (pre, post↓*#, 24 h↑*#)	60 min ECP 60 min Con	ECP—235.3 ± 26.9 mmHg

Table 1. Cont.

Draper et al. [29]/USA	RCO/2020	10 runners, endurance-trained males (38.7 ± 11.2 years)	n = 10 n = 10 exp. n = 10 con.	1 h, 24 h, 48 h, 72 h, 96 h, 120 h post-IPC (1 h) vs. 1 h, 24 h, 48 h, 72 h, 96 h, 120 h post-Placebo therapy (1 h)	2 × 20 mile runs at 70% VO2 max separated by 3 or 4 weeks	CRP, VAS (pre, post, and 24 h, 48 h, 72 h, 96 h, 120 h post)	CRP (pre-, post-run ↔, 24 h↑*, 48 h↑, 72 h↑, 96 h↔, 120 h↔). Main effect of time VAS (pre, post-run↑*, 24 h↑*, 48 h↑*, 72 h↑, 96 h↑, 120 h↔ pre-run)	6 h IPC 6 h Con	IPC—90 mmHg for cell 1 (distal) and cell 5 (proximal) and 100 mmHg for cells 2–4 (compression 30 s)
Northey et al. [30]/AU	RCO/2016	12 strength-trained male (24.0 ± 6.3 years)	n = 12 n = 12 exp. n = 12 con.	1 h post-exercises SIPC (45 min) vs. Placebo therapy (45 min)	10 sets × 10 rep. of back squats at 70% 1 repetition maximum	VAS, CON (peak of quadriceps), SJ, CMJ (Pre, post, 1 h, 24 h)	CON peak (pre, post↓*, 1 h↓*, 24 h↔) SJ (pre, post↓*, 1 h↓*, 24 h↓*) CMJ (pre, post↓*, 1 h↓*, 24 h↓) VAS (pre, post↑*, 1 h↑*, 24 h↑↑)	12 min OCC -2 sets × 3 min (per leg) 45 min SIPC 45 min Con	SIPC—80 mmHg (deflation—15 s) OCC 220 mmHg (inflation 3 min)
Heapy et al. [31]/NZ	RCT/2018	56 ultra-marathoners (con. = 19; 42 ± 9 years), (IPC = 18; 41 ± 8 years), (Massage = 19; 43 ± 9 years), men	n = 56 n = 18 exp. (IPC) n = 19 exp. (Massage) n = 19 con.	Post-race, 24 h, 48 h, 72 h post-race IPC (20 min), post-race, 24 h, 48 h, 72 h post-race Massage (25 min) vs. Placebo therapy (20 min)	Run race—three distance options of 62.7 km, 87.4 km, and 102.8 km	400 m run times (pre-race 1, pre-race 2, post-race at 72 h, 120 h, 168 h, and 336 h), VAS, Fatigue Scores (pre, post, day 24–168 h post and 336 h post)	400 m run times (pre-race 1, pre-race 2↔, 72 h↑, 120 h↑, 168 h↔, 336 h↔) Time effect* (No group, or interaction effect) VAS (pre-race, post-race↑*, 24 h↑*, 48 h↑, 72 h↑, 96 h↑, 120 h↑, 144 h↔, 168 h↔, 336 h↔) Time effect* (No group or interaction effect) Muscle Fatigue (pre-race, post-race↑*, 24 h↑*, 48 h↑*, 72 h↑*#, 96 h↑#, 120 h↑#, 144 h↔, 168 h↔, 336 h↔) Time and interaction effect* (No group effect)	80 min IPC 100 min Massage 80 min Con.	IPC—80 mmHg
Chleboun et al. [19]/USA	RCT/1995	22 college women students (21.7 ± 0.7 years)	n = 22 n = 22 exp. (IPC) n = 10 con. (passive rest)	Post-exercise, 24 h, 48 h, 72 h, 96 h, 120 h post IPC (20 min) vs. Placebo therapy (20 min)	3 sets of ECC exercise performed with weights equal to 90%, 80%, and 70% of the ISO MVC	Pain (five-point pain-rating scale), Swelling (post, day 1 to 5), Stiffness, and Isometric Strength (pre-exercise, pre-, post-IPC days 1 to 5)	Pain (post, 24 h↑, 48 h↑, 72 h↑, 96 h↑, 120 h↑) Swelling (post, pre IPC (post IPC), 24 h↑ (24 h↑*), 48 h↑ (96 h↑), 72 h↑ (72 h↑*), 96 h↑ (96 h↑), 120 h↑ (120 h↑*)) Stiffness (post-, pre-IPC, (post-IPC), 24 h↑ (24 h↑), 48 h↑ (48 h↓*), 72 h↓ (72↓*), 96 h↓ (96 h↓), 120 h↓ (120 h↓)) Strength (post-, pre-IPC (post-IPC) 24 h↓ (24 h↓), 48 h↓ (48 h↓), 72 h↓ (72 h↓), 96 h↑ (96 h↑), 120 h↑ (120 h↑))	120 min IPC	IPC—60 mmHg (inflation 40 s/deflation 20 s)

Table 1. Cont.

Study	Design/Year	Participants	Sample	Intervention	Exercise	Outcomes	Results	Protocol	Device/Pressure
Velanzuela et al. [32]/ES	RCO/2018	10 healthy participants (27 ± 4 years), 7 men, 3 females	$n = 10$ $n = 10$ exp. $n = 10$ con.	Post-exercises, 24 h post-EECP (30 min) vs. Placebo therapy (30 min)	Plyometric exercise bout (10 sets of 10 jumps)	Muscle Soreness (VAS), CK, CMJ, RSI (pre and 24 and 48 h post)	Muscle Soreness (pre, 24 h post↑, 48 h post↑) CK (pre, 24 h post↑, 48 h post↓) CMJ (pre, 24 h post↓, 48 h post↔) RSI (pre, 24 h post↓, 48 h post↔)	60 min EECP 60 min Con.	EECP—80 mmHg
Haun C.T. et al. [11]/USA	RCT/2017	20 resistance-trained male (21.6 ± 2.4 years)	$n = 10$ $n = 10$ exp. (EPC) $n = 10$ con.	48 h, 72 h, 96 h, 120 h, 144 h post-EPC (1 h) vs Placebo therapy (1 h)	10 sets of five rep. at 80% of back squat 1 RM	CK, Flexibility (pre, 48–168 h post) CRP (pre, 8–168 h post)	CK (pre, 72 h↑*, 120 h↑*, 144 h↓, 168 h↑) Flexibility (pre, 72 h↑*#, 96 h↑, 120 h↑*, 144 h↑, 168 h↓) CRP (pre, 48 h↑, 72 h↑, 96 h↑, 120 h↑, 144 h↑, 168 h↑)	5 h EPC 5 h Con.	EPC—70 mmHg (inflation—30 s/deflation—30 s)
Oliver et al. [33]/NZ	RCO/2021	11 well-trained wheelchair basketball and rugby athletes (33 ± 10 years), men	$n = 11$ $n = 11$ exp. $n = 11$ con.	post exercises ISPC (20 min) vs. Placebo therapy (30 min)	10 wheelchair court sprints (28 m). Ten times figure of eight agility drill (the 30 s). Ten sprints (28 m) immediately followed by three medicine ball chest throws	Medicine Ball Throw (m), Wheelchair Sprint, 5, 10, 15 (m) (pre-ex, post-ex, post-rec) Muscle Soreness 0–10 scale and Muscle Fatigue 0–10 scale (pre-ex, post-ex, post-rec, 24 h post-rec) Blood Lactate (post-ex, post-rec)	Medicine Ball Throw (pre-ex, post-ex↓, post-rec↑), Wheelchair Sprint: (5 m) (pre-ex, post-ex↑, post-rec↑) (10 M) (pre-ex, post-ex↑, post-rec↑) (15 m) (pre-ex, post-ex↑, pot-rec↑) Muscle Soreness (pre-ex, post-ex↑, post-rec↑, 24 h post↑) Muscle Fatigue (pre-ex, post-ex↑, post-rec↑) Blood Lactate (post-ex, post-rec↓)	20 min ISPC 30 min Con.	ISPC—80 mmHg (inflation 30 s/deflation 15 s)

Table 1. Cont.

Study	Design/Year	Participants	Groups	Intervention	Measurements	Results
Cranston et al. [34]	RCT/2020	50 resistance-trained athletes (27 ± 4 years), 37 men, 13 females	n = 50 n = 25 exp. n = 25 con.	post exercises ISPC (30 min) vs. Placebo therapy (30 min)	Fatiguing Exercise Circuit (consisted of five different exercises): 1. Reverse grip battle rope waves (the 60 s) 2. 20 m Farmers carry (20 kg for women and 30 kg for men) 3. Chin-ups (maximum number of repetitions) 4. Chin-up bar hangs (long as possible with their hands in a pronated grip) 5. Handgrip crushers (as many times as possible) Grip Strength Dynamometer (kg), Single-Arm Medicine Ball Throw (m), Preacher Bench Bicep Curls - max repetitions (pre-ex, post-ex, post-rec)	Grip Strength Dynamometer (pre-ex, post-ex↓, post-rec↓), Single-Arm Medicine Ball Throw (pre-ex, post-ex↓, post-rec↑), Max. Rep. Preacher Bench Bicep Curls (pre-ex, post-ex↓, post-rec↓), Triceps Brachii Long Head Soreness (pre-ex, post-ex↑, post-rec↓#, 24 h post-rec↑#), Biceps Brachii Soreness (pre-ex, post-ex↑, post-rec↓#, 24 h post-rec↑#), Extensor Digitorum Soreness (pre-ex, post-ex↑, post-rec↓#, 24 h post-rec↑#), Flexor Carpi Radialis Soreness (pre-ex, post-ex↑, post-rec↓#, 24 h post-rec↑#)	30 min ISPC 30 min Con.	ISPC—80 mmHg (inflation—26 s / deflation—15 s)

Abbreviations: PCD (pneumatic compression device), CS (compression sleeve), PC (pneumatic compression), EPC (external pneumatic compression), ECP (External counterpulsation), EECP (Enhanced external counterpulsation), IPC (intermittent pneumatic compression), ISPC (intermittent sequential pneumatic compression), OCC (evaluate vascular occlusion), SIPC (sequential intermittent pneumatic compression), VJ (vertical jump), SJ (squat jump), CK (creatine kinase), LDH (lactate dehydrogenase), ISO (isometric), CON (concentric), ECC (eccentric), HIIT (high intensity interval training), HIE (high-intensity exercise), CMJ (countermovement jump), DEC (deceleration), AMRAP (as much repetitions as possible), ALAP (as long as possible), WAnT (Wingate anaerobic test), THB (total hemoglobin), O2HB (oxyhemoglobin), HHB (deoxyhemoglobin), ROM (range of motion), C (cortisol), T (testosterone), IgA (immunoglobulin-A), sAA (salivary alpha-amylase), CRP (C-reactive protein), PkP (peak power), AP (average power), FI (fatigue index), BLa (blood lactate concentration), NRS (numeric rating scale), CWI (cold water immersion), MuscleMechFx (muscle mechanical function), RPE (rate of perceived exertion), DM (Muscle radial deformation), TC (time of contraction), BF (biceps femoris), RF (rectus femoris), RSI (reactive strength index). #—significant difference between groups, * $p < 0.05$, ↑—significant increase, ↓—significant decrease, ↔—no significant change.

3.3. Characteristics of the Exercise Protocols, Therapies and Outcomes

To induce muscle damage exercise protocols encompassed in running and other activities, five used run [11,12,28,29,31]. One of these types of exercise was sprint [28], another one was middle—6 km [11]—and three of the remaining five were long-distance run 62.7 [31]; 87.4 [31]; 102.8 [31]; 2 × 20 mile [29]; 161 km [12]. Two studies used back squats, 10 sets × 10 rep [30], and 10 sets of five repetitions [27]. Another way to induction DOMS intervention was ECC exercise on Biodex system [18], eccentric exercise performed with weight [19], plyometric exercise bout [32], countermovement jump (CMJ) [28], and wheelchair court sprints [33]. One study used specific training: Reverse grip battle rope waves, Farmers carry, Chin-ups, Bar hangs, Handgrip crushers [34]. Table 1 gives a detailed overview of the conducted exercise protocols.

Considerable variation was observed in therapy parameters among the studies. Intermittent sequential pneumatic compression (ISPC) was used in three studies [12,33,34]. Time of therapy was 2 min [2], 30 s/15 s [33], or 26 s/15 s [34]. External pneumatic compression (EPC) was used in three studies [11,27,28], two authors used the same parameters 70 mmHg inflation—30 s, deflation—30 s [11,27], and one study used 235 mmHg pressure [28]. The most popular therapy was IPC [18,19,29,31].

There was a different time of experimental and control condition; the majority performed therapy post-exercise, and after 24 h. The average therapy session was 30 min. The shortest time was 6 min [30] and the maximum was 1 h [11,27,29]. Total therapeutic exposition time varied from 20 to 30 min. [12,33,34] to longer times of 80 min to 6 h [18,19,31].

Outcome variables and time of measurement varied depending on the study. The period of measurement keeps on from Po-E [12,19,28–30,33,34] to 336 h after exercise [31]. The average time of access outcomes was 48 h. Muscle pain soreness and (CK) were the most-often measured. Six studies investigated CK [11,18,27,28,32], five MS [11,12,32–34], and eight pain Visual analogue scale (VAS) [11,12,19,28–32]. Other authors access Over Fatigue [12], Flexibility [11], Muscle Dynamometry and vertical jump (VJ) [18,19] C-reactive protein (CRP) [27,29], countermovement jump (CMJ), reactive strength index (RSI) [28,30,32], cortisol, testosterone, alpha-amylase, and immunoglobulin [28]. Detailed information about the measured parameters can be observed in Table 1.

Main effects were measured Po-E through to 336 h after. CK increased Po-E to 24 h [28], 72 h [18] and 168 h [27]. Haun (2017) concluded that after 168 h there was no significant change. Significant effect was observed after 24 h [18,28] and 96 h [11,27] and 120 h [27]

Muscle Pain increased Po-E to 24 h [28,30], 96 h [29], 120 h [19,31] and 168 h [12]. Significant effect was observed after one hour [30], 24 h [28,30,31], 48 h [29], 96 h [12]. In one study, an increase was observed Po-E to 144 h but with no significant changes [19].

Muscle soreness had a heterogeneous direction of changes. Some authors observed decreasing after exercise from 72 h to 144 h and significant changes were measured after 72 h and 120 h [11,31]. The majority observed significantly increasing MS Po-E and after 24 h to 96 h [12]. Velanzuela (2018) observed increasing MS after 24 and 48 h but without any significant changes [32]. Oliver (2021) observed increasing MS Po-E, post-recovery, and after 24 h and also without any significant changes [33]. Cranston (2020) observed increasing Po-E in all four muscle groups, post-recovery decreasing in three groups with significant differences between groups, and after 24 h increasing in all four muscle groups, with significant differences between groups [34].

Hoffman (2016) observed that muscle fatigue increases post-race, post-treatment significantly and reached significant difference between groups post-race 24–168 h [12]. Two other authors analyzed the change of these parameters [31,33] and Heapy (2018) observed changes post-race, 24–168 h, and 336 h after exercise, and post-race, the 24–72 h increase was significant [31]. Furthermore, there was a significant difference between the groups of 72 h, 96 h, and 120 h. In Oliver et al (2021) muscle fatigue Po-E, post-recovery, and 24 h Po-E remained unchanged [33].

Two studies assess muscle flexibility parameters [11,27]. Both observed increasing after 72 h and decreasing after 168 h. Swelling and stiffness were observed by Chleboun et al (1995) after 24–96 h and 120 h [19]. The stiffness increased after 24 and 48 h and then decreased to 120 h.

Two studies measured isometric strength [18,19]. Cochrane (2013) observed decreased peak isometric strength after 24 h and increased after 48 and 72 h—all changes were significant [18]. Chleboun (1995) observed a decrease after 24–72 h and an increase after 96 and 120 h [19].

Cochrane et al (2013) measured a few dynamometry parameters: Peak concentric 30°—decreased after 24, 48, and 72 h; peak concentric 180° decreased similar to previous parameters; peak ECC 30° and 180°—decreased after 24 h and increased after 48 and 72 h [18]. Other parameters: Average concentric 30°, 180° decreased after 24–72 h; average ECC 30°, 180° decreased after 24 h and increased after 48–72 h [18]. Northey et al. (2016) also measured concentric peak and he observed decreased post and after 1 h and then no significant changes [30].

Collins et al. (2019) assessed blood test results: cortisol, testosterone, immunoglobulin—increased Po-E and decreased after 24 h; Alpha-amylase—significant changes post and 24 h and between groups [28]. Oliver et al. (2021) measured blood lactate—post-recovery it decreased. C-reactive protein was measured in two studies [27,29] and remained unchanged after 24–144 h and 168 h [33].

Some authors used exercises to measure the main effect. Hoffman et al. (2016) and Heapy et al. (2018) used 400 m runs with increased time after 72 h [12] and 120 h [31], and decreased time after 120 h [12]. Another activity to measure effects was a 6 km run after 168 h Po-E. In a countermovement jump (CM) [28,30,32] heterogenous results were observed: decreased post and increased after 24 h—significant changes between groups [28]. Decreased post, 1 and 24 h post and 1 h showed significant changes [30]. After 24 h, it decreased and after 48 h there were no significant changes [32]. Valenzuela et al. (2018) also measured reactive strength index and had the same results as in the CMJ case [32]. Cochrane et al (2013) observed changes in vertical jump height—it decreased after 24 h and increased after 48 h and 72 h; vertical jump peak power—decreased after 24–72 h [18]. Northey et al. (2016) used squat jump (SJ) to measure the main effect and noted only decreased post and after 1 and 24 h [30]. Oliver et al. (2021) used a medicine ball throw test and wheelchair sprint on 5, 10, and 15 m, and observed decrease with post-recovery increase [33]. Sprint on every distance was increased. Cranston et al. (2020) used exercises: Grip strength dynamometer—decreased Po-E and post-recovery; Single-arm medicine ball throw—Po-E it decreased and then post-recovery increased; Max repetition single-arm preacher biceps curls—Po-E and recovery it decreased [34].

3.4. Subgroup Analysis

3.4.1. Muscle Soreness

There was moderate and statistically significant reduction in MS in overall effect from 24 to 96 h after DOMS induction in pressotherapy intervention (Standard Mean Difference (SMD) = -0.33, 95% CI -0.49, -0.18; $p < 0.0001$; $I^2 = 7\%$). In the Subgroup 24 h Po-E (participants = 311; studies = nine) there was moderate but NS reduction in MS (SMD = -0.28, 95% CI -0.60, 0.04; $p = 0.09$; $I^2 = 43\%$), 48 h Po-E (participants = 144; studies = nine) there was moderate and significant reduction in MS (SMD = -0.40, 95% CI -0.73, 0.07; $p = 0.02$; $I^2 = 0\%$), 72 h Po-E (participants = 124; studies = four) there was moderate but NS reduction in MS (SMD = -0.37, 95% CI -0.79, 0.05; $p = 0.08$; $I^2 = 24\%$) and 96 h Po-E (participants = 124; studies = four) there was moderate but NS reduction in MS. In overall effect from 24 to 96 h heterogeneity was small ($I^2 = 7\%$; $\chi^2 = 22.6$, df = 21; $p = 0.96$). Only in the subgroup 24 h Po-E we detected NS heterogeneity ($I^2 = 43\%$; $\chi^2 = 14.16$, df = 8; $p = 0.08$). After 48–96 h, heterogeneity was low. Subgroup analysis from 24 h to 96 h did not reveal a statistically significant difference ($p = 0.96$) (Figure 4).

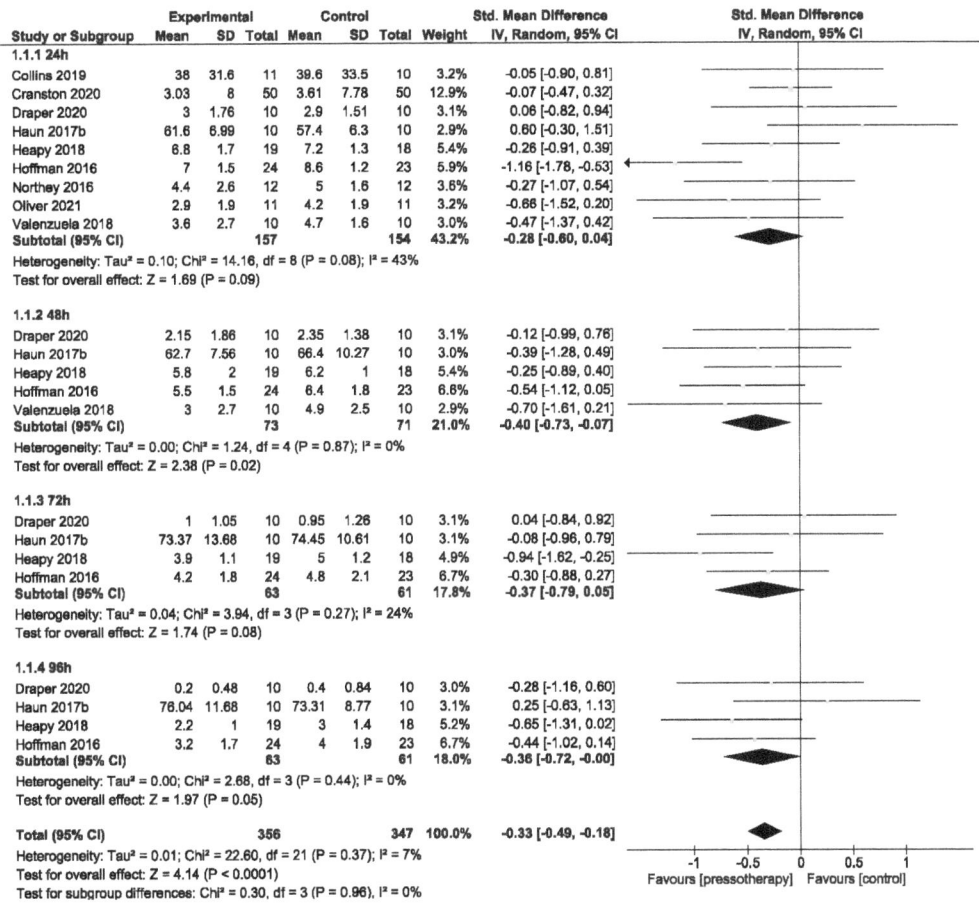

Figure 4. Effects of pressotherapy on muscle soreness from 24 h to 96 h after exercise.

3.4.2. Jump Performance

In 24 h Po-E (participants = 84; studies = 4; SMD = −0.05, 95% CI −0.47, −0.38; $p = 0.99$; $I^2 = 0\%$), 48 h Po-E (participants = 40; studies = 2; SMD = −0.01, 95% CI −0.61, 0.63; $p = 0.77$; $I^2 = 0\%$), and 72 h Po-E (participants = 20; studies = 1; SMD = −0.10, 95% CI −0.98, 0.78; $p = 0.82$; I^2 = not applicable) there was a small statistically NS effect of pressotherapy on jump height. In overall effect from 24 to 72 h (SMD = −0.04, 95% CI −0.36, −0.29; $p = 0.82$) heterogeneity was small ($I^2 = 0\%$; $\chi^2 = 0.25$, df = 21; $p = 1.00$).

Subgroup analysis from 24 h to 96 h did not reveal a statistically significant difference ($p = 0.98$) (Figure 5).

3.4.3. Creatine Kinase

There was an NS increase in serum CK activity in overall effect from 24 to 96 h after DOMS induction in pressotherapy intervention (SMD = 0.41, 95% CI −0.07, 0.89; $p = 0.09$; $I^2 = 63\%$). In the subgroup 24 h Po-E (participants = 81; studies = four; SMD = 0.14, 95% CI −0.30, 0.58; $p = 0.54$; $I^2 = 0\%$), 48 h Po-E (participants = 60; studies = three; SMD = 0.52, 95% CI −0.77, 1.81; $p = 0.43$; $I^2 = 82\%$), 72 h Po-E (participants = 40; studies = two; SMD = 0.49, 95% CI −1.25, 2.23; $p = 0.58$; $I^2 = 85\%$) there were small (24 h) and moderate (48–72 h) but NS increases in serum CK activity. In the 96 h Po-E group (participants = 20; studies =one) there was large and significant increase in CK activity for the pressotherapy group (SMD = 1.26, 95% CI 0.28, 2.23; $p = 0.01$; I^2 = not applicable).

Overall, the heterogeneity in effects from 24 to 96 h was moderate ($I^2 = 63\%$; $\chi^2 = 24.47$, df = 9; $p = 0.004$). Only in the subgroup 24 h Po-E we detected homogeneity ($I^2 = 0\%$; $\chi^2 = 2.44$, df = 3; $p = 0.49$). 48 h ($I^2 = 82\%$; $\chi^2 = 11.05$, df = 2; $p = 0.004$) and 72 h ($I^2 = 85\%$; $\chi^2 = 6.78$, df = 1; $p = 0.009$) heterogeneity was large. Subgroup analysis from 24 h to 96 h did not reveal a statistically significant difference ($p = 0.23$) (Figure 6).

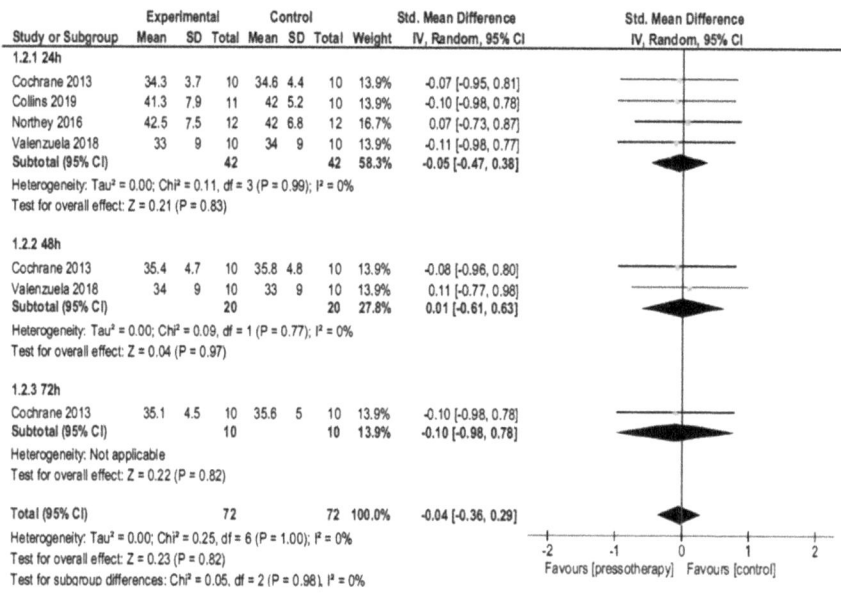

Figure 5. Effects of pressotherapy on jump performance from 24 h to 96 h after exercise. SMDs are calculated from CMJ, VJ, etc.

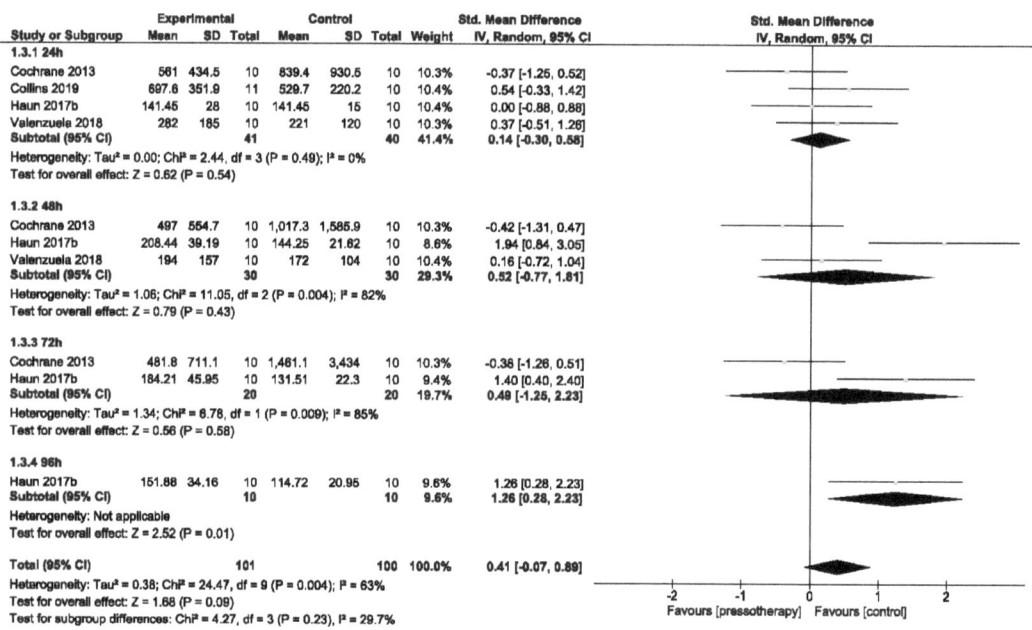

Figure 6. Effects of pressotherapy on serum CK activity from 24 h to 96 h after exercise.

4. Discussion

4.1. Brief Study Informations: Purposes, Direction, and Possible Main Outcomes

Most of the studies used a one-time protocol to assess the time of post-workout regeneration. The most reliable method would be to use it multiple times under different conditions to maximize result accuracy [35].

The best methods of post-workout recovery are sleep and a proper diet [36,37]. Additional methods can only be supplementary. For the assessment of the credibility of the studies, we recommend that the information on whether pressotherapy was the primary method or an addition to the more comprehensive scheme should be included in the research Methodology section.

Maximizing the efficiency of post-workout adaptation is crucial for athletes to maintain an appropriate performance level throughout the season and during the pre-competition preparation periods [38,39]. This is especially important in sports with a high frequency of competitions (i.e., team sports such as soccer and basketball), as well as in disciplines where the athlete prepares for a long time for one event in which their organism achieves peak performance (i.e., individual disciplines such as sprinting or swimming).

We stipulate that pressotherapy does NS affect post-workout regeneration and can only supplement a complex protocol.

4.2. Serum CK Level

The blood level of CK is an indicator of the status of muscle damage and of change in both pathological and normal conditions [40]. An increase in this enzyme may predict a state of microscopic tissue impairment after acute and prolonged injuries. Variables in CK level are also observed under physiological conditions in athletes after demanding training. The highest CK growth is observed after prolonged exercise, i.e., triathlon events and demanding strength exercises, or activities that include an eccentric muscle contraction phase, i.e., downhill running [41,42]. In our study, we saw an improvement in this parameter, which suggests that pressotherapy improves regeneration. However, its impact was not statistically significant in any case except the 96 h Po-E group, which had the lowest number of participants. In addition, a significant result was observed in the longest period after the training was performed, which leaves some ambiguity as CK activity decreases with time and it is a natural process [43]. Not without relevance is also the fact that a significant result was observed by Haun et al., who investigated CK levels on a group of trained high-volume endurance athletes, who underwent over 70 h of exertion per week for 3 months. Although significant results have been observed, previous studies suggest that CK levels naturally decline between days 4 and 10 after exercise [44]. The characteristics of the test group (endurance athletes) and testing protocol could also affect the results, as resting CK levels are higher in the trained population [45,46] and everyday strenuous workouts may cause persistent blood rise of CK [47]. Therefore, the potential outcome of pressotherapy on a different group of people would not be so important. To summarize, in the current state of knowledge, pressotherapy should not be recommended as the basic method of recovery after exercise, because there is a large heterogeneity of previous research results.

4.3. DOMS

DOMS is a regular experience for advanced or beginner athletes. Its manifestations can range from muscle stiffness to severe excruciating pain [48]. DOMS is most prevalent at the beginning of the sporting season when athletes are returning to training following a period of reduced activity [49]. DOMS is also common when athletes are first introduced to certain types of activities regardless of the time of year. DOMS can negatively attenuate athletic performance [50]. Possible mechanisms include a reduction in joint ROM, peak torque, and a feeling of pain [48]. Compensation methods may raise the probability of further injury [51,52] when participants try to return to activity too early without completing the full recovery process. Therefore, it is of high importance to search for new methods of the most effective regeneration and reduction of MS. Commonly described in the literature are pressotherapy [48], stretching [53], cryotherapy [54], and massage, mainly considered as self-foam rolling. It has been the most often assessed parameter in selected studies. Although pressotherapy is one of the methods of DOMS reduction, our results indicate that its use for this purpose remains questionable. Only when MS was measured after 48 h, was a a significant effect of pressotherapy observed. This method also significantly alleviates DOMS when considering the whole population and all protocols. On the other hand, no significant reduction in MS was found in the remaining groups. Taking into account the previously mentioned methods of therapy, which are easily available (stretching or foam-rolling), as well as low-cost (cryotherapy and water immersion) or self-applicable and physiologic (i.e., rest), there are few arguments in favor of the wide use of pressotherapy in the current state of knowledge. High prices and limited availability suggest other forms as a method of choice and first-line treatment strategy. However, pressotherapy has shown some positive effects, mainly limited to the 48 h Po-E period, so while the above-mentioned factors are not a barrier, it can be used in some circumstances [55] (e.g., in professional athletes as a supplemental method).

4.4. Jump Performance

The level of muscle power in the lower limbs is a vital factor in numerous disciplines, such as sprinting [56,57] or in decisive moments of team sports [58,59]. In a widespread view, the research has demonstrated that jump heigh is an applicable index to characterize power output, mainly described by the association found between them [60]. It is meaningful that upright jump may be easily evaluated and hereafter used by team staff and physical trainers to categorize the level of athletes' muscle power within a wider group of participants [61,62]. Due to the great practical importance of jump performance in the overall assessment of an athlete's fitness and the development of motor skills, it is crucial to properly place this type of activity in the training plan and the microcycle [63,64]. Effective recovery after jumping efforts would be of key importance, hence the influence of pressotherapy on jump performance was also assessed in this meta-analysis. In our review, we did not observe any significant effect of pressotherapy on jump ability performed at various intervals from the previous exercise. Further investigation is needed to specify whether and in what population this method will be an effective approach for improving jump performance and overall power generation.

4.5. Practical Implications

This study has several practical implications and contributes significantly to the actual state of knowledge in this research area. It can be used by motor preparation specialists and physiotherapy professionals in the prescription of individualized, advanced recovery strategies. This is especially important when maximizing the effectiveness of post-exercise regeneration is necessary (e.g., for elite athletes during the beginning of the season or directly before competitive event).

5. Conclusions

The conducted systematic review and meta-analysis assessed 12 randomized controlled studies investigating the outcome of pressotherapy on the recovery of absolute (i.e., physiological), and subjective (i.e., perceptual) outcomes. The findings indicate only moderate benefits of using pressotherapy as a recovery intervention, dependent on the type of exercise and used protocol. A reduction in DOMS, changes in CK level, and improvements in perceived recovery were observed after pressotherapy, although they were usually not significant. Dose–response relationships emerged for several variables indicating that different duration protocols may improve the efficacy of pressotherapy if applied after exercise. We recommend further, and continuing, research on various populations and broadening tested protocols to obtain the highest possible homogeneity of results and to facilitate the creation of a consensus statement on whether pressotherapy seems to be an effective method in minimizing exercise-induced negative effects.

6. Limitations

Although, this paper has a few limitations. Firstly, we performed a comprehensive literature investigation, where we excluded articles that were not published in English. However, from an actual point of view, we suppose this will have a minor effect on our outcomes [65]. Nevertheless, we conducted a reasonable attitude to overwhelm these barriers and attempted to stick to principles of open science. Secondly, the protocols used and the study groups differed between the selected articles. Third, the time of outcome evaluation from the preliminary endpoint was not identical in all trials. Fourth, the particular subgroup analyses were conceivably underpowered due to their small participant number and should be interpreted carefully. To enhance the validity of results in similar research, future randomized studies should concentrate on better conducting and reporting of applied protocol and methodology, intention-to-treat examination, assessor blinding, random sequence generation, control group observation, and reporting of adverse events or the possible other influencing factors. Moreover, not all databases (i.e., EMBASE) were searched.

Author Contributions: Conceptualization, S.W. and M.C.; methodology, S.W., P.W.; writing—original draft preparation, P.W., S.W., P.S.K., M.C., and W.P.; software and statistics, S.W., writing—review and editing, M.J., M.C., B.M., P.S.K., and W.P.; supervision, S.W. and P.S.K. All authors have read and agreed to the published version of the manuscript.

Funding: This research received no external funding.

Institutional Review Board Statement: Not applicable.

Informed Consent Statement: Not applicable.

Data Availability Statement: Data are available from the corresponding author upon reasonable request.

Conflicts of Interest: The authors declare there are no conflict of interest.

References

1. Howatson, G.; van Someren, K.A. The Prevention and Treatment of Exercise-Induced Muscle Damage. *Sport. Med.* **2008**, *38*, 483–503. [CrossRef]
2. McAnulty, S.; McAnulty, L.; Nieman, D.; Morrow, J.; Dumke, C., Henson, D. Effect of NSAID on Muscle Injury and Oxidative Stress. *Int. J. Sports Med.* **2007**, *28*, 909–915. [CrossRef]
3. Kim, J.; Lee, J. A review of nutritional intervention on delayed onset muscle soreness. Part I. *J. Exerc. Rehabil.* **2014**, *10*, 349–356. [CrossRef]
4. Monedero, J.; Donne, B. Effect of Recovery Interventions on Lactate Removal and Subsequent Performance. *Int. J. Sports Med.* **2000**, *21*, 593–597. [CrossRef]
5. Tanner, R.K.; Fuller, K.L.; Ross, M.L.R. Evaluation of three portable blood lactate analysers: Lactate Pro, Lactate Scout and Lactate Plus. *Eur. J. Appl. Physiol.* **2010**, *109*, 551–559. [CrossRef]
6. Mair, J.; Mayr, M.; Mullet, E.; Koller, A.; Haid, C.; Artner-Dworzak, E.; Calzolari, C.; Larue, C.; Puschendorf, B. Rapid Adaptation to Eccentric Exercise-Induced Muscle Damage. *Int. J. Sports Med.* **1995**, *16*, 352–356. [CrossRef]
7. Lieber, R.L.; Fridén, J. Morphologic and Mechanical Basis of Delayed-Onset Muscle Soreness. *J. Am. Acad. Orthop. Surg.* **2002**, *10*, 67–73. [CrossRef]
8. Gaitanos, G.C.; Williams, C.; Boobis, L.H.; Brooks, S. Human muscle metabolism during intermittent maximal exercise. *J. Appl. Physiol.* **1993**, *75*, 712–719. [CrossRef]
9. Machado, A.F.; Ferreira, P.H.; Micheletti, J.K.; de Almeida, A.C.; Lemes, Í.R.; Vanderlei, F.M.; Netto Junior, J.; Pastre, C.M. Can Water Temperature and Immersion Time Influence the Effect of Cold Water Immersion on Muscle Soreness? A Systematic Review and Meta-Analysis. *Sport. Med.* **2016**, *46*, 503–514. [CrossRef]
10. Cochrane, D.J. Effectiveness of using wearable vibration therapy to alleviate muscle soreness. *Eur. J. Appl. Physiol.* **2017**, *117*, 501–509. [CrossRef]
11. Haun, C.T.; Roberts, M.D.; Romero, M.A.; Osburn, S.C.; Mobley, C.B.; Anderson, R.G.; Goodlett, M.D.; Pascoe, D.D.; Martin, J.S. Does external pneumatic compression treatment between bouts of overreaching resistance training sessions exert differential effects on molecular signaling and performance-related variables compared to passive recovery? An exploratory study. *PLoS ONE* **2017**, *12*, e0180429. [CrossRef]

12. Hoffman, M.D.; Badowski, N.; Chin, J.; Stuempfle, K.J. A Randomized Controlled Trial of Massage and Pneumatic Compression for Ultramarathon Recovery. *J. Orthop. Sport. Phys. Ther.* **2016**, *46*, 320–326. [CrossRef]
13. Field, A.; Harper, L.D.; Chrismas, B.C.R.; Fowler, P.M.; McCall, A.; Paul, D.J.; Chamari, K.; Taylor, L. The use of recovery strategies in professional soccer: A worldwide survey. *Int. J. Sports Physiol Perform.* **2021**, *1*, 1804–1815. [CrossRef]
14. Sands, W.A.; Murray, M.B.; Murray, S.R.; McNeal, J.R.; Mizuguchi, S.; Sato, K.; Stone, M.H. Peristaltic Pulse Dynamic Compression of the Lower Extremity Enhances Flexibility. *J. Strength Cond. Res.* **2014**, *28*, 1058–1064. [CrossRef]
15. Sands, W.A.; McNeal, J.R.; Murray, S.R.; Stone, M.H. Dynamic Compression Enhances Pressure-to-Pain Threshold in Elite Athlete Recovery. *J. Strength Cond. Res.* **2015**, *29*, 1263–1272. [CrossRef]
16. Muluk, S.C.; Hirsch, A.T.; Taffe, E.C. Pneumatic Compression Device Treatment of Lower Extremity Lymphedema Elicits Improved Limb Volume and Patient-reported Outcomes. *Eur. J. Vasc. Endovasc. Surg.* **2013**, *46*, 480–487. [CrossRef]
17. Martin, J.S.; Friedenreich, Z.D.; Borges, A.R.; Roberts, M.D. Acute Effects of Peristaltic Pneumatic Compression on Repeated Anaerobic Exercise Performance and Blood Lactate Clearance. *J. Strength Cond. Res.* **2015**, *29*, 2900–2906. [CrossRef]
18. Cochrane, D.; Booker, H.; Mundel, T.; Barnes, M. Does Intermittent Pneumatic Leg Compression Enhance Muscle Recovery after Strenuous Eccentric Exercise? *Int. J. Sports Med.* **2013**, *34*, 969–974. [CrossRef]
19. Chleboun, G.S.; Howell, J.N.; Baker, H.L.; Ballard, T.N.; Graham, J.L.; Hallman, H.L.; Perkins, L.E.; Schauss, J.H.; Conatser, R.R. Intermittent pneumatic compression effect on eccentric exercise-induced swelling, stiffness, and strength loss. *Arch. Phys. Med. Rehabil.* **1995**, *76*, 744–749. [CrossRef]
20. Zuj, K.A.; Prince, C.N.; Hughson, R.L.; Peterson, S.D. Enhanced muscle blood flow with intermittent pneumatic compression of the lower leg during plantar flexion exercise and recovery. *J. Appl. Physiol.* **2018**, *124*, 302–311. [CrossRef]
21. Kevin Stetter, E.H. An Intermittent Pneumatic Compression Device Reduces Blood Lactate Concentrations More Effectively Than Passive Recovery after Wingate Testing. *J. Athl. Enhanc.* **2013**, *2*, 18–25. [CrossRef]
22. Waller, T.; Caine, M.; Morris, R. *Intermittent Pneumatic Compression Technology for Sports Recovery in The Engineering of Sport 6*; Springer: New York, NY, USA, 2006; pp. 391–396.
23. Brown, D. A Review of the PubMed PICO Tool: Using Evidence-Based Practice in Health Education. *Health Promot. Pract.* **2020**, *21*, 496–498. [CrossRef] [PubMed]
24. Moher, D.; Liberati, A.; Tetzlaff, J.; Altman, D.G. Preferred Reporting Items for Systematic Reviews and Meta-Analyses: The PRISMA Statement. *PLoS Med.* **2009**, *6*, e1000097. [CrossRef] [PubMed]
25. Sterne, J.A.C.; Savović, J.; Page, M.J.; Elbers, R.G.; Blencowe, N.S.; Boutron, I.; Cates, C.J.; Cheng, H.-Y.; Corbett, M.S.; Eldridge, S.M.; et al. RoB 2: A revised tool for assessing risk of bias in randomised trials. *BMJ* **2019**, *366*, l4898. [CrossRef]
26. *Review Manager (RevMan) [Computer Program]*; Version 5.4.1; The Cochrane Collaboration: London, UK, 2020.
27. Haun, C.T.; Roberts, M.D.; Romero, M.A.; Osburn, S.C.; Healy, J.C.; Moore, A.N.; Mobley, C.B.; Roberson, P.A.; Kephart, W.C.; Mumford, P.W.; et al. Concomitant external pneumatic compression treatment with consecutive days of high intensity interval training reduces markers of proteolysis. *Eur. J. Appl. Physiol.* **2017**, *117*, 2587–2600. [CrossRef]
28. Collins, R.; McGrath, D.; Horner, K.; Eusebi, S.; Ditroilo, M. Effect of External Counterpulsation on Exercise Recovery in Team Sport Athletes. *Int. J. Sports Med.* **2019**, *40*, 511–518. [CrossRef]
29. Draper, S.N.; Kullman, E.L.; Sparks, K.E.; Little, K.; Thoman, J. Effects of Intermittent Pneumatic Compression on Delayed Onset Muscle Soreness (DOMS) in Long Distance Runners. *Int. J. Exerc. Sci.* **2020**, *13*, 75–86.
30. Northey, J.M.; Rattray, B.; Argus, C.K.; Etxebarria, N.; Driller, M.W. Vascular Occlusion and Sequential Compression for Recovery After Resistance Exercise. *J. Strength Cond. Res.* **2016**, *30*, 533–539. [CrossRef]
31. Heapy, A.M.; Hoffman, M.D.; Verhagen, H.H.; Thompson, S.W.; Dhamija, P.; Sandford, F.J.; Cooper, M.C. A randomized controlled trial of manual therapy and pneumatic compression for recovery from prolonged running—An extended study. *Res. Sport. Med.* **2018**, *26*, 354–364. [CrossRef]
32. Valenzuela, P.L.; Montalvo, Z.; Torrontegi, E.; Sánchez-Martínez, G.; Lucia, A.; de la Villa, P. Enhanced External Counterpulsation and Recovery From a Plyometric Exercise Bout. *Clin. J. Sport Med.* **2018**, *30*, 416–419. [CrossRef]
33. Oliver, A.; Driller, M. The Use of Upper-Body Intermittent Sequential Pneumatic Compression Arm Sleeves on Recovery From Exercise in Wheelchair Athletes. *Am. J. Phys. Med. Rehabil.* **2021**, *100*, 65–71. [CrossRef]
34. Cranston, A.W.; Driller, M.W. Investigating the Use of an Intermittent Sequential Pneumatic Compression Arm Sleeve for Recovery After Upper-Body Exercise. *J. Strength Cond. Res.* **2020**. [CrossRef]
35. Wiecha, S.; Jarocka, M.; Wiśniowski, P.; Cieśliński, M.; Price, S.; Makaruk, B.; Kotowska, J.; Drabarek, D.; Cieśliński, I.; Sacewicz, T. The efficacy of intermittent pneumatic compression and negative pressure therapy on muscle function, soreness and serum indices of muscle damage: A randomized controlled trial. *BMC Sports Sci. Med. Rehabil.* **2021**, *13*, 144. [CrossRef] [PubMed]
36. Halson, S.L. Nutrition, sleep and recovery. *Eur. J. Sport Sci.* **2008**, *8*, 119–126. [CrossRef]
37. Kerksick, C.M.; Arent, S.; Schoenfeld, B.J.; Stout, J.R.; Campbell, B.; Wilborn, C.D.; Taylor, L.; Kalman, D.; Smith-Ryan, A.E.; Kreider, R.B.; et al. International society of sports nutrition position stand: Nutrient timing. *J. Int. Soc. Sports Nutr.* **2017**, *14*, 33. [CrossRef] [PubMed]
38. Davis, J.K.; Oikawa, S.Y.; Halson, S.; Stephens, J.; O'Riordan, S.; Luhrs, K.; Sopena, B.; Baker, L.B. In-Season Nutrition Strategies and Recovery Modalities to Enhance Recovery for Basketball Players: A Narrative Review. *Sport. Med.* **2021**, *36*, 1–23. [CrossRef] [PubMed]

39. Kovacs, M.S.; Baker, L.B. Recovery interventions and strategies for improved tennis performance. *Br. J. Sports Med.* **2014**, *48*, i18–i21. [CrossRef]
40. Brancaccio, P.; Maffulli, N.; Limongelli, F.M. Creatine kinase monitoring in sport medicine. *Br. Med. Bull.* **2007**, *81–82*, 209–230. [CrossRef]
41. Noakes, T.D. Effect of Exercise on Serum Enzyme Activities in Humans. *Sport. Med.* **1987**, *4*, 245–267. [CrossRef]
42. Malm, C.; Sjödin, B.; Sjöberg, B.; Lenkei, R.; Renström, P.; Lundberg, I.E.; Ekblom, B. Leukocytes, cytokines, growth factors and hormones in human skeletal muscle and blood after uphill or downhill running. *J. Physiol.* **2004**, *556*, 983–1000. [CrossRef]
43. Baird, M.F.; Graham, S.M.; Baker, J.S.; Bickerstaff, G.F. Creatine-Kinase- and Exercise-Related Muscle Damage Implications for Muscle Performance and Recovery. *J. Nutr. Metab.* **2012**, *2012*, 960363. [CrossRef] [PubMed]
44. Ehlers, G.G.; Ball, T.E.; Liston, L. Creatine Kinase Levels are Elevated During 2-A-Day Practices in Collegiate Football Players. *J. Athl. Train.* **2002**, *37*, 151–156. [PubMed]
45. Fallon, K.E.; Sivyer, G.; Sivyer, K.; Dare, A. The biochemistry of runners in a 1600 km ultramarathon. *Br. J. Sports Med.* **1999**, *33*, 264–269. [CrossRef] [PubMed]
46. Hortobágyi, T.; Denahan, T. Variability in Creatine Kinase: Methodological, Exercise, and Clinically Related Factors. *Int. J. Sports Med.* **1989**, *10*, 69–80. [CrossRef]
47. Kratz, A.; Lewandrowski, K.B.; Siegel, A.J.; Chun, K.Y.; Flood, J.G.; Van Cott, E.M.; Lee-Lewandrowski, E. Effect of Marathon Running on Hematologic and Biochemical Laboratory Parameters, Including Cardiac Markers. *Am. J. Clin. Pathol.* **2002**, *118*, 856–863. [CrossRef]
48. Cheung, K.; Hume, P.A.; Maxwell, L. Delayed Onset Muscle Soreness. *Sport. Med.* **2003**, *33*, 145–164. [CrossRef]
49. Armstrong, R.B. Mechanisms of exercise-induced delayed onset muscular soreness: A brief review. *Med. Sci. Sports Exerc.* **1984**, *16*, 529–538. [CrossRef]
50. Hamill, J.; Freedson, P.S.; Clarkson, P.M.; Braun, B. Muscle Soreness during Running: Biomechanical and Physiological Considerations. *Int. J. Sport Biomech.* **1991**, *7*, 125–137. [CrossRef]
51. Orchard, J.; Marsden, J.; Lord, S.; Garlick, D. Preseason Hamstring Muscle Weakness Associated with Hamstring Muscle Injury in Australian Footballers. *Am. J. Sports Med.* **1997**, *25*, 81–85. [CrossRef]
52. Edgerton, V.R.; Wolf, S.L.; Levendowski, D.J.; Roy, R.R. Theoretical basis for patterning EMG amplitudes to assess muscle dysfunction. *Med. Sci. Sport. Exerc.* **1996**, *28*, 744–751. [CrossRef]
53. Wessel, J.; Wan, A. Effect of Stretching on the Intensity of Delayed-Onset Muscle Soreness. *Clin. J. Sport Med.* **1994**, *4*, 83–87. [CrossRef]
54. Gulick, D.T.; Kimura, I.F. Delayed Onset Muscle Soreness: What Is It and How Do We Treat It? *J. Sport Rehabil.* **1996**, *5*, 234–243. [CrossRef]
55. Vairo, G.L.; Miller, S.J.; Rier, N.M.C.I.; Uckley, W.B.I. Systematic Review of Efficacy for Manual Lymphatic Drainage Techniques in Sports Medicine and Rehabilitation: An Evidence-Based Practice Approach. *J. Man. Manip. Ther.* **2009**, *17*, 80E–89E. [CrossRef] [PubMed]
56. Harrison, A.J.; Keane, S.P.; Coglan, J. Force-Velocity Relationship and Stretch-Shortening Cycle Function in Sprint and Endurance Athletes. *J. Strength Cond. Res.* **2004**, *18*, 473. [CrossRef] [PubMed]
57. Loturco, I.; Pereira, L.A.; Cal Abad, C.C.; D'Angelo, R.A.; Fernandes, V.; Kitamura, K.; Kobal, R.; Nakamura, F.Y. Vertical and Horizontal Jump Tests Are Strongly Associated With Competitive Performance in 100-m Dash Events. *J. Strength Cond. Res.* **2015**, *29*, 1966–1971. [CrossRef]
58. Sattler, T.; Hadžić, V.; Dervišević, E.; Markovic, G. Vertical Jump Performance of Professional Male and Female Volleyball Players. *J. Strength Cond. Res.* **2015**, *29*, 1486–1493. [CrossRef]
59. Castagna, C.; Castellini, E. Vertical Jump Performance in Italian Male and Female National Team Soccer Players. *J. Strength Cond. Res.* **2013**, *27*, 1156–1161. [CrossRef]
60. Kons, R.L.; Ache-Dias, J.; Detanico, D.; Barth, J.; Dal Pupo, J. Is Vertical Jump Height an Indicator of Athletes' Power Output in Different Sport Modalities? *J. Strength Cond. Res.* **2018**, *32*, 708–715. [CrossRef]
61. Canavan, P.K.; Vescovi, J.D. Evaluation of Power Prediction Equations: Peak Vertical Jumping Power in Women. *Med. Sci. Sports Exerc.* **2004**, *36*, 1589–1593. [CrossRef]
62. Potteiger, J.A.; Lockwood, R.H.; Haub, M.D.; Dolezal, B.A.; Almuzaini, K.S.; Schroeder, J.M.; Zebas, C.J.; Lockwood, R.; Dolezal, B.; Almuzaini, K.; et al. Muscle Power and Fiber Characteristics Following 8 Weeks of Plyometric Training. *J. Strength Cond. Res.* **1999**, *13*, 275–279.
63. Bobbert, M.F. Drop Jumping as a Training Method for Jumping Ability. *Sports Med.* **1990**, *9*, 7–22. [CrossRef]
64. Markovic, G.; Markovic, G. Does Plyometric Training Improve Vertical Jump Height? A Meta-Analytical Review. *Br. J. Sports Med.* **2007**, *41*, 349–355. [CrossRef] [PubMed]
65. Morrison, A.; Polisena, J.; Husereau, D.; Moulton, K.; Clark, M.; Fiander, M.; Mierzwinski-Urban, M.; Clifford, T.; Hutton, B.; Rabb, D. The Effect of English-Language Restriction on Systematic Review-Based Meta-Analyses: A Systematic Review of Empirical Studies. *Int. J. Technol. Assess. Health Care* **2012**, *28*, 138–144. [CrossRef] [PubMed]

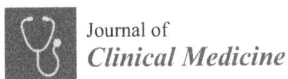

Article

Differences in Adiposity Profile and Body Fat Distribution between Forwards and Backs in Sub-Elite Spanish Female Rugby Union Players

Dolores Escrivá [1,2], Jordi Caplliure-Llopis [2,3], Inmaculada Benet [2,4], Gonzalo Mariscal [2], Juan Vicente Mampel [5] and Carlos Barrios [2,*]

1 Intensive Care Unit, La Fe Polytechnic and University Hospital, 46026 Valencia, Spain; descpei@gmail.com
2 Institute for Research on Musculoskeletal Disorders, School of Medicine, Valencia Catholic University, 46001 Valencia, Spain; jordi.kaliu@hotmail.com (J.C.-L.); inmabenet@yahoo.es (I.B.); gonzalo.mariscal@mail.ucv.es (G.M.)
3 Primary Health Care Services, La Ribera University Hospital, 46600 Alzira, Spain
4 Surgical Emergency Facilities, Valencia University Hospital, 46010 Valencia, Spain
5 Department of Physiotherapy, Catholic University of Valencia San Vicente Mártir, 46001 Valencia, Spain; juan.vicente@ucv.es
* Correspondence: carlos.barrios@ucv.es; Tel.: +34-610-408-001; Fax: +34-963-944-590

Abstract: The purpose of this study was to analyze the adiposity profile and the body fat distribution in 56 sub-elite female rugby union players involved in the Spanish National Women's Rugby Union Championships. The participants included in this study, which was the first to analyze sub-elite players, show thinner skinfolds, lower fat mass, and lesser fat percentage than previously reported for elite female rugby union players. Forwards were heavier and had higher body mass index (BMI) and fat mass, thicker skinfolds, and higher fat percentage than back players. Forwards also possessed significantly greater total fat-free mass than backs. All these differences were applicable only to players under 25 years of age. A negative correlation between age and both abdominal and lower extremity fat was found in forward players but not in the backs. Both Yuhasz and Faulkner equations tended to underestimate fat percentage in comparison to Reilly equation. Although Yuhasz equation provided higher systematic error, random error was lower in comparison to Faulkner equation. This study shows the relevance of analyzing and monitoring adiposity in female rugby union players to optimize adaptation to the sports requirements of different playing positions and age.

Keywords: women's rugby; anthropometry; body composition; adiposity; somatotype

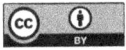

1. Introduction

Rugby union is a highly demanding contact team sport that requires participants to be in exceptionally good physical condition, which includes muscle strength and power, agility, reaction ability, and sprinting speed, among other qualities [1,2]. In addition to frequent heavy impacts, matches combine intermittent periods of high-intensity physical tasks (i.e., sprinting, scrummaging, etc.) with periods of less intensity (i.e., walking, jogging, etc.). In the past, rugby was a male sport, but in recent years, the involvement of women in rugby competitions at different levels has grown markedly all around the world [3]. Rugby requirements for women are also challenging. Using global positioning system tracking technology, the distance covered by elite female rugby union players during a match was found to be 5820 ± 512 m, with a maximum heart rate of more than 90% of their base rate during 50% of the match [4].

In Rugby union, the 15 players on the field assume different playing positions that require specific physical and anthropometric qualities [1,2]. Classically, participants are categorized into forward and back players. Forwards are involved in offensive and defensive collisions, scrums, and ball retention during lineouts and mauls. For better completion of these tasks, forwards usually have greater total body and fat mass than back players [1,5–7]. On the contrary, conditioning demands for back players include agility, speed, and reaction ability [8]. To satisfactorily perform their role, backs should be lighter and leaner than forwards and avoid having excess fat.

For more than two decades, differences in anthropometry and body composition between forward and back male players have been extensively addressed in the literature [9–13]. Despite the impact of anthropometry on the performance level of males, there is limited information and lack of consensus on the anthropometric profile of female rugby union players with special reference to adiposity. Some reports describe anthropometric differences between female forward and back rugby union players comparable to those found in male players [7,14,15]. However, other authors did not detect any significant differences among female forwards and backs in both the anthropometric and physical performance measurements [16,17]. Both type of reports, in favor of or against anthropometric and body composition differences between female forwards and backs, only focused on elite rugby union players and did not analyze deeply the impact of adiposity on females. To our knowledge, there are no other studies on sub-elite female rugby union players.

The influence of body composition on physical condition and performance has already been addressed both in male and female players of league rugby, another popular modality of this sport [1,18–20]. Specifically, total body fat was negatively correlated with fitness characteristics and performance tests in female rugby league players [15]. The particular and cyclic hormonal environment of women suggests that the monitoring of the body fat component should be relevant in female athletes since there is a close relationship between performance and body fat parameters. Therefore, the aim of this study was to analyze the effect of age (i.e., <21 years, 21–25 years, and >25 years) and players position (i.e., forwards and backs) on body fat distribution (i.e., abdominal fat and lower body fat) and adiposity profile (i.e., sum 7 skinfolds and body fat percentage) in sub-elite female rugby union players. In addition, other objective of the present study was to compare three equations used to estimate the fat mass percentage and analyze the limit of agreement between two of the most widely used equations, Yuhasz and Faulkner vs. Reilly equation, specifically proposed for soccer players [21]. Both rugby and soccer are team sports with similar physiologic demands related to the position played that condition comparable anthropometric characteristics [1,6,22,23]. A deeper knowledge of the body composition profile of these athletes, particularly adiposity, could help to develop specific training programs and physical performance standards for rugby players according to their anthropometric characteristics and the requirements of their playing position. Our hypothesis is that female rugby union forward and back players differ in their adiposity characteristics only during their first years (i.e., younger players) of involvement in competition. After a certain number of years of playing rugby, differences in anthropometry and body composition become less evident.

2. Methods

2.1. Design

Analytical cross-sectional study of anthropometric data of female rugby union players involved in the sub-elite Spanish National Rugby Championships. Data were recorded at the end of the 2019–2020 season, just prior to the training sessions before the last two matches of the competition.

2.2. Participants

A total of 56 female players took part in this study. For analysis and comparison, players were categorized into two groups depending on their position: forwards ($n = 26$) and backs ($n = 30$). The average values of the total sample in terms of age, stature, and body mass were 23.7 ± 6.4 years, 163.5 ± 7.1 cm, and 65.7 ± 10.0 kg, respectively. Regarding age, there were 18 rugby union players under 21 years, 24 players from 21 to 25 years, and 14 players above 25 years.

All participants had at least two years of experience in rugby training in a structured and organized manner by a sports entity and one year of experience at a professional rugby club. None of the participants received any payment for involvement in the sport. Most of them were university students or generated income through employment outside of rugby.

At the time of assessment, players trained at least three times a week with sessions lasting over 90 min. These last in-season micro-cycles included a general physical conditioning workout combined with plyometric exercises in the first day of training after the match day. The other two days were devoted to strength and speed training, technical skills, and tactic aspects. We added this information in the manuscript. Competition matches took place on the weekends. The sample was recruited from the players of different rugby teams (UCV, CAU, Les Abelles, and Tecnidex) from the region of Valencia, Spain. Players who did not participate in any activity for more than six weeks due to a sporting injury and those who did not take part in at least six of the last ten competition matches were excluded from the study.

Both managers of each club and participants were informed of the objectives, procedures, and possible benefits or risks of the study. Informed consent was obtained from all participants as a previous requirement to access the study. The study was conducted in accordance with the Declaration of Helsinki 1961 (reviewed in Edinburgh, 2000) and approved by the Research Ethics Committee of the Catholic University of Valencia (reference: UCV/2019-2020/017).

2.3. Anthropometry and Instruments

All general anthropometric measurements of stature, weight, and thickness of seven skinfolds (biceps, triceps, subscapular, abdominal, suprailiac, thigh, and calf) were taken in accordance with the recommendations from the International Society for the Advancement of Kinanthropometry (ISAK) [24]. To homogenize the hydration status, participants were encouraged to drink at least 1 L of water 30 min before the anthropometric assessment. Each participant's body mass and stature were measured and recorded with the same equipment, which was regularly calibrated for clinical use. Before a normal training session, all participants were measured and weighed without wearing shoes, with minimal clothing, and with an empty bladder. Regarding precision, stature was measured to the nearest 0.1 cm (SECA 225, SECA, Hamburg, Germany), and weight was measured to the nearest 0.1 kg (SECA 861, SECA, Hamburg, Germany). BMI was calculated as weight (in kilograms) divided by the square of their height (in meters).

Skinfold thicknesses were measured from the right side of the body with a Holtain Tanner/Whitehouse skinfold caliper (Holtain Ltd., Crymmych, UK). The circumferences of the arms, thighs, and legs were also measured in centimeters. The bi-styloid diameter and both intercondylar diameters in the distal humerus and femur were also measured. All measurements were taken by the same well-trained investigator (ISAK level 2 certified). Each measurement was repeated three times at the same evaluation, and the average value was calculated. The technical measurement error was within the recommended limits by ISAK [24].

Body fat percentage were calculated from measurements of two common skinfold equations for the general population, the Yuhasz [25] and the Faulkner equation, which was modified by Slaughter et al. [26]. Since rugby union players have comparable characteristics to soccer players, the Reilly equation, a specific body-fat-predicting equation for soccer players, was also used to test its reliability in our sample [21] (Table 1). Total fat mass was calculated by multiplying the total mass by fat percentage. Fat-free mass was obtained by subtracting from total weight the total fat mass in kilograms. The somatotype components (endomorphy, mesomorphy, and ectomorphy) of each participant were assessed by the Heath–Carter method [27].

Table 1. Skinfold equation used to estimate body fat percentage (%BF) in females.

Author	Equation	Ref.
Reilly	%BF = 5.174 + (0.124 × thigh) + (0.147 × abdominal) + (0.196 × triceps) + (0.130 × calf)	[21]
Faulkner (Slaughter's modification)	(Triceps + subscapular < 35 mm) %BF = 1.33 (triceps + subscapular) − 0.013 (triceps + subscapular)^2 − 2.5 (Triceps + subscapular > 35 mm) %BF = 0.546 (triceps + subscapular) + 9.7	[26]
Yuhasz	%BF = 0.1548 (triceps + subscapular + suprailiac + abdominal + thigh + calf) + 3.580	[27]

2.4. Statistical Analyses

All variables were expressed as mean ± standard deviation (SD) and 95% confident interval ($CI_{95\%}$). Normal distribution was assessed using Kolmogorov–Smirnov Test. Due to the wide range of the players' ages, three different age groups were arbitrarily defined for comparison: under 21 years, from 21 to 25, and older than 25. To analyze the effect of age (i.e., under 21 years, 21–25 years, and older than 25 years) and players position (i.e., forwards and backs), a between-groups analysis of variance (ANOVA) was performed. Bonferroni post-hoc corrections were performed to account for type I error. Within age groups, the differences between forwards and backs were analyzed using the nonparametric Mann–Whitney U test, as recommended by the literature for limited samples [28]. To compare the differences between the three equations to estimate fat percentage, a one-way repeated measures ANOVA was performed. The effect sizes were calculated using g Hedges method with the following thresholds: small = 0.20 to 0.49, medium = 0.50 to 0.79, and large >0.80. The associations between anthropometric parameters were described using Pearson correlation coefficient. To account systematic and random error, Bland–Altman plot was used to assess the mean difference and limits of agreement between the Faulkner and Yuhasz equations vs. Reilly equation. Statistical significance was $p < 0.05$. All statistical analyses were performed with the statistical package (Rstudio, v 1.3.959, for MacOS).

2.5. Ethical Approval

The study was conducted in accordance with the Declaration of Helsinki 1961 (reviewed in Edinburgh, 2000) and approved by the Research Ethics Committee of the Catholic University of Valencia (reference: UCV/2019-2020/017).

2.6. Data Availability

The datasets generated during and/or analyzed during the current study are available from the corresponding author on reasonable request.

3. Results

Tables 2 and 3 include the general anthropometric characteristics, including adiposity parameters, of the sample. Regarding adiposity profile (i.e., sum of seven skinfolds), the between groups ANOVA showed statistically significant differences in main effect of players position ($F_{(1,50)} = 22.43$, $p < 0.001$) and *age* ($F_{(2,30)} = 6.49$, $p = 0.003$) variables. However, no significant differences were found at interaction effect of player position x age ($F_{(2,50)} = 2.57$, $p = 0.087$). Bonferroni post-hoc comparison revealed a mean difference (MD) and 95% of confident interval ($CI_{95\%}$) of 46.47 mm (26.76 to 66.18) between forwards and backs ($p < 0.001$). Regarding age variable, no significant differences were found between <21 years group vs. 21–25 years group (MD = 12.95 mm (−15.01 to 40.93), $p = 0.770$). However, statistically significant differences were found between <21 years group vs. >25 years group and 21–25 years group vs. >25 years group (MD = 45.11 mm (13.24 to 77.03), $p = 0.003$, MD = 32.19 mm (2.96 to 61.52), $p = 0.027$), respectively. See Tables 2 and 3 and Figures 1 and 2 for more information regarding the other variables.

Table 2. General anthropometric data, skinfold thickness (mm), fat mass, fat-free mass parameters, and body composition profile of the female rugby players included in the study. Differences according to player position are also indicated.

	Whole Equoationsample	Forwards (n = 26)	Backs (n = 30)	p-Value [§]	g Hedges (CI$_{95\%}$)
Age (years)	23.7 ± 6.4	24.8 ± 7.2	22.7 ± 5.5	0.230	0.32 (−0.21 to 0.85)
		General anthropometric data			
Stature (cm)	163.5 ± 7.1	164.0 ± 9.3	163.0 ± 4.6	0.603	0.14 (−0.39 to 0.66)
Weight (kg)	65.7 ± 10.0	71.5 ± 10.2	60.6 ± 6.5	0.001 **	1.28 (0.70 to 1.85)
BMI	24.7 ± 4.4	26.8 ± 5.3	22.8 ± 4.4	0.001 **	1.03 (0.46 to 1.58)
Body surface (m^2)	1.91 ± 0.15	1.99 ± 0.15	1.84 ± 0.11	0.001 **	0.98 (0.42 to 1.54)
		Skinfolds			
Triceps (mm)	16.8 ± 6.3	19.5 ± 7.1	14.4 ± 4.3	0.002 **	0.87 (0.32 to 1.42)
Biceps (mm)	8.6 ± 5.1	10.6 ± 6.3	6.8 ± 2.8	0.002 **	0.78 (0.23 to 1.33)
Subscapular (mm)	14.3 ± 7.3	18.1 ± 8.2	10.9 ± 4.1	0.001 **	1.10 (0.53 to 1.66)
Abdominal (mm)	20.3 ± 8.9	24.9 ± 9.1	16.2 ± 6.4	0.001 **	1.10 (0.52 to 1.65)
Suprailiac (mm)	14.8 ± 7.9	18.3 ± 9.4	11.7 ± 4.4	0.001 **	0.90 (0.35 to 1.45)
Thigh (mm)	27.5 ± 8.8	29.6 ± 9.8	25.7 ± 7.6	0.101	0.44 (−0.09 to 0.97)
Leg (mm)	18.1 ± 7.2	21.9 ± 7.6	14.8 ± 4.9	0.000 **	1.11 (0.54 to 1.67)
		Fat Mass			
Total Fat Mass (kg)	10.7 ± 4.6	13.3 ± 5.3	8.5 ± 2.2	0.001 **	1.18 (0.60 to 1.74)
FMI	4.1 ± 1.9	5.1 ± 2.3	3.2 ± 0.8	0.001 **	1.10 (0.53 to 1.66)
%BF—Yuhasz	14.3 ± 4.2	16.5 ± 4.7	12.4 ± 2.5	0.001 **	1.08 (0.51 to 1.64)
%BF—Faulkner	15.9 ± 4.2	18.2 ± 4.8	13.9 ± 2.4	0.001 **	1.13 (0.56 to 1.69)
%BF—Reilly	17.2 ± 3.9	19.1 ± 4.3	15.5 ± 2.6	0.001 **	1.03 (0.46 to 1.58)
		Fat-Free Mass			
Fat Free Mass (FFM)	58.9 + 7.5	63.3 ± 7.4	55.3 ± 5.2	0.001 **	1.24 (0.67 to 1.82)
		Body composition			
Endomorphy	4.68 ± 1.74	5.56 ± 1.97	3.92 ± 1.05	0.001 **	1.04 (0.48 to 1.60)
Mesomorphy	2.74 ± 1.43	3.13 ± 1.79	2.39 ± 0.91	0.054	0.52 (−0.02 to 1.05)
Ectomorphy	1.71 ± 1.08	1.22 ± 1.23	2.12 ± 0.72	0.001 **	−0.89 (−1.42 to −0.33)

BMI, body mass index; FMI, fat mass index; %BF body fat percentage; CI$_{95\%}$, confident interval at 95%; [§] Mann−Whitney U test ** ($p < 0.01$).

Table 3. General anthropometric data, adiposity parameters, and lean measurements of forward and back players of the three age groups.

	Under 21 Years			From 21 to 25 Years			More than 25 Years		
	Forwards (n = 6)	Backs (n = 12)	p-Value § (g Hedges)	Forwards (n = 12)	Backs (n = 12)	p-Value § (g Hedges)	Forwards (n = 8)	Backs (n = 6)	p-Value § (g Hedges)
				General anthropometry					
Body mass (kg)	74.2 ± 11.7	58.9 ± 5.8	0.011 * (1.78)	73.4 ± 11.4	63.4 ± 7.2	0.035 * (1.02)	66.8 ± 5.7	58.5 ± 5.2	0.014 * (1.40)
BMI	31.4 ± 8.1	22.6 ± 1.9	0.031 * (1.75)	26.7 ± 3.9	23.2 ± 2.2	0.026 * (1.08)	23.7 ± 2.1	22.3 ± 1.8	0.302 (0.66)
Fat-Free Mass (kg)	65.0 ± 7.8	53.8 ± 4.8	0.009 ** (1.81)	64.3 ± 8.4	57.5 ± 5.7	0.038 * (0.53)	60.5 ± 56.3	53.7 ± 4.7	0.033 * (1.43)
				Adiposity parameters					
Abdominal Fat (mm)	50.3 ± 22.9	28.7 ± 9.9	0.049 * (1.34)	46.4 ± 16.6	27.9 ± 11.1	0.006 * (1.23)	33.2 ± 11.6	26.5 ± 9.9	0.219 (0.57)
Lower Extremity Fat (mm)	65.7 ± 20.5	41.5 ± 9.9	0.015 * (1.63)	52.0 ± 13.6	43.1 ± 11.2	0.183 (0.68)	40.3 ± 7.8	33.3 ± 14.2	0.272 (0.60)
Total Fat mass (kg)	15.9 ± 6.9	8.3 ± 1.8	0.031 * (1.76)	14.4 ± 5.4	9.2 ± 2.6	0.005 ** (1.18)	9.8 ± 1.4	7.8 ± 2.0	0.039 * (1.09)
FMI	6.7 ± 3.0	3.2 ± 0.7	0.025 * (1.93)	5.2 ± 1.9	3.4 ± 0.9	0.004 ** (1.18)	3.5 ± 0.6	3.0 ± 0.8	0.156 (0.65)
%BF—Yuhasz	19.7 ± 6.0	12.5 ± 1.8	0.011 * (1.87)	17.2 ± 4.1	13.0 ± 2.8	0.018 * (1.16)	12.9 ± 1.5	11.2 ± 3.1	0.121 (0.69)
%BF—Slaugther	20.7 ± 6.1	13.9 ± 2.0	0.035 * (1.72)	17.2 ± 4.1	14.3 ± 2.7	0.005 ** (1.30)	12.9 ± 1.5	13.2 ± 2.5	0.121 (0.60)
%BF—Reilly	22.4 ± 5.4	15.7 ± 19	0.015 * (1.86)	19.7 ± 3.9	16.2 ± 2.9	0.033 * (1.00)	15.9 ± 1.2	13.7 ± 2.9	0.053 (1.01)

§ Mann–Whitney U test * ($p < 0.05$); ** ($p < 0.01$).

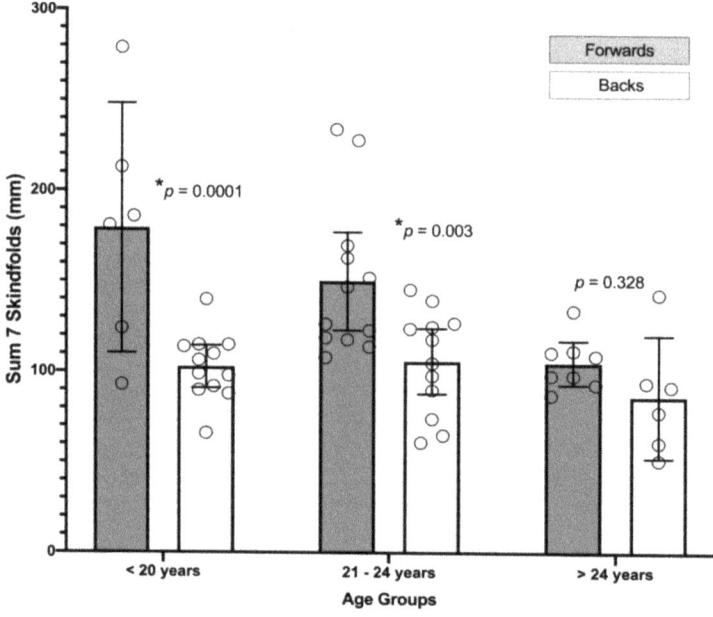

Figure 1. Sum of the seven skinfolds thickness (mm) in the three age-groups regarding players position (i.e., forwards and backs) and age (i.e., <21 years, 21–25 years, and >25 years). Bars represent the mean and 95% of confident interval. * Asterisk represent significant differences ($p < 0.05$).

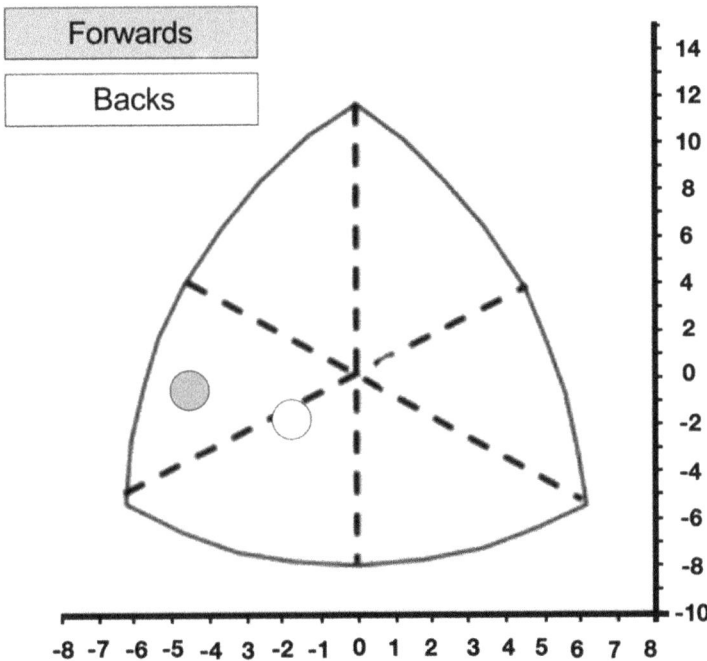

Figure 2. Body composition diagram of the two groups of female rugby players according to Carter and Heath charts.

Forwards had a fat-free mass significantly higher than back players (Table 2). Regarding somatotype, a significantly higher endomorphic component and a lower ectomorphic component were observed in the group of forward players when compared to the backs ($p < 0.01$) (Table 2). Figure 2 displays the body composition diagram of the two groups of female rugby players according to Carter and Heath charts.

Regarding body fat distribution, in abdominal fat, the between groups ANOVA showed statistical significant differences in main effect of players position ($F_{(1,50)} = 16.11$, $p < 0.001$), but no significant differences were found in age variable ($F_{(2,30)} = 6.49$, $p = 0.003$). Bonferroni post-hoc comparison revealed a MD and $CI_{95\%}$ of 15.56 mm (7.77 to 23.34) between forwards and backs ($p < 0.001$). In relation to age, no significant differences were found at any comparison level ($p > 0.05$). However, statistically significant differences were found in the interaction effect of players position x age: <21 years, forwards vs. backs (MD = 21.58 mm (7.71 to 35.45)) and 21–25 years group, forwards vs. backs (MD = 18.42 mm (7.01 to 29.75)). No significant differences were found in >25 years group, forwards vs. backs (MD = 6.67 mm (−8.83 to 21.65)) (Figure 3).

On the other hand, statistically significant differences were found in the interaction effect of players position x age: <21 years, forwards vs. backs (MD = 24.17 mm (11.43 to 36.90), $p < 0.001$). No significant differences were found between forwards vs. back in 21–25 years group ($p = 0.094$) and >25 years group ($p = 0.313$) (Figure 3).

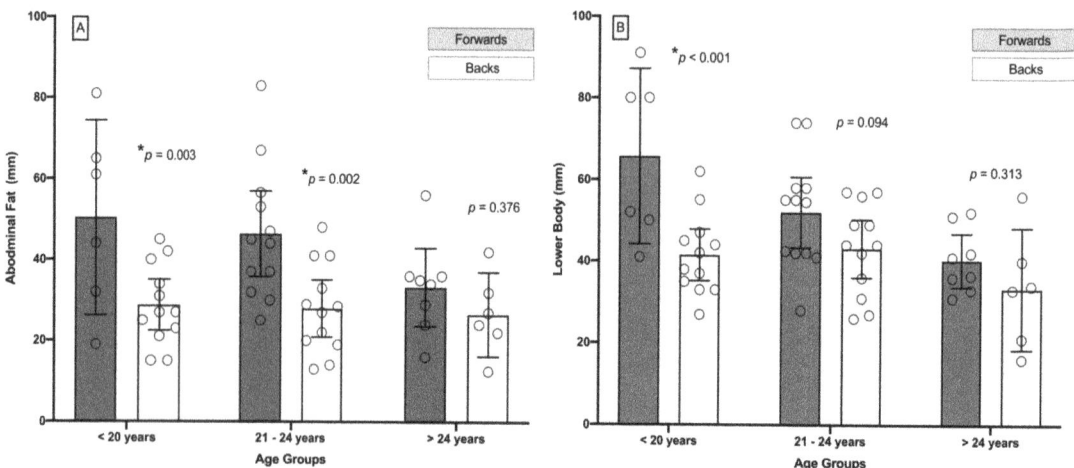

Figure 3. (**A**) Abdominal fat (mm) and (**B**) lower extremity fat (mm) in the three age groups regarding players position (i.e., forwards and backs) and age (i.e., <21 years, 21–25 years, and >25 years). Bars represent the mean and 95% of confident interval. * Asterisk represent significant differences ($p < 0.05$).

Total fat mass and fat percentages calculated with the different equations were significantly higher in forwards (Table 2). Total fat mass was 56.4% higher in forward than in back players ($p < 0.001$, g Hedges = 1.18 (0.60–1.74)). The Yuhasz equations provided the lowest values of body fat percentage, and the Reilly's equation yielded the highest values. Differences between these two equations were statistically significant (MD ± SE = 2.9 ± 1.9; $p = 0.003$; g Hedges = 0.72). When three equations were compared, the one-way RM ANOVA showed significant differences ($F_{(1.16, 63.68)} = 153$, $p < 0.0001$). Bonferroni post-hoc corrections revealed significant differences between Yuhasz vs. Faulkner equations (MD = −1.57% (−1.93 to −1.22), $p < 0.0001$, g Hedges = −1.47 (−1.84 to −1.08)), Yuhasz vs. Reilly equations (MD = −2.88% (−3.14 to −2.62), $p < 0.0001$, g Hedges = −3.62 (−4.34 to −2.89)) and Faulkner vs. Reilly equations (MD = −1.31% (−1.71 to −0.91), $p < 0.0001$, g Hedges = −0.78 (−1.08 to −0.48)). Reilly's equation, a specific body fat percentage estimation for soccer players, detected the lowest difference in body fat percentage between forwards and backs (3.7 ± 0.9%). Body fat percentage estimations for all three equations were well correlated (see Figure 4). There was also a strong correlation between the fat mass index and the body fat percentage values of the three equations (Faulkner: $r = 0.979$, $p > 0.001$; Reilly: $r = 0.818$, $p > 0.001$) for both forwards and backs. Mean differences and limits of agreement between of Yuhasz equation vs. Reilly equation and Faulkner equation vs. Reilly equation correspond to −2.88% (−4.43 to −1.33) and −1.31% (−0.459 to 1.97), respectively, as shown in Figure 4B,C.

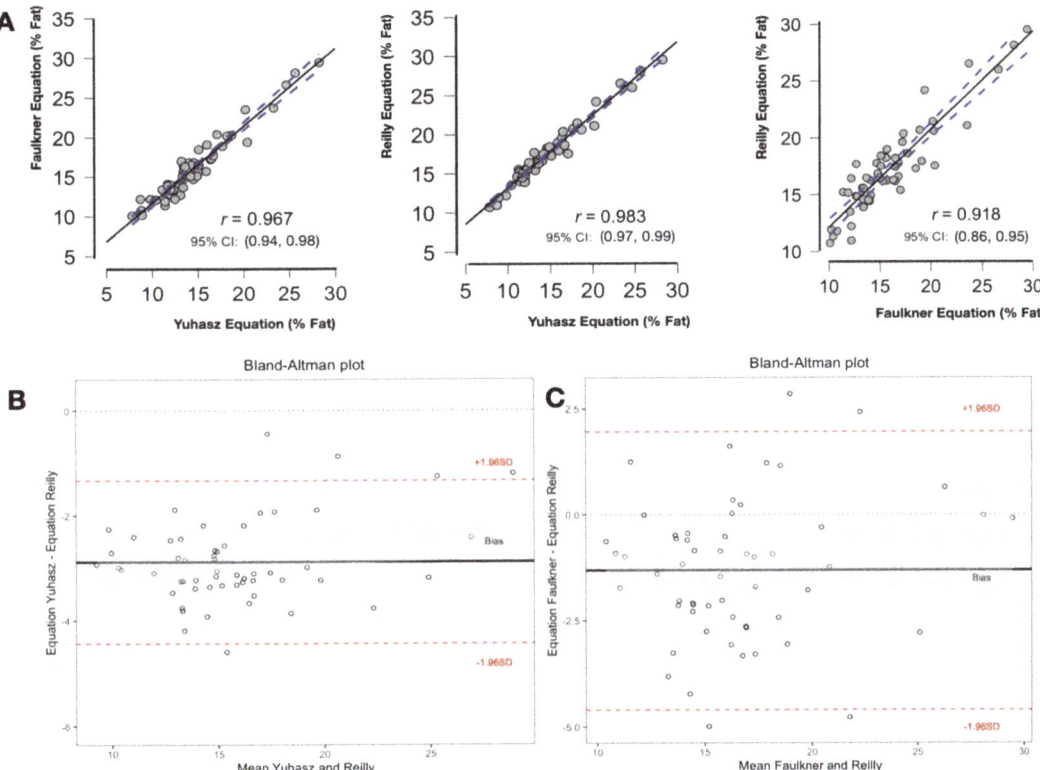

Figure 4. (**A**) Relationships between three fat percentage equations (i.e., Faulkner, Yuhasz, and Reilly). Bland–Altman plot comparing the mean differences and limits of agreement between (**B**) Yuhasz and Reilly equations and (**C**) Faulkner and Reilly equations.

4. Discussion

The main objective of this study was to analyze the effect of age and players position on body fat distribution and adiposity profile in a sample of sub-elite female rugby union players. In addition, the second objective of this study was to compare three equations used to obtain the fat mass percentage and analyze the limit of agreement between Yuhasz and Faulkner equations vs. Reilly equation. Results obtained showed that there was considerable variation in the anthropometric profile, especially in fat mass and somatotype, which showed a significantly higher body mass, BMI, and adiposity levels in the forwards. In terms of somatotype characteristics, compared to back players, forwards had a predominant endomorphic component with statistical differences. Backs had a significantly lower fat percentage, which mainly defines an ectomorphic somatotype. Fat percentage equations revealed statistical differences between equations. Both Yuhasz and Faulkner equations tended to underestimate fat percentage in comparison to Reilly equation. Although Yuhasz equation provided higher systematic error, random error was more stable. These data provide valuable information in designing specific training programs in accordance with players' positions and adapting diets to the players' needs.

To our knowledge, the literature addressing the anthropometry characteristics of female rugby union players is limited to five studies, four of which evaluated elite players (7, 14, 16, 17) and one of which focused on collegiate athletes (22). All these reports come from countries with long traditions in rugby. Nevertheless, the studies covered limited samples of elite players that became fewer when players were discriminated by playing position. The current study described the largest and most unique study so far done on a series of forward and back female rugby union players that focused on sub-elite or non-professional female European players. The current sample revealed lower total body mass, fat mass, and fat percentage in both forwards and backs as compared to data from elite female rugby union players reported in previous studies [14,16,29]. These sub-elite rugby union players had markedly thinner skinfolds than in previous studies, as shown by comparison of the sum of the usual seven skinfold assessments [16,29]. Regarding fat percentage, the estimation for forwards in previous studies varied from a mean of 21.2% (English players) to 30.8% (South Africans). Fat percentage in backs oscillated from 20.2% (English players) to 26.1% (South African players). Our figures were considerably lower: 19.1% and 15.5% for forwards and backs, respectively. Differences found among the six studies could be most likely related to the variety of body composition assessment methods. Even using the DXA, the method shown the lowest variability and greatest accuracy, two of the previously reported studies exhibit quite different results [7,30].

Both forwards and backs in our sample were almost similar in mean age and total body mass to those in Kirby's study reported in 1993 [14]. Besides the similarities, back players from Spain showed statistically significant lower fat percentages than their English counterparts. The difference cannot be attributed to changes in dietary styles along the last 30 years since body fat percentage in the forward groups was quite similar. In any case, body composition differences between forwards and backs in the current series were coherent with previous research [7,14,16,17,29,30].

The most recent data reporting total body and fat mass in female rugby union players were obtained from a New Zealand cohort of elite players. Although there were no differences in the mean age of players as compared to our series, both New Zealand forwards and backs were significantly heavier (more than 15 kg of mean total mass), had greater fat mass (more than 9 kg of mean fat mass), and showed an estimated higher body fat percentage (more than 6% of the total mass) than sub-elite female players from Spain. These huge differences in the two contemporary series are difficult to explain and may only be attributed to cultural and ethnicity differences between European and Oceanic countries. In fact, different distribution patterns of fat and lean mass have been described in elite male Polynesian rugby union players and in Caucasians [6,12].

The wide range of age of female rugby union players in our sample reflects the current situation of the different teams involved in the Spanish National Women's Rugby Union Championships. Some players were engaged for several years in competition and had no chance to upgrade to the elite category and continued to play at the sub-elite level. Therefore, players in our sample were discriminated by three different age groups. When the forwards and backs in the three groups were compared, some interesting findings were detected. As hypothesized, forwards' anthropometric and body composition profiles tended to change with increasing age and progressively showed less total body mass and BMI, and they become thinner (less skinfold thickness and body fat percentage). However, the back players showed almost constant anthropometric and body composition parameters in the three age groups. Among younger players (under 21 years), the differences in body composition profiles between forwards and backs were clear. However, in older players (more than 25 years), there were minimal differences, including lower total body mass and fat mass in backs, between the two groups.

Our findings about the older players conflict with those reported by Nyberg and Penpraze [17], which, in a sample of 19 elite Scottish female rugby union players, found no significant differences between forwards and backs with regards to total body and fat mass. The mean age of their sample was 27.7 ± 7.8 years. In our group of older players (mean age 32.0 ± 7.8 years), forwards still had a heavier body mass (both fat mass and total fat-free mass) than the back players. However, as in the Nyberg and Penpraze series, our forward and back players' body fat percentages were not significantly different. The difference with respect to Nyberg and Penpraze's data is that, even in younger participants, our female rugby union players had a much lower body fat percentage. Again, this difference could be likely due in part to the different methods used to estimate body fat percentage. Nyberg and Penpraze used the BOD POD Body Composition System, a method that measures body volume by air displacement to calculate body density and estimate body fat percentage. BOB POD has shown to overestimate body fat percentage as compared to skinfold equations [31]. This fact could confirm our hypothesis regarding the differences between Nyberg and Penpraze's findings and our current results.

In male rugby union players, total body mass and lean mass increase as their playing level increases [32]. Skinfold thickness and body fat percentage showed the opposite trend and decreased as their playing level improved. According to the current results, female rugby union players revealed a similar tendency. Abdominal, supriliac, and lower extremity skinfold thickness progressively decreased in the three age-groups analyzed. Consequently, body fat mass also decreased with age. This applied specifically to forwards. Opposite of the previously reported findings in male players [32], total body mass also decreased with age in female forwards. It seems that, in female rugby union players, being heavier has no relevant impact on performance, which has been determined to be the opposite for male players during some of the Rugby World Cups [33,34].

Although this study provides new data to the literature, there are inherent limitations as a direct consequence of the cross-sectional design. As the participants were sub-elite players, many of them did not have a fixed or defined position and were versatile (within their group of forward or back players). Players were only measured once during the season, and it is well documented that anthropometric profiles can change during this time [29]. In addition, no data were collected regarding the eating habits of each player. Furthermore, the estimation of body fat percentage was evaluated through skinfold thickness measurements. It is already known that fat-prediction skinfold equations offer a limited ability to estimate body fat percentage as compared to the standard reference provided by DEXA assessment [35]. Nevertheless, the Reilly equation used in the current study has shown consistency in the fat estimations in sports similar to rugby and was defined as the most suitable equation to evaluate elite male rugby union players [35].

Maintaining optimal body composition is positively related to athletic development in athletes. Depending on the sport, high levels of fat percentage, insufficient levels of fat-free mass, and high BMI can affect performance and health [36]. The research conducted so far agrees that there is no ideal fat value for rugby players. Till et al. [37] conducted a retrospective study in which it was shown that United Kingdom Academy players with lower skinfolds showed long-term progression in their professional sports careers. As a result, evaluating body fat could be the best way to monitor individual changes in diet and/or personalized training as well as other changes [38,39]. In the rugby union case, anthropometric determinations could also be used as a valuable tool for coaches when assessing the profile or position in the game for each player. It seems important to plan training sessions and design a diet in relation to the position of each player on the field to optimize and improve the sporting life of athletes. Finally, an interesting aspect that requires further research is the relation of the somatotype and anaerobic resistance, as the forwards have a higher BMI and must perform strong physical exercises of running short distances at higher speeds.

5. Conclusions

This study shows that the adiposity parameters of athletes involved in the sub-elite Spanish National Women's Rugby Union Championships are related with the player's position and can vary according to age. Forward players were heavier, had a higher BMI and fat mass, and had thicker skinfolds and a higher fat percentage than back players. Forwards also possessed significantly greater total fat-free mass than backs. All these differences applied only for players under 25 years of age. Female rugby union players included in this study showed thinner skinfolds, lower fat mass, and lesser fat percentage than previously reported for elite female rugby union players versus females of comparable age in other sports. Both Yuhasz and Faulkner equations tended to underestimate fat percentage in comparison to Reilly equation. Although Yuhasz equation provided higher systematic error, random error was lower in comparison to Faulkner equation. These changes could be related to differences in dietary habits and/or the culture of the different countries. This study shows the importance of analyzing and monitoring adiposity in female rugby union players to optimize their adaptation to the requirements of different playing positions.

Author Contributions: Conceptualization, C.B.; Data curation, D.E., J.C.-L. and I.B.; Formal analysis, J.C.-L., G.M., J.V.M. and C.B.; Investigation, G.M.; Methodology, D.E., I.B. and J.V.M.; Software, G.M.; Writing—original draft, J.C.-L. and C.B.; Writing—review & editing, D.E., I.B., G.M., J.V.M. and C.B. All authors have read and agreed to the published version of the manuscript.

Funding: This research received no external funding.

Institutional Review Board Statement: The study was conducted in accordance with the Declaration of Helsinki 1961 (re-viewed in Edinburgh, 2000) and approved by the Research Ethics Committee of the Catholic University of Valencia (reference: UCV/2019-2020/017).

Informed Consent Statement: Informed consent was obtained from all participants as a previous requirement to access the study.

Data Availability Statement: Data are available upon request to the corresponding author.

Conflicts of Interest: The authors declare no conflict of interest.

References

1. Duthie, G.; Pyne, D.; Hooper, S. Applied physiology and game analysis of rugby union. *Sports Med.* **2003**, *33*, 973–991. [CrossRef] [PubMed]
2. Gabbett, T.J.; Seibold, A.J. Relationship between tests of physical qualities, team selection, and physical match performance in semiprofessional rugby league players. *J. Strength Cond. Res.* **2013**, *27*, 3259–3265. [CrossRef]
3. King, D.; Hume, P.; Cummins, C.; Pearce, A.; Clark, T.; Foskett, A.; Barnes, M. Match and training injuries in women's rugby union: A systematic review of published studies. *Sports Med.* **2019**, *49*, 1559–1574. [CrossRef] [PubMed]
4. Suarez-Arrones, L.; Portillo, J.; Pareja-Blanco, F.; Sáez der Villareal, E.; Sánchez-Medina, L.; Mungía-Izquierdo, D. Match-play activity profile in elite women's rugby union players. *J. Strength Cond. Res.* **2014**, *28*, 452–458. [CrossRef] [PubMed]
5. Gabbett, T.; Kelly, J.; Pezet, T. Relationship between physical fitness and playing ability in rugby league players. *J. Strength Cond. Res.* **2007**, *21*, 1126–1133.
6. Zemski, A.J.; Slater, G.J.; Broad, E.M. Body composition characteristics of elite Australian rugby union athletes according to playing position and ethnicity. *J. Sports Sci.* **2015**, *33*, 970–978. [CrossRef] [PubMed]
7. Posthumus, L.; Macgregor, C.; Winwood, P.; Tout, J.; Morton, L.; Driller, M.; Gill, N. The Physical Characteristics of Elite Female Rugby Union Players. *Int. J. Environ. Res. Public Health* **2020**, *17*, 6457. [CrossRef] [PubMed]
8. Smart, D.; Hopkins, W.G.; Quarrie, K.L.; Gill, N. The relationship between physical fitness and game behaviours in rugby union players. *Eur. J. Sport. Sci.* **2014**, *14*, S8–S17. [CrossRef] [PubMed]
9. Duthie, G.M.; Pyne, D.B.; Hopkins, W.G.; Livingstone, S.; Hooper, S.L. Anthropometry profiles of elite rugby players: Quantifying changes in lean mass. *Br. J. Sports Med.* **2006**, *40*, 202–207. [CrossRef] [PubMed]
10. Cheng, H.L.; O'Connor, H.; Kay, S.; Cook, R.; Parker, H.; Orr, R. Anthropometric characteristics of Australian junior representative rugby league players. *J. Sci. Med. Sport* **2014**, *17*, 546–551. [CrossRef] [PubMed]
11. Lees, M.J.; Oldroyd, B.; Jones, B.; Brightmore, A.; O'Hara, J.; Barlow, M.J.; Till, K.; Hind, K. Three-Compartment Body Composition Changes in Professional Rugby Union Players Over One Competitive Season: A Team and Individualized Approach. *J. Clin. Densitom.* **2017**, *20*, 50–57. [CrossRef] [PubMed]
12. Zemski, A.J.; Keating, S.E.; Broad, E.M.; Marsh, D.J.; Hind, K.; Slater, G.J. Preseason body composition adaptations in elite white and polynesian rugby union athletes. *Int. J. Sport Nutr. Exerc. Metab.* **2019**, *29*, 9–17. [CrossRef]
13. Posthumus, L.; Macgregor, C.; Winwood, P.; Darry, K.; Driller, M.; Gill, N. Physical and Fitness Characteristics of Elite Professional Rugby Union Players. *Sports* **2020**, *8*, 85. [CrossRef]
14. Kirby, W.J.; Reilly, T. Anthropometric and fitness profiles of elite female rugby union players. In *Science and Football*; Reilly, T., Ed.; E & FN Spon: London, UK, 1993; pp. 62–72.
15. Jones, B.; Emmonds, S.; Hind, K.; Nicholson, G.; Rutherford, Z.; Till, K. Physical Qualities of International Female Rugby League Players by Playing Position. *J. Strength Cond. Res.* **2016**, *30*, 1333–1340. [CrossRef]
16. Hene, N.M.; Bassett, S.H.; Andrews, B.S. Physical fitness profiles of elite women's rugby union players. *Afr. J. Phys. Health Edu. Recreat. Dance* **2011**, *17*, 1–8.

17. Nyberg, C.C.; Penpraze, V. Determination of Anthropometric and Physiological Performance Measures in Elite Scottish Female Rugby Union Players. *Int. J. Res. Ex. Phys.* **2016**, *12*, 10–16.
18. Gabbett, T.J. Physiological and anthropometric characteristics of elite women rugby league players. *J. Strength Cond. Res.* **2007**, *21*, 875–881.
19. Till, K.; Cobley, S.; O'Hara, J.; Brightmore, A.; Cooke, C.; Chapman, C. Using anthropometric and performance characteristics to predict selection in junior UK Rugby League players. *J. Sci. Med. Sport* **2011**, *14*, 264–269. [CrossRef]
20. Morehen, J.C.; Routledge, H.E.; Twist, C.; Morton, J.P.; Close, G.L. Position specific differences in the anthropometric characteristics of elite European Super League rugby players. *Eur. J. Sport Sci.* **2015**, *15*, 523–529. [CrossRef] [PubMed]
21. Reilly, T.; George, K.; Marfell-Jones, M.; Scott, M.; Sutton, L.; Wallace, J.A. How well do skinfold equations predict percent body fat in elite soccer players? *Int. J. Sports Med.* **2009**, *30*, 607–613. [CrossRef] [PubMed]
22. Roberts, S.P.; Trewartha, G.; Higgitt, R.J.; El-Abd, J.; Stokes, K.A. The physical demands of elite English rugby union. *J. Sports Sci.* **2008**, *26*, 825–833. [CrossRef]
23. Leão, C.; Camões, M.; Clemente, F.M.; Nikolaidis, P.T.; Lima, R.; Bezerra, P.; Rosemann, T.; Knechtle, B. Anthropometric Profile of Soccer Players as a Determinant of Position Specificity and Methodological Issues of Body Composition Estimation. *Int. J. Environ. Res. Public Health* **2019**, *16*, 2386. [CrossRef] [PubMed]
24. Marfell-Jones, M.; Stewart, A.; Olds, T. *Kinanthropometry IX*; International Society for the Advancement of Kinanthropometry (ISAK): Potchefstroom, South Africa, 2006; pp. 61–75.
25. Carter, J.E.L.; Yuhasz, M.S. Skinfolds and body composition of olympic athletes. In *Physical Structure of Olympic Athletes*; Part II, Kinanthropometry of olympic athletes; Carter, J.E.L., Ed.; Karger: Basilea, Switzerland, 1984.
26. Slaughter, M.H.; Lohman, T.G.; Boileau, R.A.; Horswill, C.A.; Sillman, R.J.; Van Loan, M.D.; Bemben, D.A. Skinfold equations for estimation of body fatness in children and youth. *Hum. Biol.* **1988**, *60*, 709–723.
27. Carter, J.E.L.; Heath, B. *Somatotyping Development and Applications*; Cambridge University Press: Cambridge, UK, 1990.
28. Smalheiser, N.R. Nonparametric Test. In *Data Literacy. How to Make your Experiments Robust and Reproducible*; Academic Press: New York, NY, USA, 2017; pp. 157–167.
29. Hene, N.M.; Bassett, S. Changes in the physical fitness of elite women's rugby union players over a competition season. *S. Afr. J. Sports Med.* **2013**, *25*, 47–50. [CrossRef]
30. Harty, P.S.; Zabriskie, H.A.; Stecker, R.A.; Currier, B.S.; Moon, J.M.; Richmond, S.R.; Jagim, A.R.; Kerksick, C.M. Position-Specific Body Composition Values in Female Collegiate Rugby Union Athletes. *J. Strength Cond. Res.* **2021**, *35*, 3158–3163. [CrossRef]
31. Bentzur, K.; Kravitz, L.; Lockner, D.W. Evaluation of the BOD POD for Estimating Percent Body Fat in Collegiate Track and Field Female Athletes: A Comparison of Four Methods. *J. Strength Cond. Res.* **2008**, *22*, 1985–1991. [CrossRef]
32. Smart, D.J.; Hopkins, W.G.; Gill, N.D. Differences and changes in the physical characteristics of professional and amateur rugby union players. *J. Strength Cond. Res.* **2013**, *27*, 3033–3044. [CrossRef] [PubMed]
33. Sedeaud, A.; Marc, A.; Schipman, J.; Tafflet, M.; Hager, J.P.; Toussaint, J.F. How they won Rugby World Cup through height, mass and collective experience. *Br. J. Sports Med.* **2012**, *46*, 580–584. [CrossRef]
34. Barr, M.J.; Newton, R.U.; Sheppard, J.M. Were height and mass related to performance at the 2007 and 2011 Rugby World Cups? *Int. J. Sports Sci. Coach.* **2014**, *9*, 671–680. [CrossRef]
35. Zemski, A.J.; Broad, E.M.; Slater, G.J. Skinfold Prediction Equations Fail to Provide an Accurate Estimate of Body Composition in Elite Rugby Union Athletes of Caucasian and Polynesian Ethnicity. *Int. J. Sport Nutr. Exerc. Metab.* **2018**, *28*, 90–99. [CrossRef]
36. Thomas, D.T.; Erdman, K.A.; Burke, L.M. American College of Sports Medicine Joint Position Statement. Nutrition and Athletic Performance. *Med. Sci. Sports Exerc.* **2016**, *48*, 543–568. [PubMed]
37. Till, K.; Cobley, S.; O'Hara, J.; Morley, D.; Chapman, C.; Cooke, C. Retrospective analysis of anthropometric and fitness characteristics associated with long-term career progression in Rugby League. *Sci. Med. Sport* **2015**, *18*, 310–314. [CrossRef]
38. Farley, J.B.; Stein, J.; Keogh, J.; Woods, C.T.; Milne, N. The Relationship Between Physical Fitness Qualities and Sport-Specific Technical Skills in Female, Team-Based Ball Players: A Systematic Review. *Sports Med. Open* **2020**, *6*, 18. [CrossRef] [PubMed]
39. Sánchez-Díaz, S.; Yanci, J.; Castillo, D.; Scanlan, A.T.; Raya-González, J. Effects of Nutrition Education Interventions in Team Sport Players. A Systematic Review. *Nutrients* **2020**, *12*, 3664. [CrossRef] [PubMed]

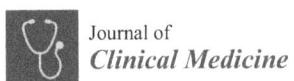

Review

Criteria for Return-to-Play (RTP) after Rotator Cuff Surgery: A Systematic Review of Literature

Marco Bravi [1,2], Chiara Fossati [2,*], Arrigo Giombini [2], Andrea Macaluso [2], José Kawazoe Lazzoli [3], Fabio Santacaterina [1], Federica Bressi [1], Ferruccio Vorini [4], Stefano Campi [4], Rocco Papalia [4] and Fabio Pigozzi [2]

1. Department of Physical and Rehabilitation Medicine, Università Campus Bio-Medico, 00128 Rome, Italy; m.bravi@policlinicocampus.it (M.B.); f.santacaterina@policlinicocampus.it (F.S.); f.bressi@policlinicocampus.it (F.B.)
2. Department of Movement, Human and Health Sciences, University of Rome "Foro Italico", 00135 Rome, Italy; arrigo.giombini@uniroma4.it (A.G.); andrea.macaluso@uniroma4.it (A.M.); fabio.pigozzi@uniroma4.it (F.P.)
3. Biomedical Institute, Medical School, Fluminense Federal University, Niterói 24220-008, Brazil; jklazzoli@uol.com.br
4. Department of Orthopaedic and Trauma Surgery, Università Campus Bio-Medico, 00128 Rome, Italy; f.vorini@unicampus.it (F.V.); s.campi@policlinicocampus.it (S.C.); r.papalia@policlinicocampus.it (R.P.)
* Correspondence: chiara.fossati@uniroma4.it

Abstract: This systematic review of the literature aimed to highlight which criteria are described in the literature to define when a patient, after rotator cuff repair (RCR), is ready for return-to-play (RTP), which includes return to unrestricted activities, return to work, leisure, and sport activities. An online systematic search on the US National Library of Medicine (PubMed/MEDLINE), SCOPUS, Web of Science (WOS), and the Cochrane Database of Systematic Reviews, was performed with no data limit until December 2021. A total of 24 studies that reported at least one criterion after RCR were included. Nine criteria were identified and among these, the most reported criterion was the time from surgery, which was used by 78% of the studies; time from surgery was used as the only criterion by 54% of the studies, and in combination with other criteria, in 24% of the studies. Strength and ROM were the most reported criteria after time (25%). These results are in line with a previous systematic review that aimed to identify RTP criteria after surgical shoulder stabilization and with a recent scoping review that investigated RTP criteria among athletes after RCR and anterior shoulder stabilization. Compared to this latest scoping review, our study adds the methodological strength of being conducted according to the Prisma guidelines; furthermore, our study included both athletes and non-athletes to provide a comprehensive view of the criteria used after RCR; moreover, ten additional recent manuscripts were examined with respect to the scoping review.

Keywords: return-to-play; rotator cuff repair; shoulder injuries; shoulder surgery; shoulder assessment

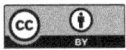

1. Introduction

Rotator cuff injuries are common shoulder injuries that often cause pain and subsequent dysfunction and require surgical repair. The supraspinatus tendon is the most frequently involved, but isolated lesions of the supraspinatus tendon only occur in 40% of cases [1]. Rotator cuff repair (RCR) is currently considered as definitive treatment for rotator cuff tears and no differences have been found between arthroscopic repair and mini-open technique, which are the two main surgical techniques [2]. In the general population, the estimated prevalence of rotator cuff tears varies between 9.7% and 62% in patients aged 20 and 80, respectively [3]. Among athletes, rotator cuff injuries are quite common: the study by Kaplan et al. [4] reported that 12% of competitive collegiate American football players had a history of rotator cuff injuries. Furthermore, athletes who play overhead sports are at greater risk of injury than other athletes due to the repetitive stresses imposed on the shoulder, while athletes who play contact sports have an additional increased risk of acute traumatic injuries [5]. These injuries can be highly impacting for professional athletes and can compromise career opportunities [6,7]; therefore, it is crucial not to delay the return-to-play (RTP) in safe conditions.

The decision-making process related to RTP after RCR is complex and requires a multidisciplinary approach involving the injured athlete, physicians, physiotherapists, and the athletic training staff. However, there are currently no clear criteria to precisely define when and whether an athlete is safely ready to RTP after rotator cuff repair. One of the reasons could be the lack of reliable and valid quantitative tests and indices that can guide the choices of clinicians regarding progression through the different phases of the rehabilitation process [8,9].

A systematic review by Ciccotti et al. [10] identified seven criteria that have been used to determine whether patients, after another shoulder condition, the anterior stabilization surgery, are ready or not to RTP, and 75% of studies used the time from surgery as the only criterion. A recent scoping review by Griffith et al. [11] confirmed the results of Ciccotti et al. [10] with regard to anterior stabilization surgery, and showed the same trend in RCR studies.

The literature lacks a systematic review regarding RTP criteria used after RCR. Therefore, the aim of this systematic review of the literature is to analyze and describe what are the currently reported criteria for RTP after RCR.

2. Materials and Methods

2.1. Systematic Literature Search

An online systematic search on the US National Library of Medicine (PubMed/MEDLINE), SCOPUS, Web of Science (WOS), and the Cochrane Database of Systematic Reviews, was performed with no data limit until December 2021, according to the Preferred Reporting Items for Systematic Reviews and Meta-analysis (PRISMA) guidelines [12]. The Population Intervention Comparison and Outcome (PICO) model was adopted to conduct an evidence-based practice literature search, [13] (Table 1). The review protocol has been registered on PROSPERO (registration number: CRD42022306254).

Table 1. PICO model.

Population	Intervention	Comparison	Outcome
Patients with rotator cuff tear	Rotator cuff repair Rotator cuff surgery	-	Return to play criteria, return to unrestricted activity criteria

The search strategy (Table 2) used a combination of medical subject heading (MeSH) terms and free-text terms adjusted according to each database characteristics; in addition, we performed a manual and a reference lists search.

Table 2. Search strategy.

Database	Search Terms
PubMed	("rotator cuff repair" [All Fields] OR "rotator cuff surger *" [All Fields] OR "rotator cuff tear" [All Fields] OR "Rotator Cuff Injuries" [MeSH Terms] OR "Rotator Cuff" [MeSH Terms]) AND ("return to sport" [All Fields] OR "return to play" [All Fields] OR "unrestricted activity" [All Fields] OR "full activity" [All Fields])
SCOPUS	ALL ("rotator cuff repair" OR "rotator cuff surger *" OR "rotator cuff tear" OR "Rotator Cuff") AND ("return to sport" OR "return to play" OR "unrestricted activity" OR "full activity")
Cochrane	(rotator cuff repair OR rotator cuff surger OR rotator cuff tear) AND (return to sport OR return to play OR unrestricted activity OR full activity)
WOS	(ALL = ("rotator cuff repair" OR "rotator cuff surger *" OR "rotator cuff tear" OR "Rotator Cuff")) AND ALL = ("return to sport" OR "return to play" OR "unrestricted activity" OR "full activity")

* asterisk is added to perform truncation search.

2.2. Eligibility Criteria and Data Extraction

The articles that were included in this systematic review had to meet the following inclusion criteria: (1) English language full-text articles; (2) Level I to IV studies of patients undergoing surgical repair of rotator cuff tear; (3) population of patients aged ≥13 years); (4) describe criteria to RTP.

According to Ciccotti et al. [10] we defined RTP also as the return to full and/or unrestricted activity including sports, work, etc. We excluded (1) studies lacking explicit return to play criteria; (2) review articles, biomechanical studies, technical notes; (3) studies in which surgical procedures were not described.

Firstly, duplicated references were checked and excluded through the Rayyan web app [14] for systematic reviews. Eligible articles were identified independently by two reviewers (MB, CF) by screening title and abstracts, then the inclusion of all articles was discussed by the two reviewers. Subsequently, both reviewers screened the full text of the selected articles to verify if they met inclusion criteria.

Data of eligible studies were extracted, including the name of the first author, year of publication, study inclusion criteria, participants' description; surgery technique, mean time to RTP in months, RTP criteria. Discrepancies were discussed with a third reviewer (SC). Incomplete data were treated as follows: firstly, we tried to contact the corresponding author; in case of non-response, we verified the presence of the data of interest published in other systematic reviews.

2.3. Quality Assessment

The methodological quality of included studies were assessed according to Ma et al. [15]. The MINORS (Methodological Index for Nonrandomized Studies) checklist [16], a specific tool developed to assess the quality of non-randomized surgical studies, was used to assess non-randomized studies. Two independent reviewers (FS, FV) assessed included studies and if discrepancies were not resolved by discussion, a third reviewer (FB) was consulted.

3. Results

A total of 1.751 records were found, including 84 from PubMed, 1.444 from SCOPUS, 111 from the Cochrane Library, and 112 from WOS. Additionally, 24 records were found through citation searching, of which 13 records were excluded because they did not report RTP criteria. A total of 24 articles [17–40] were included in systematic review (Figure 1). The quality of the included studies is reported in Table S1; all the studies were non-comparative studies, for this reason only the items from 1 to 8 of the MINORS check list were rated according to Slim et al. [16]. Details of the included studies are summarized in Table S2.

3.1. Patients' Characteristics

This systematic review included in total 847 participants (301 female and 544 male). The mean age of the participants was reported in all studies except in the study by Mazoue et al. [24] in which, however, the age of each single participant was reported and it was therefore possible to calculate mean age and standard deviation. Therefore, the mean age of the participants was of 42.8 ± 14.62 years.

Regarding the type of sport practiced, it was not possible to draw a satisfactory summary as only 11 studies [17,18,24,28,30,32,33,35,36,38,39] out of 24 accurately reported the type of sport that was practiced. Azzam et al. [29] described all sports practiced by participants; however, the number of sports exceeded the total number of patients, since some participants practiced two or three sports at the same time. Similarly, Liem et al. [23] reported that two patients practiced two sports. Among these studies, baseball is the sport most practiced by patients undergoing RCR with 88 participants (22%), followed by tennis (15%) and swimming (13%).

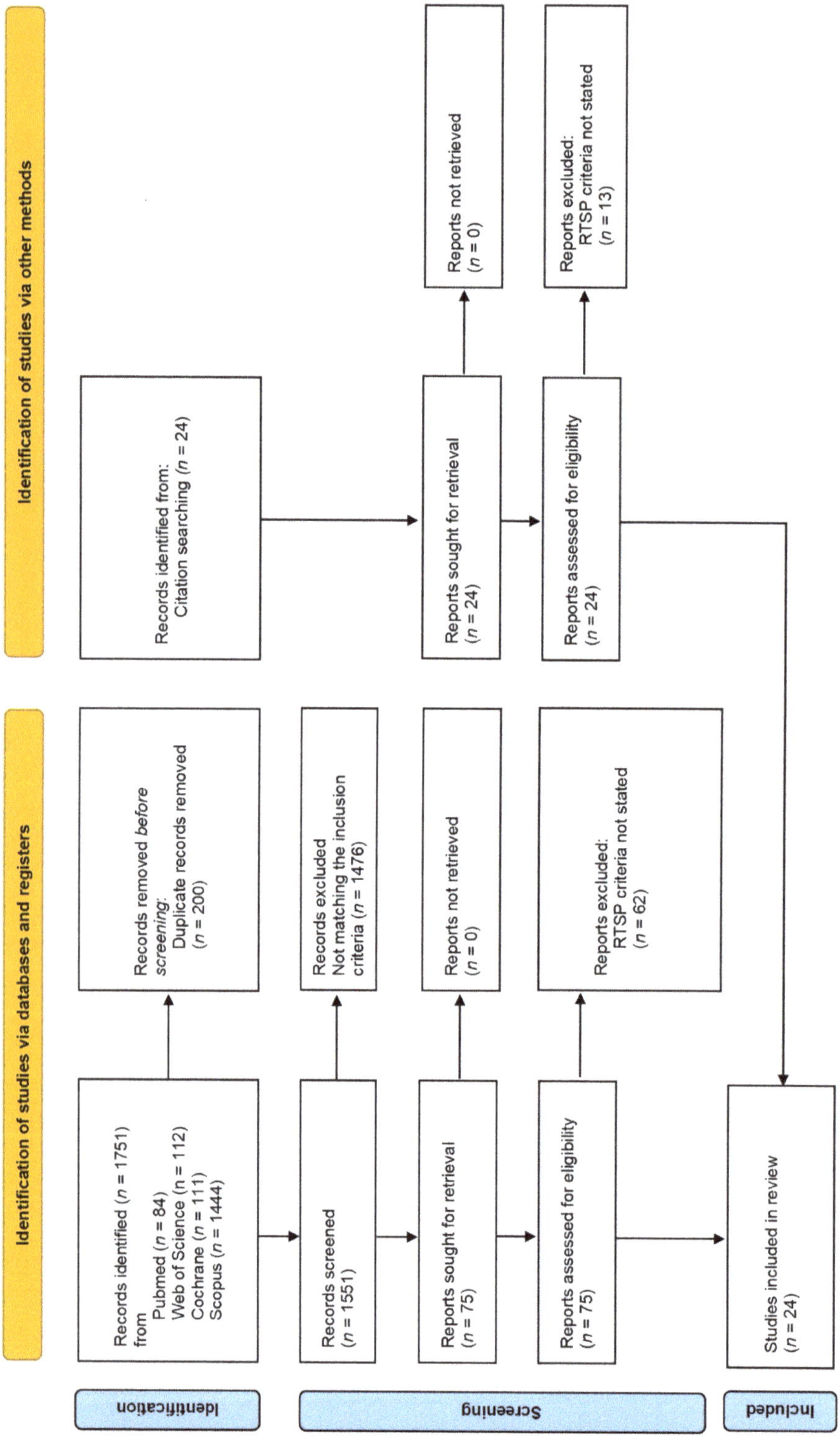

Figure 1. PRISMA Flowchart. From [41].

3.2. Surgical Procedures

In most of the studies [17,18,20,22,23,26–32,35,37–40] the arthroscopic technique for RCR was adopted (17/24; 70.8%). In one study [21] both techniques were used depending on the lesion size: arthroscopic rotator cuff repair was performed on most patients and open rotator cuff repair was chosen when tear size was >3 cm. In one study [25] the removal of calcifications was associated with the arthroscopic technique. In four studies [19,33,34,36], the open repair technique was used; among these, in the study by Bartl et al. [34], the open technique was used for the repair of the subscapularis muscle. Mazoue et al. [24] used a mini-open repair technique.

3.3. Return to Play Rates, Time and Criteria

All but one study (23/24; 95.8%) reported information on RTP rates for a total of 712 patients. The average RTP rate was 88.4 ± 10.6% (range, 100% to 58.3%); 19 out of 24 studies [17,18,20,22,23,25–33,36–40] reported a RTP rate >80%, 3 studies [19,34,35] reported an RTP rate >60% and only 1 study [24] reported a rate <60%.

The time to RTP was indicated by 13 studies [18,20,21,23–25,27,28,32,33,38–40] (13/24; 54.1%) for a total of 509 patients. The mean RTP time was 7.78 ± 3.20 months (range, 14 to 4.5 months).

Regarding the surgical procedures and the RTP, in 10 studies [18,20,23,25,27,28,32,38–40] arthroscopic repair was performed and RTP time was on average 6.8 ± 1.7 months; in one study [21], both techniques were used depending on lesion size (see Section 3.2), and an average RTP time of 14 months was reported; in another study [24], the mini-open technique was used, and an average RTP time of 4.5 months was reported; the study by Tibone et al. [33], in which the open technique was used, reported a RTP time ranging from 12 to 18 months for baseball pitchers. The year of publication did not show any correlation with the time of RTP.

All 24 included studies stated at least one RTP criterion. A total of nine different criteria were reported including: time, surgeon agreement, patients' desire for RTP, sport-specific training program, range of motion, muscle strength, pain, functional recovery, and proprioception. Fourteen studies [17,19,21–23,30,31,33,34,36–40] reported only one criterion (time); four studies [20,28,29,35] reported a combination of two criteria; four studies [18,25–27] used a combination of three RTP criteria; two studies [24,32] reported a combination of four criteria. All the combinations of RTP criteria are reported in Table 3.

Table 3. Combinations of RTP criteria among included studies.

Combination of RTP Criteria	Number of Studies (%)
Time	14 (58%)
Time, sport specific training program	1 (4%)
Time, ROM	1 (4%)
Time, strength	1 (4%)
Time, functional recovery	1 (4%)
Time, surgeon agreement, patients' desire	1 (4%)
ROM, strength, pain	3 (13%)
ROM, strength, pain, sport specific training program	1 (4%)
Time, ROM, strength, proprioception	1 (4%)

3.3.1. Time

Time from surgery alone or in combination with other criteria was the most used RTP criterion. Six studies [18,20,32,35,37,40] reported that at least 3 months is the minimum time required to RTP after surgery. Two studies [17,19] reported at least 4 months and two studies [23,29] at least 5 months. Most of the studies [21,28,30,31,33,34,36,38,39] (10/20 reported time as an RTP criterion) indicated at least 6 months: among these, in two studies [33,36], RTP increased to at least 12 months for specific sport activities (serving in tennis and pitching in baseball).

3.3.2. Strength

Shoulder muscle strength was indicated as a criterion for RTP in six studies [20,24–27,32]. The definition of strength level is described in a variable way: shoulder strength restoration [20], satisfactory muscle strength [24], shoulder strength near to 100% [25], shoulder strength near the same as pre-injury [26,27], and satisfactory isokinetic strength (not clearly specified) [32].

3.3.3. Pain

A total of four studies [24–27] used pain as a criterion for RTP (always in combination with other criteria). Pain was defined as "non-painful ROM" [24] and "pain free" [25–27].

3.3.4. Range of Motion

We found that six studies [24–27,32,35] reported ROM as a RTP criterion, which was used always in combination with other criteria. The ROM was defined as follows: full non-painful ROM [24], full shoulder ROM [25–27], satisfactory ROM (not clearly specified) [32], and Bhatia et al. [35] reported kinematic progress that we interpreted as ROM restoration.

3.3.5. Specific Training Programs

Two studies [24,29] reported completion of the sport-specific training program as an RTP criterion in combination with other criteria. Azzam et al. [29] reported that patients needed to complete a sport-specific rehabilitation progression or interval training program, depending on the sport involved, to be released to full unrestricted activity. Mazoue et al. [24] reported specific criteria for pitchers (completion of two-phase interval throwing program flat-ground program and throwing from the mound), and for position players (completion of flat ground throwing program).

3.3.6. Other Criteria

Tambe et al. [32] reported satisfactory proprioception (not better specified) as another criterion used to determine when the patient is ready to RTP. Antoni et al. [18] reported willingness to return and surgeon agreement as additional RTP criteria. Finally, Shimada et al. [28] reported a not better specified "functional recovery" to state readiness for RTP.

3.3.7. Return to Preinjury Level and Retear

We analyzed the percentage of athletes who have returned to equal or higher levels of performance than preinjury in relation to RTP criteria. Among the 15 studies [17–19,21–23,30,31,33,34,36–40] that used only "time" as RTP criterion, 3 authors did not report the new level of performance, the other 12 studies reported that on average 76% (range, 42–100%) of the athletes returned to equal or higher pre-injury level. Regarding the risk of retear, four studies [36,38–40] reported no retear cases, Bartl et al. [34] reported three small retears, Hawkins et al. [19] reported two cases of retear, and Liem et al. [23] five cases of retear, while six studies [17,18,21,30,33,37] did not report data about retear. As for the studies that used ROM, strength, and pain as RTP, we found that the three studies by Ranalletta et al. [25] and Rossi et al. [26,27] reported that an average 83.7% (range, 80–91.3%) of athletes returned to an equal or higher pre-injury level with no cases of retear. The other studies combining multiple criteria for RTP reported an average return to performance of 62% (range, 21–93%), and only two studies (Azzam et al. [29] and Shimada et al. [28]) reported one case and three cases of retear, respectively.

4. Discussion

The main finding of this systematic review, which aimed at identifying criteria for RTP following rotator cuff surgery, was that nine criteria were identified and "time from surgery" was the only criterion in 54% of the studies, and was the most reported criterion in 78% of the studies, followed by "strength and ROM", which were reported in 25% of the studies. In most cases, no clear rationale is given for using certain criteria over others. Therefore, there is a need to study and validate a set of RTP objective criteria with the aim of providing evidence-based indications that can be useful in clinical practice to define patient readiness. Furthermore, when dealing with athletes, criteria about the athlete's ability to perform sport-specific gestures should also be considered. The major strength of this systematic review in comparison with previous studies is the methodological rigour in applying Prisma guidelines and the inclusion of both athletes and non-athletes.

Regarding RTP criteria, some considerations are required. The time from surgery is the most widely used criterion by the included studies, with an average of 6–7 months for RTP. We believe that time from surgery must certainly be considered during rehabilitation after RCR to guide the progression of rehabilitation treatments and exercises, but it cannot be the only criterion used to define readiness for RTP. The studies did not clarify the reason behind the choice of this interval of time for RTP, which can likely be attributed to preserving the integrity of the repaired tendon. However, Sonnabend et al. [42], in a study on a primate model, showed that after 15 weeks the bone-tendon junction was almost mature indicating that up to 15 weeks rehabilitation programs should protect surgical repair. Therefore, after an adequate safety time has been exceeded, other criteria such as strength, ROM, and function, should guide the choice of clinicians to define patient's readiness for RTP. Kibler et al. [43] pointed out that it would be appropriate to establish specific criteria especially for the return to sport, which require the recovery of functional capacity and should be objectively demonstrated through the measurement of ROM, strength, and through physical performance tests, rather than being evaluated solely based on time from surgery or imaging. Results from this systematic review evidenced that the included studies, published from 1986 to 2021, reported a time from surgery that remained substantially unchanged, especially if we consider the studies of the last 15 years. Therefore, despite the progress in surgery and rehabilitation fields, the "time" criterion (usually reported to be at least of 6 months) appears to be handed down over the years in a quite empirical way, and is barely supported by human and animal models.

The strength criterion, and more precisely the level of strength, has never been adequately defined; in fact, most studies do not mention how strength is assessed (i.e., maximum voluntary isometric strength, manual muscle strength testing, or isokinetic strength assessment). As a matter of fact, only the study by Tambe et al. [32] reported the use of isokinetic evaluation, without reporting the levels of strength. A recent consensus statement [44] stated that all sports with demands on the shoulder have a shoulder strength requirement and the external rotation/internal rotation (ER/IR) strength ratios should be used as a criterion for RTP. According to Thigpen et al. [45] it would be safe to assess muscle performance 4 months after surgery since several studies [5,45–47], in which strength was assessed with a handheld dynamometer after 4 months, reported no injuries. However, further studies should specify threshold absolute values of strength, as the use of the ER/IR ratio, as suggested by Schwank et al. [44,48], it would be useful to measure strength also during dynamic movements, since instrumented stacked plate resistance machines, which have a high test–retest reliability, allow muscle power to be determined, which is more strongly associated with functional abilities and sports performance than strength per se.

In accordance to the scoping review by Griffith et al. [11], our systematic review found a total absence of patient-reported outcome measures (PROMs) among RTP criteria, without a clear explanation of why PROMs were not used as RTP criteria. However, as highlighted in the recent 2022 Bern Consensus [44], it should be recommended to use shoulder-specific PROMs (i.e., Shoulder Pain and Disability Index, American Shoulder and Elbow Surgeons standardized shoulder assessment form, etc., see Appendix C of 2022 Bern Consensus Statement on Shoulder Injury Prevention, Rehabilitation, and Return to Sport for Athletes at All Participation Level), and to define cut-off levels to be used in conjunction with other criteria to determine when a patient is ready for RTP.

All the studies that have reported ROM as a criterion for RTP frequently required a full ROM recovery before allowing RTP; however, the use of this criterion can limit a timely return to sport, since although the overhead athletes need full ROM before return to sport, there is no need of full ROM restoration for collision athletes [44]. Therefore, it would be desirable that future studies be more specific in the use of this criterion and clarify the reason for the choice; it may be more useful to define this criterion as sport/activity-specific functional ROM recovery rather than generic full ROM recovery.

Pain is another domain that should certainly be taken into consideration to allow the RTP, but, also for this criterion, it is necessary to make essential distinctions. In fact, the total absence of pain is not required for the general population to return to unrestricted activities, while on the contrary all the athletes who have to return to sports activities and to preinjury performances must be pain-free [44].

The study by Tambe et al. is the only one that reported an improvement of shoulder proprioception as a criterion to RTP, without specifying the assessment modality. Active shoulder proprioception [49] should be considered as a RTP criterion; as shown by Gumina et al. [50], a rotator cuff tear causes an alteration of the joint position sense, which consequently results in a reduction in the neuromuscular control, with the latter being essential for an athlete's return to competition [51]. Finally, the results of this systematic review show the total absence of psychological readiness, which is a not negligible factor, especially when deciding whether the athlete is ready for the RTP; fear of re-injury and motivation may influence treatment and readiness to RTP after an injury [52]. Therefore, some scales such as the Tampa Scale of Kinesiophobia [53] or the Injury–Psychological Readiness to Return to Sport scale (I-PRRS) [54] should be used in association with other criteria.

Finally, there is no clear correlation between the use of defined RTP criteria and return to performance after RCR. As a matter of fact, the data from the studies grouped by RTP criteria show values that are close to the total average of 73% of athletes returning to equal or higher preinjury levels. Therefore, the use of different RTP criteria does not seem to influence the ability to return to preinjury levels; indeed, as also reported by Altintas et al. [55], we believe that the ability to return to performance is multifactorial: preinjury sports participation (recreational or competitive), type of sport (overhead, collision), age, etc., can all influence the return to preinjury levels.

The following limitations of this systematic review need to be highlighted. Firstly, we are not sure that the description of the criteria has been carried out in an exhaustive way; as pointed out by Ciccotti et al. [10] and by Griffith et al. [11], it is likely that some studies have omitted more accurate criteria descriptions due to publication-related limits. Our review included both athletes and non-athletes, which allows for the inclusion of a greater number of studies, but, on the other hand, makes the sample more heterogeneous; we only included English written studies, and it is therefore likely that some studies written in a different language were not considered.

5. Conclusions

Our review identified a total of nine criteria that have been used in the literature to determine the patient's readiness to RTP after RCR. Consistently with the examined papers, we have found that the time from surgery is the most widely used standard. The use of additional criteria is desirable in future studies, as we believe that it is not enough to decide when a patient is ready for the RTP solely on time and strength criteria. Future studies should strive to use criteria about shoulder function and proprioception, since emerging technologies now offer clinicians low-cost precise and reliable measurement tools (i.e., wearable magneto-inertial sensors, dynamometers, and load cells), which allow a complete assessment of the shoulder function to be easily performed [56]. Finally, when dealing with an athlete, the athlete's perception and psychological readiness should be included among RTP criteria, as psychologic factors are associated with longer duration of symptoms and higher levels of disability [57] that can negatively impact shoulder function during sport-specific gestures. This will hopefully lead to the determination of a set of activity/sport-specific conditions that can be used to correctly establish readiness for RTP, ensuring the safety of patients and avoiding reinjuries.

The following bullets points summarize the results of this systematic review:
- "Time from surgery" is the most used criterion to define readiness for RTP.
- Strength recovery is rarely used and poorly detailed.
- Preinjury performance levels and injury rates do not appear to be related to the use of specific RTP criteria
- Despite their importance, no clinical studies have used specific PROMS and psychological readiness assessment as RTP criteria.

Supplementary Materials: The following supporting information can be downloaded at: https://www.mdpi.com/article/10.3390/jcm11082244/s1, Table S1: Quality assessment; Table S2: Details of included studies.

Author Contributions: Conceptualization, M.B., C.F., R.P. and F.P.; methodology, M.B., A.G., A.M. and R.P.; data curation, F.S., F.V. and S.C.; writing—original draft preparation, M.B. and C.F.; writing—review and editing, A.G., A.M. and J.K.L.; supervision, F.P., F.B. and R.P.; All authors have read and agreed to the published version of the manuscript.

Funding: This research received no external funding.

Institutional Review Board Statement: Not applicable.

Conflicts of Interest: The authors declare no conflict of interest.

References

1. Pulici, L.; Zanini, B.; Carrai, L.; Menon, A.; Compagnoni, R.; Randelli, P. Return to play after rotator cuff surgery. In *Return to Play in Football*; Springer: Berlin/Heidelberg, Germany, 2018; pp. 313–320. ISBN 9783662557136.
2. Ji, X.; Bi, C.; Wang, F.; Wang, Q. Arthroscopic versus mini-open rotator cuff repair: An up-to-date meta-analysis of randomized controlled trials. *Arthrosc. J. Arthrosc. Relat. Surg.* **2015**, *31*, 118–124. [CrossRef] [PubMed]
3. Teunis, T.; Lubberts, B.; Reilly, B.T.; Ring, D. A systematic review and pooled analysis of the prevalence of rotator cuff disease with increasing age. *J. Shoulder Elb. Surg.* **2014**, *23*, 1913–1921. [CrossRef] [PubMed]
4. Kaplan, L.D.; Flanigan, D.C.; Norwig, J.; Jost, P.; Bradley, J. Prevalence and variance of shoulder injuries in elite collegiate football players. *Am. J. Sports Med.* **2005**, *33*, 1142–1146. [CrossRef] [PubMed]
5. Mueller, M.; Hoy, G.; Branson, R. Management of in-season concurrent rotator cuff tear with shoulder instability in professional contact football athletes; respect the career goals! *Asian J. Sports Med.* **2016**, *7*, e28377. [CrossRef] [PubMed]
6. Headey, J.; Brooks, J.H.M.; Kemp, S.P.T. The epidemiology of shoulder injuries in English professional rugby union. *Am. J. Sports Med.* **2007**, *35*, 1537–1543. [CrossRef]
7. Namdari, S.; Baldwin, K.; Ahn, A.; Huffman, G.R.; Sennett, B.J. Performance after rotator cuff tear and operative treatment: A case-control study of major league baseball pitchers. *J. Athl. Train.* **2011**, *46*, 296–302. [CrossRef]
8. Cools, A.M.J.; Struyf, F.; De Mey, K.; Maenhout, A.; Castelein, B.; Cagnie, B. Rehabilitation of scapular dyskinesis: From the office worker to the elite overhead athlete. *Br. J. Sports Med.* **2014**, *48*, 692–697. [CrossRef]
9. Creighton, D.W.; Shrier, I.; Shultz, R.; Meeuwisse, W.H.; Matheson, G.O. Return-to-play in sport: A decision-based model. *Clin. J. Sport Med.* **2010**, *20*, 379–385. [CrossRef]
10. Ciccotti, M.C.; Syed, U.; Hoffman, R.; Abboud, J.A.; Ciccotti, M.G.; Freedman, K.B. Return to play criteria following surgical stabilization for traumatic anterior shoulder instability: A systematic review. *Arthroscopy* **2018**, *34*, 903–913. [CrossRef]
11. Griffith, R.; Fretes, N.; Bolia, I.K.; Murray, I.R.; Meyer, J.; Weber, A.E.; Gamradt, S.C.; Petrigliano, F.A. Return-to-sport criteria after upper extremity surgery in athletes—A scoping review, part 1: Rotator cuff and shoulder stabilization procedures. *Orthop. J. Sport. Med.* **2021**, *9*, 23259671211021827. [CrossRef]
12. Page, M.J.; McKenzie, J.E.; Bossuyt, P.M.; Boutron, I.; Hoffmann, T.C.; Mulrow, C.D.; Shamseer, L.; Tetzlaff, J.M.; Akl, E.A.; Brennan, S.E.; et al. The PRISMA 2020 statement: An updated guideline for reporting systematic reviews. *Int. J. Surg.* **2021**, *88*, 105906. [CrossRef] [PubMed]
13. Brown, D. A review of the pubmed PICO tool: Using evidence-based practice in health education. *Health Promot. Pract.* **2020**, *21*, 496–498. [CrossRef] [PubMed]
14. Ouzzani, M.; Hammady, H.; Fedorowicz, Z.; Elmagarmid, A. Rayyan—A web and mobile app for systematic reviews. *Syst. Rev.* **2016**, *5*, 210. [CrossRef] [PubMed]
15. Ma, L.L.; Wang, Y.Y.; Yang, Z.H.; Huang, D.; Weng, H.; Zeng, X.T. Methodological quality (risk of bias) assessment tools for primary and secondary medical studies: What are they and which is better? *Mil. Med. Res.* **2020**, *7*, 1–11. [CrossRef]
16. Slim, K.; Nini, E.; Forestier, D.; Kwiatkowski, F.; Panis, Y.; Chipponi, J. Methodological index for non-randomized studies (MINORS): Development and validation of a new instrument. *ANZ J. Surg.* **2003**, *73*, 712–716. [CrossRef]
17. Andrews, J.R.; Broussard, T.S.; Carson, W.G. Arthroscopy of the shoulder in the management of partial tears of the rotator cuff: A preliminary report. *Arthroscopy* **1985**, *1*, 117–122. [CrossRef]

18. Antoni, M.; Klouche, S.; Mas, V.; Ferrand, M.; Bauer, T.; Hardy, P. Return to recreational sport and clinical outcomes with at least 2 years follow-up after arthroscopic repair of rotator cuff tears. *Orthop. Traumatol. Surg. Res.* **2016**, *102*, 563–567. [CrossRef]
19. Hawkins, R.J.; Morin, W.D.; Bonutti, P.M. Surgical treatment of full-thickness rotator cuff tears in patients 40 years of age or younger. *J. Shoulder Elb. Surg.* **1999**, *8*, 259–265. [CrossRef]
20. Ide, J.; Maeda, S.; Takagi, K. Arthroscopic transtendon repair of partial-thickness articular-side tears of the rotator cuff: Anatomical clinical study. *Am. J. Sports Med.* **2005**, *33*, 1672–1679. [CrossRef]
21. Kim, H.J.; Kim, J.Y.; Rhee, Y.G. When do patients return to previous daily activity after arthroscopic rotator cuff repair? *Clin. Orthop. Relat. Res.* **2019**, *477*, 403–413. [CrossRef]
22. Krishnan, S.G.; Harkins, D.C.; Schiffern, S.C.; Pennington, S.D.; Burkhead, W.Z. Arthroscopic repair of full-thickness tears of the rotator cuff in patients younger than 40 years. *Arthrosc. J. Arthrosc. Relat. Surg.* **2008**, *24*, 324–328. [CrossRef] [PubMed]
23. Liem, D.; Lichtenberg, S.; Magosch, P.; Habermeyer, P. Arthroscopic rotator cuff repair in overhead-throwing athletes. *Am. J. Sports Med.* **2008**, *36*, 1317–1322. [CrossRef] [PubMed]
24. Mazoué, C.G.; Andrews, J.R. Repair of full-thickness rotator cuff tears in professional baseball players. *Am. J. Sports Med.* **2006**, *34*, 182–189. [CrossRef] [PubMed]
25. Ranalletta, M.; Rossi, L.A.; Sirio, A.; Bruchmann, G.; Maignon, G.D.; Bongiovanni, S.L. Return to sports after arthroscopic treatment of rotator cuff calcifications in athletes. *Orthop. J. Sport. Med.* **2016**, *4*, 26–30. [CrossRef] [PubMed]
26. Rossi, L.A.; Atala, N.A.; Bertona, A.; Bongiovanni, S.; Tanoira, I.; Maignon, G.; Ranalletta, M. Long-term outcomes after in situ arthroscopic repair of partial rotator cuff tears. *Arthrosc. J. Arthrosc. Relat. Surg.* **2019**, *35*, 698–702. [CrossRef]
27. Rossi, L.A.; Atala, N.; Bertona, A.; Tanoira, I.; Bongiovanni, S.; Maignon, G.; Ranalletta, M. Return to sports after in situ arthroscopic repair of partial rotator cuff tears. *Arthrosc. J. Arthrosc. Relat. Surg.* **2019**, *35*, 32–37. [CrossRef]
28. Shimada, Y.; Sugaya, H.; Takahashi, N.; Matsuki, K.; Tokai, M.; Morioka, T.; Ueda, Y.; Hoshika, S.; Hamada, H.; Inoue, S.; et al. Return to sport after arthroscopic rotator cuff repair in middle-aged and elderly swimmers. *Orthop. J. Sport. Med.* **2020**, *8*, 2325967120922203. [CrossRef]
29. Azzam, M.G.; Dugas, J.R.; Andrews, J.R.; Goldstein, S.R.; Emblom, B.A.; Cain, E.L. Rotator cuff repair in adolescent athletes. *Am. J. Sports Med.* **2018**, *46*, 1084–1090. [CrossRef]
30. Simon, M.; Popp, D.; Lutter, C.; Schöffl, V. Functional and sports-specific outcome after surgical repair of rotator cuff tears in rock climbers. *Wilderness Environ. Med.* **2017**, *28*, 342–347. [CrossRef]
31. Spencer, E.E. Partial-thickness articular surface rotator cuff tears: An all-inside repair technique. *Clin. Orthop. Relat. Res.* **2010**, *468*, 1514–1520. [CrossRef]
32. Tambe, A.; Badge, R.; Funk, L. Arthroscopic rotator cuff repair in elite rugby players. *Int. J. Shoulder Surg.* **2009**, *3*, 8. [CrossRef] [PubMed]
33. Tibone, J.E.; Elrod, B.; Jobe, F.W.; Kerlan, R.K.; Carter, V.S.; Shields, C.L.; Lombardo, S.J.; Yocum, L. Surgical treatment of tears of the rotator cuff in athletes. *J. Bone Jt. Surg. Am.* **1986**, *68*, 887–891. [CrossRef]
34. Bartl, C.; Scheibel, M.; Magosch, P.; Lichtenberg, S.; Habermeyer, P. Open repair of isolated traumatic subscapularis tendon tears. *Am. J. Sports Med.* **2011**, *39*, 490–496. [CrossRef] [PubMed]
35. Bhatia, S.; Greenspoon, J.A.; Horan, M.P.; Warth, R.J.; Millett, P.J. Two-year outcomes after arthroscopic rotator cuff repair in recreational athletes older than 70 years. *Am. J. Sports Med.* **2015**, *43*, 1737–1742. [CrossRef]
36. Bigiliani, L.U.; Kimmel, J.; McCann, P.D.; Wolfe, I. Repair of rotator cuff tears in tennis players. *Am. J. Sports Med.* **1992**, *20*, 112–117. [CrossRef]
37. Burns, J.P.; Snyder, S.J. Arthroscopic rotator cuff repair in patients younger than fifty years of age. *J. Shoulder Elb. Surg.* **2008**, *17*, 90–96. [CrossRef]
38. Carbone, S.; Candela, V.; Gumina, S. High rate of return to crossfit training after arthroscopic management of rotator cuff tear. *Orthop. J. Sport. Med.* **2020**, *8*, 2325967120911039. [CrossRef]
39. Carbone, S.; Castagna, V.; Passaretti, D.; Candela, V.; Cerciello, S.; Sante, E.D.; Gumina, S. Supraspinatus repair and biceps tenodesis in competitive CrossFit athletes allow for a 100% of return to sport. *Knee Surg. Sport. Traumatol. Arthrosc.* **2021**, *29*, 3929–3935. [CrossRef]
40. Davey, M.S.; Hurley, E.T.; Scanlon, J.P.; Gaafar, M.; Pauzenberger, L.; Mullett, H. Excellent clinical outcomes and rates of return to play after arthroscopic rotator cuff repair for traumatic tears in athletes aged 30 years or less. *Arthrosc. Sport. Med. Rehabil.* **2021**, *3*, e667–e672. [CrossRef]
41. Page, M.J.; McKenzie, J.E.; Bossuyt, P.M.; Boutron, I.; Hoffmann, T.C.; Mulrow, C.D.; Shamseer, L.; Tetzlaff, J.M.; Akl, E.A.; Brennan, S.E.; et al. The PRISMA 2020 statement: An updated guideline for reporting systematic reviews *BMJ* **2021**, *372*. [CrossRef]
42. Sonnabend, D.H.; Howlett, C.R.; Young, A.A. Histological evaluation of repair of the rotator cuff in a primate model. *J. Bone Joint Surg. Br.* **2010**, *92*, 586–594. [CrossRef] [PubMed]
43. Kibler, B.W.; Siascia, A. Rehabilitation following rotator cuff repair. In *Shoulder Surgery Rehabilitation: A Teamwork Approach*; Springer: Cham, Germany, 2016; pp. 1–202. ISBN 9783319248561.
44. Schwank, A.; Blazey, P.; Asker, M.; Møller, M.; Hägglund, M.; Gard, S.; Skazalski, C.; Andersson, S.H.; Horsley, I.; Whiteley, R.; et al. 2022 bern consensus statement on shoulder injury prevention, rehabilitation, and return to sport for athletes at all participation levels. *J. Orthop. Sports Phys. Ther.* **2022**, *52*, 11–28. [CrossRef] [PubMed]

45. Thigpen, C.A.; Shaffer, M.A.; Gaunt, B.W.; Leggin, B.G.; Williams, G.R.; Wilcox, R.B. The American Society of Shoulder and Elbow Therapists' consensus statement on rehabilitation following arthroscopic rotator cuff repair. *J. Shoulder Elb. Surg.* **2016**, *25*, 521–535. [CrossRef] [PubMed]
46. Sgroi, T.A.; Cilenti, M. Rotator cuff repair: Post-operative rehabilitation concepts. *Curr. Rev. Musculoskelet. Med.* **2018**, *11*, 86–91. [CrossRef] [PubMed]
47. Rokito, A.S.; Zuckerman, J.D.; Gallagher, M.A.; Cuomo, F. Strength after surgical repair of the rotator cuff. *J. Shoulder Elb. Surg.* **1996**, *5*, 12–17. [CrossRef]
48. Pigozzi, F.; Giombini, A.; Macaluso, A. Do current methods of strength testing for the return to sport after injuries really address functional performance? *Am. J. Phys. Med. Rehabil.* **2012**, *91*, 458–460. [CrossRef]
49. Lubiatowski, P.; Ogrodowicz, P.; Wojtaszek, M.; Kaniewski, R.; Stefaniak, J.; Dudziński, W.; Romanowski, L. Measurement of active shoulder proprioception: Dedicated system and device. *Eur. J. Orthop. Surg. Traumatol.* **2013**, *23*, 177–183. [CrossRef]
50. Gumina, S.; Camerota, F.; Celletti, C.; Venditto, T.; Candela, V. The effects of rotator cuff tear on shoulder proprioception. *Int. Orthop.* **2019**, *43*, 229–235. [CrossRef]
51. Myers, J.B.; Lephart, S.M. The Role of the Sensorimotor System in the Athletic Shoulder. *J. Athl. Train.* **2000**, *35*, 351.
52. Cools, A.M.; Maenhout, A.G.; Vanderstukken, F.; Declève, P.; Johansson, F.R.; Borms, D. The challenge of the sporting shoulder: From injury prevention through sport-specific rehabilitation toward return to play. *Ann. Phys. Rehabil. Med.* **2021**, *64*, 101384. [CrossRef]
53. Tkachuk, G.A.; Harris, C.A. Psychometric properties of the Tampa Scale for Kinesiophobia-11 (TSK-11). *J. Pain* **2012**, *13*, 970–977. [CrossRef] [PubMed]
54. Glazer, D.D. Development and preliminary validation of the Injury-Psychological Readiness to Return to Sport (I-PRRS) scale. *J. Athl. Train.* **2009**, *44*, 185–189. [CrossRef] [PubMed]
55. Altintas, B.; Anderson, N.; Dornan, G.J.; Boykin, R.E.; Logan, C.; Millett, P.J. Return to sport after arthroscopic rotator cuff repair: Is there a difference between the recreational and the competitive athlete? *Am. J. Sports Med.* **2020**, *48*, 252–261. [CrossRef] [PubMed]
56. Carnevale, A.; Longo, U.G.; Schena, E.; Massaroni, C.; Lo Presti, D.; Berton, A.; Candela, V.; Denaro, V. Wearable systems for shoulder kinematics assessment: A systematic review. *BMC Musculoskelet. Disord.* **2019**, *20*, 1–24. [CrossRef] [PubMed]
57. Thorpe, A.M.; O'Sullivan, P.B.; Mitchell, T.; Hurworth, M.; Spencer, J.; Booth, G.; Goebel, S.; Khoo, P.; Tay, A.; Smith, A. Are psychologic factors associated with shoulder scores after rotator cuff surgery? *Clin. Orthop. Relat. Res.* **2018**, *476*, 2062. [CrossRef]

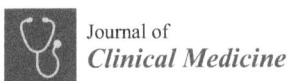

Article

Effects of Physical Activity on Daily Physical Function in Chinese Middle-Aged and Older Adults: A Longitudinal Study from CHARLS

Yuge Tian and Zhenguo Shi *

School of Physical Education, Shandong University, Jinan 250061, China
* Correspondence: 202015334@mail.sdu.edu.cn

Abstract: Objective: Impaired daily physical function has become a common health problem among Chinese middle-aged and elderly people. The aim of this study was to investigate the effects of physical activity on daily physical function in Chinese middle-aged and older adults. Methods: Data from 9056 participants in the China Health and Retirement Longitudinal Study (CHARLS) from 2011 to 2018 were included in this study. Physical activity levels were expressed as metabolic equivalents, and the impairment of daily physical function was determined in a self-reported format by the Activities of Daily Living Scale and the Instrumental Activities of Daily Living Scale. The association between different levels of physical activity and impaired daily physical function was analyzed using Cox proportional hazards regression models. Results: During a mean follow-up period of 6.73 years, 1379 middle-aged and older adults had impaired physical function. After adjusting for all covariates, participants with a physical activity volume (PAV) $\geq$ 600 MET-minutes/week had a 61% lower risk of impaired daily physical function than those who were physically inactive (HR = 0.39, 95% CI 0.35–0.44). Participants with a PAV of 1800–2999 MET-minutes/week had the lowest risk of impaired daily physical function (HR = 0.33, 95% CI 0.26–0.42). Subgroup analysis showed that participants with a PAV $\geq$ 600 MET-minutes/week had a greater reduction in the risk of impaired daily physical function among participants who were male, older than or equal to 65 years, and without respiratory disease compared to participants who were physically inactive. Conclusions: This study showed that a PAV $\geq$ 600 MET-minutes/week could reduce the risk of impaired daily physical function in Chinese middle-aged and elderly people. However, a higher PAV is not better; a PAV in the range of 1800–2999 MET-minutes/week can be more effective in preventing daily physical function impairment in Chinese middle-aged and elderly people.

Keywords: physical activity; daily physical function; middle-aged and older adults; CHARLS

Citation: Tian, Y.; Shi, Z. Effects of Physical Activity on Daily Physical Function in Chinese Middle-Aged and Older Adults: A Longitudinal Study from CHARLS. *J. Clin. Med.* **2022**, *11*, 6514. https://doi.org/10.3390/jcm11216514

Academic Editors: Mario Bernardo-Filho, Redha Taiar and Ana Cristina Rodrigues Lacerda

Received: 10 October 2022
Accepted: 31 October 2022
Published: 2 November 2022

Publisher's Note: MDPI stays neutral with regard to jurisdictional claims in published maps and institutional affiliations.

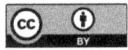

Copyright: © 2022 by the authors. Licensee MDPI, Basel, Switzerland. This article is an open access article distributed under the terms and conditions of the Creative Commons Attribution (CC BY) license (https://creativecommons.org/licenses/by/4.0/).

1. Introduction

Physical function has been defined as the integration and translation of physiological stimuli into muscular actions [1], such as walking, maintaining balance, and staying standing. Physical function in middle-aged and older adults is an important determinant in maintaining and improving their functional capacity [2]. However, physical functions such as muscle strength, postural balance, and aerobic capacity continue to decline in middle-aged and older adults as they age [3,4]. Many studies have shown that impaired daily physical function has become a common health problem among middle-aged and elderly people [5]. In addition, impaired physical function was strongly associated with individual disability [6] and increased risk of mortality [7,8] and can also affect the ability of middle-aged and older adults to care for themselves and live independently [9], as they often require more daily assistance and health care [10,11]. Related research data showed that by 2020, the elderly population with impaired physical function in China had reached 43.75 million, and it is expected to rise to more than 90 million by 2050 [12]. China has become the world's largest population of older adults with impaired physical function [13].

The serious harm caused by impaired physical function has brought a huge economic and social burden to society and has become a major public health problem [5].

Previous studies have shown that physical activity is an effective intervention to prevent impaired physical function in middle-aged and older adults, that higher levels of physical activity (PA) help maintain physical function in community-dwelling older adults [14–18], and that PA is also effective in delaying the progression of physical functional limitations or disability [19,20]. Results from several large epidemiological studies also showed that PA had a beneficial effect on the assessment of measures of physical functional performance such as balance [21], strength [22], and mobility [23]. Performing 5 min of moderate or vigorous physical activity was strongly associated with a 2% increase in physical function levels [15]. Related studies have shown that middle-aged and elderly people, who usually suffer from multiple chronic diseases, can benefit from PA on a regular basis even with physical functional limitations [24].

However, despite the widespread interest in the effectiveness of physical activity in avoiding or delaying impaired physical function, related studies have mostly been cross-sectional in design [15,25], which may limit the causal judgments regarding the relationship between PA and impaired physical function. Most previous studies have focused on moderate- or high-intensity physical activity exercise levels and have not taken into account low-intensity physical activity [26]. Some studies have shown that low-intensity physical activity also plays an important role in slowing down impaired physical function in middle-aged and elderly people [19], and most of the physical activities in middle-aged and elderly people are low-intensity physical activities [27]; thus, the role of low-intensity physical activity in slowing down impaired physical function in middle-aged and elderly people should not be ignored. Previous studies have mostly examined PA with a single variable and also lacked the combination of PA and multiple variables to explore. Furthermore, and more importantly, although PA may have beneficial effects on physical function, there may be differences between different PAVs in how much they reduce the risk of impaired physical function in middle-aged and older adults [28], and the optimal PA intervals required to infer these effects remain to be elucidated, especially in a large sample of Chinese middle-aged and older adults. Therefore, the purpose of this study was to explore the association between different physical activity volumes and impaired physical function in Chinese middle-aged and older adults, to assess the optimal PAV intervals that would allow them to avoid impaired physical function, and to provide evidence to support the reduction in the risk of impaired physical function in Chinese middle-aged and older adults. Accordingly, the following hypotheses are proposed in this study. Hypothesis 1: A higher PAV including low-intensity physical activity can significantly reduce the rate of impaired physical function in middle-aged and older adults. Hypothesis 2: The rate of impaired physical function varies among middle-aged and older adults with different PAVs, and the existence of an optimal PAV interval could more effectively reduce the risk of impaired physical function among middle-aged and older adults in China.

2. Methods

2.1. Study Design and Participants

Data for this study were obtained from the China Health and Retirement Longitudinal Study (CHARLS), a household interview survey conducted by the National Development Institute of Peking University to investigate the social, economic, and health status of community residents aged 45 years or older in China [29]. The CHARLS national baseline survey began in 2011 and used a multi-stage stratified whole-group sampling method to cover more than 17,000 people in 150 county-level units in 28 provinces and cities in China, with three follow-up surveys in 2013, 2015, and 2018 to collect information including sociodemographic, physical, and biological assessments and health-related information. The CHARLS was approved by the Biomedical Ethics Review Committee of Peking University (IRB00001052-11015), and all study subjects signed an informed consent form.

This study combined health status and function data based on ID for a total of 4 years in 2011, 2013, 2015, and 2018. After merging, a total of 13,051 participants were selected in this study. Of these, a total of 9056 participants were ultimately included in the study analysis after those with impaired daily physical function in the 2011 baseline survey (*n* = 3064) and those with missing data for physical activity, daily physical function, and covariates (*n* = 931) were excluded (Figure 1).

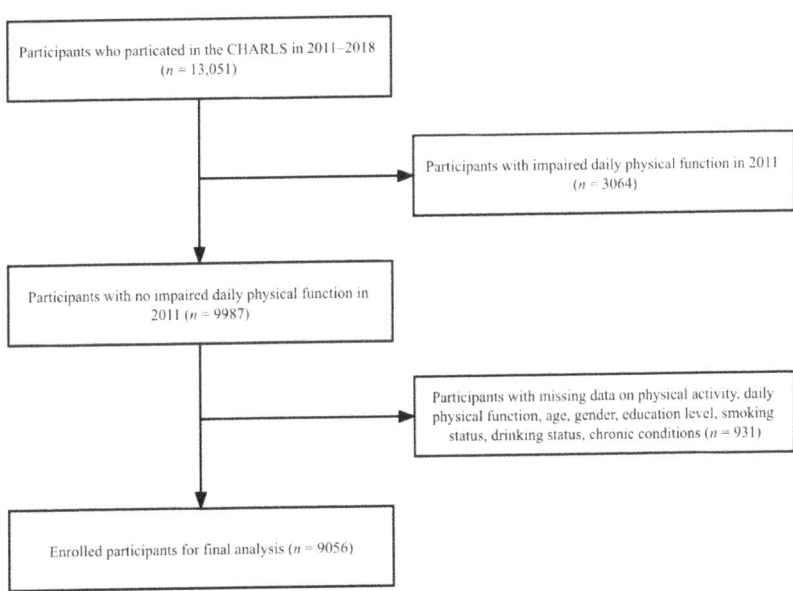

Figure 1. Flowchart of study participants.

2.2. Assessments

2.2.1. Daily Physical Function

Daily physical function (DPF) was measured by the Activities of Daily Living (ADL) and the Instrumental Activities of Daily Living (IADL) scales [30]. The ADL scale covers dressing, bathing, eating, getting into/out of bed, using the toilet, and controlling bowel movements or urination. The IADL covers money management, taking medication, shopping, meal preparation, and household chores. Each question on both scales was divided into 4 levels, where "no difficulty" = 0, "difficulty but still able to complete" = 1, "difficulty and need help" = 2, and "unable to complete" = 3. A combined ADL/IADL score ≥11 was defined as "impaired physical function" and <11 was defined as "no impaired physical function" [28]. In subsequent analyses, DPF was defined as a dichotomous variable, assigned a value of 1 if physical function was impaired and 0 otherwise. The follow-up duration was determined as the time from the participant's participation in the CHARLS (2011) to impaired physical function or to the termination of the fourth follow-up (2018), including 2 years, 4 years, and 7 years. The Cronbach's alpha coefficient for the questionnaire was 0.792.

2.2.2. Physical Activity

The questionnaire structure and statements used to measure participants' PA levels were based on the International Physical Activity Questionnaire (IPAQ). In each of the four surveys from 2011 to 2018, participants were asked whether they had performed at least 10 min of vigorous physical activity (VPA, such as carrying heavy loads, digging, plowing, aerobic exercise, fast cycling, bicycling with cargo, etc.), moderate physical activity (MPA, such as carrying light things, cycling at regular speed, mopping, tai chi, brisk walking, etc.), and low-intensity physical activity (LPA, such as walking at work or at home and walking for recreation, exercise, or leisure). If available, further questions were asked about weekly frequency (1–7 days) and time spent per day for different PA levels ($\geq$10 min and <30 min, $\geq$30 min and <2 h, $\geq$2 h and <4 h, and $\geq$4 h).

Since no specific duration was mentioned in the questionnaire, drawing on the treatment of other scholars [28], we transformed the time range by taking the middle value. That is, "$\geq$10 min and <30 min" was recorded as 20 min, "$\geq$30 min and <2 h" was recorded as 75 min, "$\geq$2 h and <4 h" was recorded as 180 min, and "$\geq$4 h" was recorded as 240 min.

The weekly duration scores for different PAs are the product of the weekly frequency of different PA levels and the time spent per day. The total physical activity volume (PAV) score can be expressed using the metabolic equivalent (MET) [31], which is calculated as follows: PAV = 8.0 × weekly vigorous physical activity duration score + 4.0 × weekly moderate physical activity duration score + 3.3 × weekly low intensity physical activity duration score. According to the IPAQ, physical inactivity (PI) was indicated if the total PAV did not reach 600 MET-minutes/week [32]. Therefore, the PAV in MET-minutes/week was divided into two major categories (0–599 and $\geq$600) and seven subcategories (0–599, 600–1199, 1200–1799, 1800–2999, 3000–5999, 6000–8999, and $\geq$9000).

2.2.3. Covariates

The covariates in this study included (1) demographic variables, such as age, gender (male or female), and education level (high school and below and college and above); (2) lifestyle behavior variables, including smoking status (current smoking, former smoking, and never smoking), and drinking status (current drinking, former drinking, and never drinking); (3) chronic disease status variables, including endocrine system diseases (no or yes), brain/nervous system diseases (no or yes), cardiovascular disease (no or yes), respiratory diseases (no or yes), orthopedic diseases (no or yes), and other diseases (no or yes).

2.3. Statistical Analysis

The baseline characteristics of the participants are expressed by frequency (n) and percentage (%). Cox proportional hazards regression models were used to calculate hazard ratios (HRs) and 95% confidence intervals (95% CIs) to determine the association between different PAV levels and impaired physical function. To assess the potential confounding effects of different covariates on the association between PAV and impaired physical function, three models were developed, and the three sets of covariates were added sequentially to the three models. The adjusted variables in Model 1 were gender and age; the adjusted variables in Model 2 were based on Model 1 with the addition of education level, smoking status, and drinking status; and the adjusted variables in Model 3 covered all covariates. The interaction between PAV and potential covariates was tested in Model 3, and subgroup analyses were conducted by gender, age, education level, smoking status, drinking status, and chronic disease status. Finally, a sensitivity analysis was performed to test the robustness of the results: the Markov chain Monte Carlo imputation method was used, assuming that the variables in the interpolated model showed a multivariate normal distribution with joint effects, specifically using predicted mean matching, binary logistic regression, and multiple logistic regression filling. The sensitivity analysis was performed on 9987 participants after five interpolations for variables with missing values.

Stata 17.0 (Stata Corporation, College Station, TX, USA) was used for all statistical analyses.

3. Results

3.1. Demographic Characteristics

Of the 9056 eligible participants included in this study, 4491 (49.59%) were men and 4565 (50.41%) were women, and the majority were younger than 65 years old (57.37%); had a high school education or less (96.41%); never smoked (56.71%); never drank alcohol

(61.75%); and did not suffer from endocrine system diseases (95.20%), brain/nervous system diseases (94.18%), cardiovascular disease (78.68%), respiratory diseases (94.14%), orthopedic diseases (93.93%), and other diseases (87.58%). The details are shown in Table 1.

Table 1. Basic characteristics of participants.

Characteristics	Overall Sample (n = 9056)	
	n	%
Age group (years)		
<65	5195	57.37
≥65	3861	42.63
Sex		
Men	4491	49.59
Women	4565	50.41
Education		
≤High school	8731	96.41
≥College	325	3.59
Smoking status		
Current	2513	27.75
Former	1407	15.54
Never	5136	56.71
Drinking status		
Current	3168	34.98
Former	296	3.27
Never	5592	61.75
Chronic conditions		
Endocrine system diseases		
No	8621	95.20
Yes	435	4.80
Brain/nervous system diseases		
No	8529	94.18
Yes	527	5.82
Cardiovascular disease		
No	7125	78.68
Yes	1931	21.32
Respiratory diseases		
No	8525	94.14
Yes	531	5.86
Orthopedic diseases		
No	8506	93.93
Yes	550	6.07
Other diseases		
No	7931	87.58
Yes	1125	12.42

3.2. Physical Activity and Physical Function Impairment Rate

A total of 1379 (15.23%) participants developed impaired physical function over the four follow-ups in the 7-year period (mean follow-up: 6.73 years) in 2011, 2013, 2015, and 2018. Tables 2 and 3 show the correlation between different metabolic equivalents of PAV and impaired physical function. In both Model 1 and Model 2, participants with a PAV ≥ 600 MET-minutes/week had a 62% lower risk of impaired physical function compared to physically inactive participants (Model 1: HR = 0.38, 95% CI 0.33–0.42; Model 2: HR = 0.38, 95% CI 0.34–0.43). In the fully adjusted model (Model 3), participants with a PAV ≥ 600 MET-minutes/week had a 61% lower risk of impaired physical function compared to participants with insufficient physical activity (HR = 0.39, 95% CI 0.35–0.44). Among them, participants with a physical activity volume of 1800–2999 MET-minutes/week had the lowest rate of impaired physical function (Table 3 and Figure 2), and their risk of impaired physical function was 67% lower than that of physically inactive participants (HR = 0.33, 95% CI 0.26–0.42).

Table 2. Associations between study participants with a PAV ≥ 600 MET-minutes/week and impaired physical function. Values are hazard ratios (95% confidence intervals) unless otherwise noted.

Variables	Events/Total	Model 1	Model 2	Model 3
PI	395/1208	1.00	1.00	1.00
≥600	984/7848	0.38 (0.33–0.42)	0.38 (0.34–0.43)	0.39 (0.35–0.44)

Note: Events indicates the number of participants who showed impaired physical function. Model 1: Adjusted for sex and age. Model 2: Model 1 + education level, smoking status, and drinking status. Model 3: Model 2 + chronic conditions. PI: Physical inactivity.

Table 3. Associations between study participants in different PAV subgroups and impaired physical function. Values are hazard ratios (95% confidence intervals) unless otherwise stated.

Variables	Events/Total	Model 1	Model 2	Model 3
PI	395/1208	1.00	1.00	1.00
600–1199	46/295	0.44 (0.33–0.60)	0.45 (0.33–0.61)	0.46 (0.34–0.63)
1200–1799	209/1283	0.48 (0.41–0.57)	0.49 (0.42–0.58)	0.50 (0.42–0.59)
1800–2999	77/676	0.33 (0.26–0.42)	0.33 (0.26–0.43)	0.33 (0.26–0.42)
3000–5999	240/1974	0.35 (0.30–0.41)	0.36 (0.31–0.43)	0.37 (0.32–0.44)
6000–8999	151/1125	0.39 (0.32–0.47)	0.40 (0.33–0.48)	0.40 (0.33–0.48)
PAV ≥ 9000	261/2495	0.33 (0.28–0.39)	0.34 (0.29–0.40)	0.35 (0.30–0.41)

Note: PI: Physical inactivity. PAV: Physical activity volume.

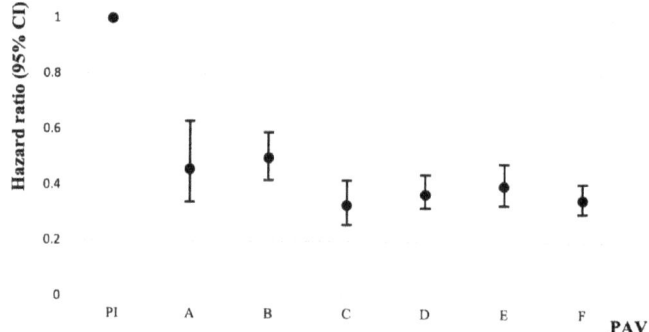

Figure 2. Plot of associations between study participants in different PAV groups and impaired physical function. Whiskers represent 95% confidence intervals. A: 600 ≤ PAV ≤ 1199. B: 1200 ≤ PAV ≤ 1799. C: 1800 ≤ PAV ≤ 2999. D: 3000 ≤ PAV ≤ 5999. E: 6000 ≤ PAV ≤ 8999. F: PAV ≥ 9000. Unit: MET-minutes/week.

3.3. Subgroup Analysis

The association between physical activity level and impaired physical function was stratified by age, sex, education level, smoking status, drinking status, presence of endocrine system diseases, presence of brain/nervous system diseases, presence of cardiovascular disease, presence of respiratory diseases, and presence of other diseases, and the results of the subgroup analysis are shown in Figure 3. In the fully adjusted model, there was a significant interaction effect of age and physical activity level on impaired physical function ($p = 0.028$). Participants with a physical activity volume greater than 600 MET-minutes/week and aged 65 years or older had a lower risk of physical function deficits (HR = 0.35) than participants younger than 65 (HR = 0.47). There was a significant interaction effect of gender and physical activity level on impaired physical function ($p = 0.01$). The risk of physical function deficits was lower in male participants with a physical activity volume greater than

600 MET-minutes/week (HR = 0.33) than in female participants (HR = 0.43). In addition, there was a significant interaction effect of respiratory disease status and physical activity level on impaired physical function (p = 0.06).

Subgroup	Total participants	PI events/total	PAV≥600MET-minutes/week events/total	Hazard Ratio (95%CI)	P for interaction
Age group (years)					0.028
<65	5195	137/583	508/4612	0.47 (0.39–0.57)	
≥65	3861	258/625	476/3236	0.35 (0.30–0.40)	
Sex					0.01
Men	4491	164/607	319/3884	0.33 (0.27–0.40)	
Women	4565	231/601	665/3964	0.43 (0.37–0.51)	
Education					0.587
≤Highschool	8731	388/1168	968/7563	0.39 (0.35–0.44)	
≥College	325	7/40	16/285	0.33 (0.13–0.85)	
Smoking status					0.17
Current	2513	88/351	174/2162	0.34 (0.26–0.44)	
Former	1407	73/199	148/1208	0.37 (0.28–0.50)	
Never	5136	234/658	662/4478	0.42 (0.36–0.49)	
Drinking status					0.76
Current	3168	69/350	242/2818	0.40 (0.31–0.53)	
Former	296	20/46	41/250	0.34 (0.19–0.59)	
Never	5592	306/812	701/4780	0.39 (0.34–0.44)	
Chronic conditions					
Endocrine system diseases					0.096
No	8621	372/1151	910/7470	0.38 (0.34–0.43)	
Yes	435	23/57	74/378	0.55 (0.34–0.89)	
Brain/nervous system diseases					0.179
No	8529	345/1123	860/7406	0.38 (0.34–0.43)	
Yes	527	50/85	124/442	0.45 (0.32–0.64)	
Cardiovascular disease					0.331
No	7125	279/929	701/6196	0.38 (0.33–0.44)	
Yes	1931	116/279	283/1652	0.42 (0.34–0.52)	
Respiratory diseases					0.006
No	8525	355/1118	896/7407	0.39 (0.35–0.44)	
Yes	531	40/90	88/441	0.41 (0.28–0.60)	
Orthopedic diseases					0.668
No	8506	366/1143	904/7363	0.40 (0.35–0.45)	
Yes	550	29/65	80/485	0.34 (0.22–0.53)	
Other diseases					0.657
No	7931	332/1057	818/6874	0.39 (0.34–0.44)	
Yes	1125	63/151	166/974	0.42 (0.31–0.57)	

Figure 3. Subgroup analysis of the association between study participants with a PAV ≥ 600 MET-minutes/week and impaired physical function.

3.4. Sensitivity Analysis

A sensitivity analysis was performed on the data to confirm the findings. The sensitivity analysis showed that excluding missing values for age, sex, education level, smoking status, drinking status, chronic conditions, and physical activity level at baseline had little effect on the risk estimate for impaired physical function (HR = 0.39, 95% CI 0.35–0.43).

4. Discussion

In this study, we found that a PAV ≥ 600 MET-minutes/week significantly reduced the risk of impaired physical function in Chinese middle-aged and elderly people. Moreover, a PAV in the range of 1800–2999 MET-minutes/week could more effectively reduce the risk of impaired physical function in Chinese middle-aged and elderly people.

This study found that higher levels of physical activity compared to physical inactivity helped to avoid or delay impairment of physical function in middle-aged and older adults. Hillsdon et al. [33] found that the decline in physical function with age was associated with low physical activity. Previous studies have also shown that aerobic exercise helps to improve cardiovascular health [34] while resistance exercise helps improve muscle strength, explosive power, flexibility, and balance [35,36], and that these improvements are essential to avoid or delay impaired physical function in middle-aged and older adults. Some studies have shown that the risk reduction from the effects of regular physical activity on various outcomes related to function is typically in the range of 30% to 50% [20]. This is generally consistent with the findings of this study that adequate physical activity can significantly reduce the risk of impaired physical function in middle-aged and older adults. Although loss of physical function is inevitable with age, early initiation of regular physical activity can reduce the age at which disability develops [37].

In order to help middle-aged and older adults engage in reasonable physical activity and promote health in this population, the World Health Organization (WHO) recommends that middle-aged and older adults should engage in at least 150 min of moderate-intensity PA or 75 min of high-intensity PA, or an equivalent combination of moderate-intensity and high-intensity aerobic PA each week [38,39]. However, most middle-aged and older adults may not meet the current recommendations [27,40]. Physical activity in middle-aged and older adults may be dominated by low-intensity physical activity, such as walking, compared to moderate- or high-intensity physical activity. It is true that meeting the WHO recommendations for physical activity plays an important role in avoiding impairment of physical function in middle-aged and older adults. However, when middle-aged and older adults are unable to meet this recommendation, our findings suggested that a PAV $\geq$ 600 MET-minutes/week, including low-intensity physical activity, can also be protective of physical function in this population. Hypothesis 1 was thus confirmed. This is consistent with previous studies showing that low-intensity physical activity can also slow the progression of physical disability in middle-aged and older adults [19,26].

It is well known that a higher PAV is not better. Previous studies have shown that excessive or high-intensity exercise impairs the immune system [41], which may adversely affect physical function in middle-aged and older adults. Several studies have also shown that overactivity is associated with reduced bone mineral density [42] and loss of muscle tissue [43]. Therefore, determining the optimal metabolic equivalent range of physical activity is essential to maintain or improve physical function. Studies have shown that for middle-aged and older adults with hypertension, PA of at least 1200 MET-minutes per week was associated with better physical function [28]. A metabolic equivalent of 1800–2999 MET-minutes per week significantly improved individual cardiopulmonary endurance, vascular endothelial function, and insulin sensitivity [44]. This is generally consistent with the findings of this study that 1800–2999 MET-minutes/week may be the optimal PAV to avoid impaired physical function in middle-aged and elderly Chinese people. Hypothesis 2 was thus confirmed. Although this study found that a PAV $\geq$ 9000 MET-minutes/week is also important for avoiding impaired physical function in middle-aged and elderly people, the possible adverse effects of excessive physical activity and the feasibility of implementing the recommended PAV in real-life situations should also be considered.

In terms of subgroup analysis, this study found that the negative association between PAV and the risk of impaired physical function in middle-aged and elderly Chinese was consistent across all subgroups. Additionally, it seemed to be more pronounced in participants who were 65 years old or older, male, and did not suffer from respiratory diseases. The reasons for this may be as follows: physical function declines gradually with age, and the effect of the decline becomes more pronounced with age, whereas physical activity counteracts the decline in physical function with age as much as possible [45]. It has been shown that middle-aged and older men are more likely to experience high-velocity muscle fatigue compared to middle-aged and older women [46], which may explain the higher reduction in the risk of impaired physical function associated with PA in middle-aged and older men than in middle-aged and older women. In addition, among middle-aged and older adults with a PAV $\geq$ 600 MET-minutes/week, those without respiratory diseases had a lower risk of impaired physical function compared to those with respiratory diseases, perhaps because the beneficial effects of physical activity were partially offset by respiratory diseases [47].

The present study has the following strengths: first, to our knowledge, it is the first study to examine the association between different physical activity levels and impaired physical function in middle-aged and older adults while considering multiple confounding factors and to explore the optimal PAV interval to avoid or mitigate impaired physical function in middle-aged and older adults in China. Second, this study was a longitudinal cohort study with a mean follow-up of 6.73 years for its sample. Third, this study used a large, nationally representative sample covering 28 provinces in mainland China, so the results of this study can be generalized to the entire Chinese middle-aged and elderly population. Furthermore, this database resource has been adopted by a large number of high-quality research institutes [48–50], with high validity and reliability. Fourth, considering the influence of confounding factors, this study added them to the model in turn, including demographic variables, life behavior variables, and chronic disease status variables. However, this study also has some limitations. First, PA was measured in a self-reported format, and self-report questionnaires are inevitably subject to recall bias. It has been shown that self-reported physical activity is on average overestimated compared to objective physical activity values measured by accelerometers [51]. For the measurement of PA, more objective measures such as the use of accelerometers are needed in the future. Second, survival time was derived from the difference between follow-up times. Since physical function was measured at the time of the questionnaire, the study could not determine the exact time of physical function impairment for individuals with impaired physical function. Therefore, only a rough estimate can be made due to the difference between the follow-up times.

5. Conclusions

Although current physical activity guidelines focus on moderate and vigorous physical activity, this study found that fulfilling a PAV $\geq$ 600 MET-minutes/week, including low-intensity physical activity (LPA, such as walking), also significantly reduced the risk of impaired physical function in Chinese middle-aged and older adults. In addition, a PAV in the range of 1800–2999 MET-minutes/week could be more effective in reducing the risk of impaired physical function in middle-aged and elderly Chinese.

Author Contributions: Conceptualization, Y.T.; methodology, Y.T.; software, Y.T.; validation, Y.T. and Z.S.; formal analysis, Y.T.; investigation, Y.T.; resources, Y.T.; data curation, Y.T.; writing—original draft preparation, Y.T. and Z.S.; writing—review and editing, Y.T. and Z.S. All authors have read and agreed to the published version of the manuscript.

Funding: This work was supported by the National Social Science Fund of China (No. 20BTY081).

Institutional Review Board Statement: The study was conducted in accordance with the Declaration of Helsinki and approved by the Biomedical Ethics Review Committee of Peking University (IRB00001052-11015).

Informed Consent Statement: Informed consent was obtained from all subjects involved in the study. Written informed consent has been obtained from the patients to publish this paper

Data Availability Statement: Publicly available datasets were analyzed in this study. These data can be found at http://charls.pku.edu.cn/, accessed on 10 October 2022.

Conflicts of Interest: The authors declare no conflict of interest.

References

1. Coelho-Junior, H.J.; Calvani, R.; Picca, A.; Gonçalves, I.O.; Landi, F.; Bernabei, R.; Cesari, M.; Uchida, M.C.; Marzetti, E. Association between dietary habits and physical function in brazilian and italian older women. *Nutrients* **2020**, *12*, 1635. [CrossRef]
2. Sugiura, Y.; Tanimoto, Y.; Watanabe, M.; Tsuda, Y.; Kimura, M.; Kusabiraki, T.; Kono, K. Handgrip strength as a predictor of higher-level competence decline among community-dwelling Japanese elderly in an urban area during a 4-year follow-up. *Arch. Gerontol. Geriatr.* **2013**, *57*, 319–324. [CrossRef]
3. Ishizaki, T.; Furuna, T.; Yoshida, Y.; Iwasa, H.; Shimada, H.; Yoshida, H.; Kumagai, S.; Suzuki, T. Declines in physical performance by sex and age among nondisabled community-dwelling older Japanese during a 6-year period. *J. Epidemiol.* **2011**, *21*, 176–183. [CrossRef]
4. Lyu, Y.; Yu, X.; Yuan, H.C.; Yi, X.R.; Dong, X.S.; Ding, M.; Lin, X.Y.; Wang, B.Z. Associations between dietary patterns and physical fitness among Chinese elderly. *Public Health Nutr.* **2021**, *24*, 4466–4473. [CrossRef]
5. Zhang, L.; Cui, H.J.; Chen, Q.Z.; Li, Y.; Yang, C.X.; Yang, Y.F. A web-based dynamic Nomogram for predicting instrumental activities of daily living disability in older adults: A nationally representative survey in China. *BMC Geriatr.* **2021**, *21*, 311. [CrossRef]

6. Guralnik, J.M.; Ferrucci, L.; Simonsick, E.M.; Salive, M.E.; Wallace, R.B. Lower-extremity function in persons over the age of 70 years as a predictor of subsequent disability. *N. Engl. J. Med.* **1995**, *332*, 556–562. [CrossRef]
7. Studenski, S.; Perera, S.; Patel, K.; Rosano, C.; Faulkner, K.; Inzitari, M.; Brach, J.; Chandler, J.; Cawthon, P.; Connor, E.B. Gait speed and survival in older adults. *Jama* **2011**, *305*, 50–58. [CrossRef]
8. Nakazawa, A.; Nakamura, K.; Kitamura, K.; Yoshizawa, Y. Association Between Activities of Daily Living and Mortality Among Institutionalized Elderly Adults in Japan. *J. Epidemiol.* **2012**, *22*, 501–507. [CrossRef]
9. Hlebichuk, J.L.; Gretebeck, R.J.; Garnier-Villarreal, M.; Piacentine, L.B.; Singh, M.; Gretebeck, K.A. Physical Activity, Inflammation, and Physical Function in Older Adults: Results From the Health & Retirement Study. *Biol. Res. Nurs.* **2022**. [CrossRef]
10. Hu, X.Q.; Zeng, Y.H.; Zhen, X.M.; Zhang, H.; Li, Y.Y.; Gu, S.Y.; Dong, H.J. Cognitive and physical function of people older than 80 years in China from 1998 to 2014. *J. Int. Med. Res.* **2018**, *46*, 2810–2827. [CrossRef]
11. Johnston, K.J.; Wen, H.F.; Hockenberry, J.M.; Maddox, K.E.J. Association Between Patient Cognitive and Functional Status and Medicare Total Annual Cost of Care Implications for Value-Based Payment. *JAMA Intern. Med.* **2018**, *178*, 1489–1497. [CrossRef] [PubMed]
12. Zhang, L.; Fang, Y. A study on the prediction of the scale of disablement and its cost of care for the elderly in urban and rural areas in China from 2020 to 2050. *Chin. J. Health Stat.* **2021**, *38*, 39–42.
13. Zhao, H. The relationship between resource endowment and quality of home care for urban elderly with disabilities. *Chin. Health Serv. Manag.* **2013**, *30*, 711–714.
14. Halaweh, H.; Willen, C.; Svantesson, U. Association between physical activity and physical functioning in community-dwelling older adults. *Eur. J. Physiother.* **2017**, *19*, 40–47. [CrossRef]
15. Hrubeniuk, T.J.; Senechal, M.; Mayo, A.; Bouchard, D.R. Association between physical function and various patterns of physical activity in older adults: A cross-sectional analysis. *Aging Clin. Exp. Res.* **2020**, *32*, 1017–1024. [CrossRef]
16. Dong, X.; Yi, X.; Ding, M.; Gao, Z.; McDonough, D.J.; Yi, N.; Qiao, W. A Longitudinal Study of a Multicomponent Exercise Intervention with Remote Guidance among Breast Cancer Patients. *Int. J. Environ. Res. Public Health* **2020**, *17*, 3425. [CrossRef]
17. Dong, X.; Yi, X.; Gao, D.; Gao, Z.; Huang, S.; Chao, M.; Chen, W.; Ding, M. The effects of the combined exercise intervention based on internet and social media software (CEIBISMS) on quality of life, muscle strength and cardiorespiratory capacity in Chinese postoperative breast cancer patients:a randomized controlled trial. *Health Qual. Life Outcomes* **2019**, *17*, 109. [CrossRef]
18. Dong, X.; Yi, X.; Huang, S.; Gao, D.; Chao, M.; Ding, M. The effects of combined exercise intervention based on Internet and social media software for postoperative patients with breast cancer: Study protocol for a randomized controlled trial. *Trials* **2018**, *19*, 477. [CrossRef]
19. Miller, M.E.; Rejeski, W.J.; Reboussin, B.A.; Ten Have, T.R.; Ettinger, W.H. Physical activity, functional limitations, and disability in older adults. *J. Am. Geriatr. Soc.* **2000**, *48*, 1264–1272. [CrossRef]
20. Paterson, D.H.; Warburton, D.E.R. Physical activity and functional limitations in older adults: A systematic review related to Canada's Physical Activity Guidelines. *Int. J. Behav. Nutr. Phys. Act.* **2010**, *7*, 38. [CrossRef]
21. Sturnieks, D.L.; St George, R.; Lord, S.R. Balance disorders in the elderly. *Neurophysiol. Clin./Clin. Neurophysiol.* **2008**, *38*, 467–478. [CrossRef] [PubMed]
22. Latham, N.K.; Bennett, D.A.; Stretton, C.M.; Anderson, C.S. Systematic review of progressive resistance strength training in older adults. *J. Gerontol. Ser. A Biol. Sci. Med. Sci.* **2004**, *59*, M48–M61. [CrossRef] [PubMed]
23. Keysor, J.J.; Jette, A.M. Have we oversold the benefit of late-life exercise? *J. Gerontol. Ser. A Biol. Sci. Med. Sci.* **2001**, *56*, M412–M423. [CrossRef] [PubMed]
24. Cheung, C.; Talley, K.M.; McMahon, S.; Schorr, E.; Wyman, J.F. Knowledge of Physical Activity Guidelines and Its Association with Physical Activity and Physical Function in Older Adults. *Act. Adapt. Aging* **2020**, *44*, 106–118. [CrossRef]
25. Morie, M.; Reid, K.F.; Miciek, R.; Lajevardi, N.; Choong, K.; Krasnoff, J.B.; Storer, T.W.; Fielding, R.A.; Bhasin, S.; LeBrasseur, N.K. Habitual Physical Activity Levels Are Associated with Performance in Measures of Physical Function and Mobility in Older Men. *J. Am. Geriatr. Soc.* **2010**, *58*, 1727–1733. [CrossRef] [PubMed]
26. Mayo, A.; Senechal, M.; Boudreau, J.; Belanger, M.; Bouchard, D.R. Potential functional benefits of a comprehensive evaluation of physical activity for aging adults: A CLSA cross-sectional analysis. *Aging Clin. Exp. Res.* **2021**, *33*, 285–289. [CrossRef]
27. Colley, R.C.; Garriguet, D.; Janssen, I.; Craig, C.L.; Clarke, J.; Tremblay, M.S. Physical activity of Canadian adults: Accelerometer results from the 2007 to 2009 Canadian Health Measures Survey. *Health Rep.* **2011**, *22*, 7.
28. Ding, M.; Jia, N.; Zhou, Y.; Li, B. The Dose-Response Relationships of Different Dimensions of Physical Activity with Daily Physical Function and Cognitive Function in Chinese Adults with Hypertension: A Cross-Sectional Study. *Int. J. Environ. Res. Public Health* **2021**, *18*, 12698. [CrossRef]
29. Zhao, Y.; Hu, Y.; Smith, J.P.; Strauss, J.; Yang, G. Cohort Profile: The China Health and Retirement Longitudinal Study (CHARLS). *Int. J. Epidemiol.* **2014**, *43*, 61–68. [CrossRef]
30. Cantwell, J.; Muldoon, O.T.; Gallagher, S. Social support and mastery influence the association between stress and poor physical health in parents caring for children with developmental disabilities. *Res. Dev. Disabil.* **2014**, *35*, 2215–2223. [CrossRef]
31. Deng, Y.; Paul, D.R. The Relationships Between Depressive Symptoms, Functional Health Status, Physical Activity, and the Availability of Recreational Facilities: A Rural-Urban Comparison in Middle-Aged and Older Chinese Adults. *Int. J. Behav. Med.* **2018**, *25*, 322–330. [CrossRef]

32. Li, X.W.; Zhang, W.D.; Zhang, W.Y.; Tao, K.; Ni, W.L.; Wang, K.; Li, Z.L.; Liu, Q.; Lin, J.H. Level of physical activity among middle-aged and older Chinese people: Evidence from the China health and retirement longitudinal study. *BMC Public Health* **2020**, *20*, 1682. [CrossRef]
33. Hillsdon, M.M.; Brunner, E.J.; Guralnik, J.M.; Marmot, M.G. Prospective study of physical activity and physical function in early old age. *Am. J. Prev. Med.* **2005**, *28*, 245–250. [CrossRef] [PubMed]
34. Fleg, J.L. Aerobic Exercise in the Elderly: A Key to Successful Aging. *Discov. Med.* **2012**, *13*, 223–228. [PubMed]
35. Hunter, G.R.; McCarthy, J.P.; Bamman, M.M. Effects of resistance training on older adults. *Sports Med.* **2004**, *34*, 329–348. [CrossRef] [PubMed]
36. Orr, R.; Raymond, J.; Singh, M.F. Efficacy of progressive resistance training on balance performance in older adults: A systematic review Randomized controlled trials. *Sports Med.* **2008**, *38*, 317–343. [CrossRef] [PubMed]
37. Manini, T.M.; Pahor, M. Physical activity and maintaining physical function in older adults. *Br. J. Sports Med.* **2009**, *43*, 28–31. [CrossRef]
38. Bull, F.C.; Al-Ansari, S.S.; Biddle, S.; Borodulin, K.; Buman, M.P.; Cardon, G.; Carty, C.; Chaput, J.-P.; Chastin, S.; Chou, R.; et al. World Health Organization 2020 guidelines on physical activity and sedentary behaviour. *Br. J. Sports Med.* **2020**, *54*, 1451–1462. [CrossRef]
39. Ding, M.; Zhou, Y.A.; Li, C.X.; Li, W.P.; Jia, N.X.; Dong, X.S. Can the WHO's recommendations of physical activity volume decrease the risk of heart disease in middle and older aged Chinese People: The evidence from a seven year longitudinal survey. *BMC Geriatr.* **2022**, *22*, 596. [CrossRef]
40. Keevil, V.L.; Cooper, A.J.M.; Wijndaele, K.; Luben, R.; Wareham, N.J.; Brage, S.; Khaw, K.T. Objective Sedentary Time, Moderate-to-Vigorous Physical Activity, and Physical Capability in a British Cohort. *Med. Sci. Sports Exerc.* **2016**, *48*, 421–429. [CrossRef]
41. Mourao, N.; Lopes, J.S.S.; Neto, A.M.M.; Perego, S.M.; Franca, A.C.H.; Franca, E.L. Behavior profile of cytokines submitted to combat sports. A systematic review. *Sci. Sports* **2022**, *37*, 244–254. [CrossRef]
42. DiMarco, N.M.; Dart, L.; Sanborn, C.B. Modified activity-stress paradigm in an animal model of the female athlete triad. *J. Appl. Physiol.* **2007**, *103*, 1469–1478. [CrossRef]
43. Steinacker, J.M.; Lormes, W.; Reissnecker, S.; Liu, Y.F. New aspects of the hormone and cytokine response to training. *Eur. J. Appl. Physiol.* **2004**, *91*, 382–391. [CrossRef]
44. Li, J.; Chang, Y.-P.; Riegel, B.; Keenan, B.T.; Varrasse, M.; Pack, A.I.; Gooneratne, N.S. Intermediate, But Not Extended, Afternoon Naps May Preserve Cognition in Chinese Older Adults. *J. Gerontol. Ser. A* **2017**, *73*, 360–366. [CrossRef]
45. Ip, E.H.; Church, T.; Marshall, S.A.; Zhang, Q.; Marsh, A.P.; Guralnik, J.; King, A.C.; Rejeski, W.J.; Investigators, L.-P.S. Physical Activity Increases Gains in and Prevents Loss of Physical Function: Results From the Lifestyle Interventions and Independence for Elders Pilot Study. *J. Gerontol. Ser. A-Biol. Sci. Med. Sci.* **2013**, *68*, 426–432. [CrossRef]
46. Senefeld, J.; Yoon, T.; Hunter, S.K. Age differences in dynamic fatigability and variability of arm and leg muscles: Associations with physical function. *Exp. Gerontol.* **2017**, *87*, 74–83. [CrossRef]
47. Breda, A.I.; Watts, A.S. Expectations Regarding Aging, Physical Activity, and Physical Function in Older Adults. *Gerontol. Geriatr. Med.* **2017**, *3*, 2333721417702350. [CrossRef]
48. Ko, P.C.; Hank, K. Grandparents Caring for Grandchildren in China and Korea: Findings From CHARLS and KLoSA. *J. Gerontol. Ser. B-Psychol. Sci. Soc. Sci.* **2014**, *69*, 646–651. [CrossRef]
49. Wang, Y.; Shen, H.; Morrow-Howell, N. Family intergenerational non-time transfers in china: New evidence from charls. *Gerontologist* **2015**, *55*, 668–669.
50. Li, J.; Alfini, A.J.; Yu, F.; Schrack, J.A.; Cotter, V.; Taylor, J.L.; Spira, A.P. Sleep duration, physical activity and cognitive decline In chinese older adults: Findings from the charls. *Sleep* **2020**, *43*, A433. [CrossRef]
51. Colley, R.C.; Butler, G.; Garriguet, D.; Prince, S.A.; Roberts, K.C. Comparison of self-reported and accelerometer-measured physical activity in Canadian adults. *Health Rep.* **2018**, *29*, 3–15.

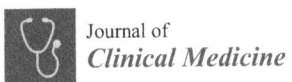

Article

Effects of an Eccentric Training Protocol Using Gliding Discs on Balance and Lower Body Strength in Healthy Adults

Juan Lopez-Barreiro *, Pablo Hernandez-Lucas, Jose Luis Garcia-Soidan and Vicente Romo-Perez

Faculty of Education and Sport Sciences, Universidade de Vigo, Campus A Xunqueira, s/n., 36005 Pontevedra, Spain; phernandez@uvigo.es (P.H.-L.); jlsoidan@uvigo.es (J.L.G.-S.); vicente@uvigo.es (V.R.-P.)
* Correspondence: juan.lopez.barreiro@uvigo.es

Abstract: Impaired balance and lower body weakness are the main causes of falls, which are considered to be the major cause of fractures and head injuries in the elderly and are recognised as a serious health problem. The aim of this study is to observe the effect of eccentric training, introducing new technologies (gliding discs), on body composition, lower body strength, balance and quality of life. A quasi-experimental study was carried out with 56 healthy participants who were divided into an experimental group (n = 31) who underwent the protocol consisting of 12 training sessions and a control group (n = 25) who did not undergo the training. Before and after the intervention, all participants underwent a measurement of body composition, the SJ jump, balance with accelerometry and quality of life with the Short Form 12 Health Survey. In the experimental group, statistically significant improvements were found in the variables balance and lower body strength. The application of this training protocol improves lower body strength and the ability to control balance in the adult population.

Keywords: lower-body strength; accelerometry; falls; quality of life; squat jump

1. Introduction

Balance impairment is considered to be responsible for 10–25% of falls [1]. Another risk factor for falls is lower extremity weakness, and according to Graafmans et al. [2], this weakness is a predictor of future falls [2].

Falls are the major cause of fractures and head injuries in the elderly, especially in women [3]. Moreover, they are recognised as a serious health problem that can cause serious injuries such as fractures or head injuries and even death [4,5].

Known risk factors are age, previous falls, arthritis, cognitive disorders, dependence in daily activities, depression, gait and balance dysfunctions, medication, muscle weakness, and visual and sensory impairments [6–8].

Elderly people with a history of falls, due to poor muscle strength, experience fear of a possible subsequent fall that could limit their activities and mobility, which directly affects their quality of life [5].

Older adults are more likely to have a higher level of quality of life in relation to an increase in the frequency and duration of physical activity [9]. On this basis, relationships are also established between physical–functional problems and loss of strength, flexibility, hearing, sight, memory and balance [9]. These factors are the same as fall risk factors. Therefore, a direct relationship can be established between balance, risk of falls and quality of life. On the other hand, in addition to the preventive role of training in young adults, the prevalence of frailty in young and middle-aged adults is similar to that of older adults living in the community [10].

Considering this, and given the rapid increase in the age of the world's population, falls prevention is of extreme importance. It is essential to establish an effective, simple, safe and low-cost method to reduce the risk of fall occurrence [11]. Knowledge of the relationship between balance, strength and power is important for the identification of individual fall risk factors, because deficits in these neuromuscular components are associated with an increased risk of injury or falls [12]. The WHO further recommends varied and multicomponent physical activity with an emphasis on functional balance and moderate- to higher-intensity muscle strength training, three or more days a week, to improve functional capacity and prevent falls [12].

Several studies have shown that training focused on eccentric muscle contractions is more effective in increasing strength and muscle mass, compared to training focused on concentric muscle contractions [13–17]. The most traditional form of eccentric training is the performance of body weight exercises with a long eccentric contraction [18], that was applied by introducing the gliding discs, which make the exercise more complicated and interesting for those who perform it as they increase the amplitude of movement [19].

Based on this, it seems necessary to design and apply appropriate interventions with programmes that are capable of delaying or reversing the limitations produced by the alteration of balance in order to improve quality of life [20].

It is for these reasons that the protocol described in this paper is presented, with the aim of testing whether it improves balance and lower body strength in a healthy adult population, and with the previous hypothesis that this eccentric training programme using gliding discs will produce positive effects on body composition, lower body strength, balance and quality of life.

2. Materials and Methods

2.1. Design

A quasi-experimental study was conducted with a control group (CG) in a convenience sample, comparing the scores on the measures of the dependent variables before and after the intervention, both in the experimental group (EG) (they followed the training protocol) and in the CG (they continued with their normal daily activity) to compare the possible effects of the programme.

2.2. Participants

A non-probabilistic purposive sampling was carried out at the Faculty of Physical Activity and Sport Sciences of the Universidade de Vigo. Eighty-four volunteers were willing to participate in the study and the following inclusion criteria were applied: (a) age between 18 and 65 years; (b) signing the informed consent form; (c) being able to attend the initial measurements (d) not taking medication or presenting any limiting pathology; exclusion: (a) missing more than two training sessions; (b) not being able to attend the final measurements; (c) varying their lifestyle in relation to physical activity, rest and nutrition.

After applying these inclusion criteria, we found 68 subjects, who were randomly assigned to the EG and CG.

There were 12 drop-outs, nine from the CG and three from the EG, with 56 subjects completing the study, leaving the final study sample comprising 31 subjects belonging to the EG and 25 to the CG as shown in the following diagram (Figure 1).

2.3. Studied Variables

2.3.1. Anthropometric variables

The anthropometric variables were measured using an OMRON BF-511 scale previously used in research [21,22] and a homologated tallimeter (Seca™ 709, Hamburg, Germany), with the subjects positioned with their heels placed together and their heads in the Frankfort plane. The measurements were taken three times and then averaged.

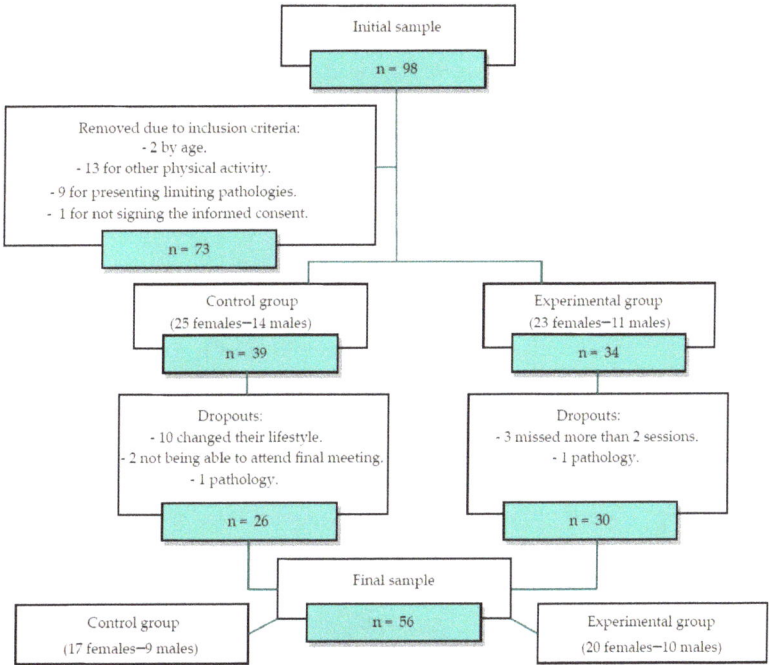

Figure 1. Sample selection flowchart.

2.3.2. Lower Body Strength

To measure lower body strength, the ErgoJump Bosco System platform was used to record jump height [23]. This device is a conductive mat (dimensions L-175 × W-70 cm) connected to an electronic timing system. The timer switches on automatically when a subject takes off and switches off as soon as a foot makes contact with the mat again. The test performed was the Squat Jump (SJ). The protocol used for the SJ was as follows: bare feet at hip width, hands on hips, knees bent at 90° and trunk upright, without downward countermovements. Again, subjects performed three jumps from which the average was found.

2.3.3. Quality of Life

The Spanish version of the Short-Form Health Survey SF-12 was used to measure the subjects' quality of life [24]. This survey was given to the subjects on paper in the measurement sessions before and after the 12 weeks of training.

2.3.4. Balance

To obtain the balance values of each subject, triaxial accelerometers model ActiGraph GT3X+® placed in the lumbar region were used following the measurement protocol described by Leirós-Rodríguez et al. [25].

2.4. Intervention

The intervention consisted of an eccentric training programme using gliding discs. It lasted eight weeks, with two sessions per week. A total of 12 training sessions were carried out, lasting approximately 45 min and two sessions to measure the different variables, one at the beginning and other at the end. The training sessions were conducted in small groups organised according to the availability of the participants. Both the measurement sessions and the training sessions were carried out in sports clothes and in an air-conditioned room at a temperature of 22 °C.

2.4.1. Assessment

The measurement sessions were structured as follows, except that the explanation of the study and the reading and signing of the consent form were not repeated in the post-test: (a) explanation of the study to the participants; (b) reading and signing of the informed consent form by the participants; (c) completing the SF-12 questionnaire by the participants; (d) taking anthropometric measurements of the participants; (e) measuring the SJ height; (f) measuring the quality of balance using accelerometry.

2.4.2. Training Sessions

The structure of each training session consisted of a warm-up, a main part and a cool-down.

The warm-up consisted of 6′ walking on a treadmill at 6 km/h with a 1% incline and performing ten repetitions of each of the following joint mobility exercises: left and right ankle internal and external ankle circling, internal and external knee rotations with semi-flexed knees, right and left hip rotations; ten repetitions of the following strength exercises using body weight: half squats, dynamic front splits with left and right leg, dynamic back splits with left and right leg and lateral splits with left and right leg.

The main part consisted of eccentric training using body weight and gliding discs, performing four sets of ten repetitions of the exercises described in Table 1. After eight sessions, the load was increased by increasing the number of repetitions of each exercise by 20%, that is, 12 repetitions.

Table 1. Main part of the training.

Exercise	Starting/Ending Position	Middle Position
Back split		
Lateral split		
Front split		

Table 1. Cont.

Exercise	Starting/Ending Position	Middle Position
Hamstring curl		

In the cool down, static stretching was performed for 15″ per muscle group, specifically: calf, soleus, quadriceps, hamstrings, psoas iliacus, gluteus, abdominal and lumbar area.

2.5. Ethics

The Research Ethics Committee of the Faculty of Education and Sport Sciences of the Universidade de Vigo evaluated and approved the study with registration 04-0721 and all procedures were designed and administered in accordance with the Declaration of Helsinki. An informed consent form was also administered prior to the start of the study.

2.6. Statistics Analysis

The normal distribution of the data was verified using the Shapiro–Wilk test and homogeneity of variance with Levene's test. Both pre-intervention groups were found to show no significant differences in the variables under study with the t-test for independent samples.

An ANOVA 2 × 2 (Group × Momentum) analysis was used to analyse the effects of the intervention for all variables of interest and the effect size was calculated using Cohen's d statistic defined as small: $d = 0.1$; medium: $d = 0.5$; large: $d = 0.8$ [26].

The significance level was set at $p < 0.05$. Analyses were performed with STATA 15.0 for MacOS® software (STATA Corporation, College Station, TX, USA).

3. Results

Table 2 details the pre-intervention values. No significant differences were found in any of the variables analysed between the groups at baseline.

Table 2. Baseline of the studied variables.

Variable	ALL (n = 56)		CG (n = 25)		EG (n = 31)		p-Value
	x̄ ± SD	Median	x̄ ± SD	P50	x̄ ± SD	Median	
Age (Years)	30.9 ± 10.5	27.5	30.6 ± 8.9	28	31.2 ± 11.8	27	0.827
Weight (Kg)	72.1 ± 12.7	71	69.8 ± 11.5	69	74 ± 13.5	71.1	0.313
Height (cm)	1.7 ± 0.1	1.7	1.7 ± 0.1	1.68	1.7 ± 0.1	1.7	0.219
BMI (Kg/m²)	24.9 ± 2.7	24.7	24.5 ± 2.4	24.62	25.2 ± 3.1	24.5	0.359
%MG	25.6 ± 7.9	23.8	24.3 ± 6.9	22.6	27.1 ± 9.1	27.7	0.207
%MM	33.1 ± 5.6	32.4	32.6 ± 5	31.5	33.3 ± 6.4	33.1	0.633
SJ	23.8 ± 6.2	23.8	22.4 ± 5.6	21.3	22.4 ± 6.7	21.9	0.987
EQUI	2.2 ± 1.1	2	2.3 ± 1.2	1.99	2.6 ± 1.2	2.4	0.339
mSF-12	50.2 ± 1.9	51	49.9 ± 2.1	51	49.6 ± 2.3	51	0.594
fSF-12	52.8 ± 2.8	53	52.1 ± 2.4	53	52.7 ± 3.3	53	0.611

SD: standard deviation; BMI: body mass index; %MG: body fat percentage; %MM: muscle mass percentage; SJ: squat jump; EQUI: capacity to control balance; fSF-12: physical dimension of the survey SF-12; mSF-12: mental dimension of the survey SF-12.

Table 3 shows the results of the descriptive analysis of the variables in both groups before and after the intervention (mean and confidence interval). The results obtained in the 2 × 2 ANOVA test and the effect size after the intervention are also shown. In the percentage improvement, it is understood that negative percentages indicate worse results and positive percentages indicate better results between the pre-test and the post-test.

Table 3. Inferential statistics of the 2 × 2 ANOVA test and effect sizes.

Variable	Group	Pre-Test Mean	95% CI	Post-Test Mean	95% CI	Cohen's d	Group	M	Group × M p-Value
%MG	CG	24.3	(21.4–27.2)	24.1	(21.2–26.9)	−0.10	0.107	0.727	0.818
	EG	27.1	(23.8–30.4)	26.2	(23.2–29.3)				
%MM	CG	32.6	(30.5–34.6)	32.8	(30.7–34.9)	0.06	0.438	0.777	0.933
	EG	33.3	(30.9–35.6)	33.7	(31.5–35.9)				
SJ	CG	22.4	(20.1–24.8)	22.6	(20.6–24.7)	0.76	0.043	0.027	0.045
	EG	22.4	(19.9–24.9)	27.2	(25.1–29.3)				
EQUI	CG	2.3	(1.8–2.8)	2.3	(1.9–2.8)	−1.11	0.226	0.010	0.008
	EG	2.6	(2.2–3)	1.5	(1.3–1.8)				
pSF-12	CG	49.9	(48.6–51.1)	49.8	(48.4–50.9)	−0.01	0.654	0.754	0.862
	EG	49.6	(48.4–50.9)	49.8	(48.5–50.7)	0.02			
fSF-12	CG	53.1	(52.1–54.1)	53	(51.9–54.1)	−0.03	0.424	0.899	0.958
	EG	52.7	(51.5–53.9)	52.6	(51.6–53.6)				

SD: standard deviation; BMI: body mass index; %MG: body fat percentage; %MM: muscle mass percentage; SJ: squat jump; EQUI: capacity to control balance; fSF-12: physical dimension of the survey SF-12; mSF-12: mental dimension of the survey SF-12.

3.1. Results of Anthropometric Variables

The results obtained for %MG shown in Figure 2, indicate that it was not significantly affected after the intervention, with respect to the factor Group $F_{(1-108)} = 2.64$, $p = 0.107$, with respect to the factor Momentum $F_{(1-108)} = 0.12$, $p = 0.727$ and with respect to the interaction (Group × Momentum) $F_{(1-108)} = 0.05$, $p = 0.818$.

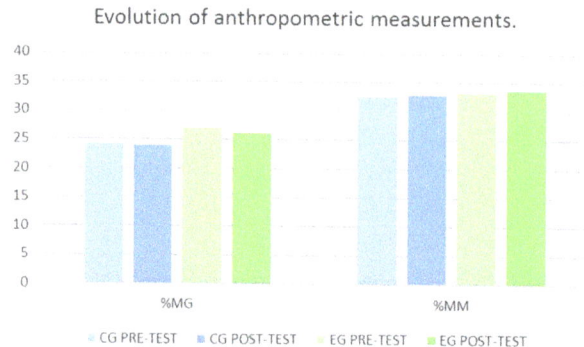

Figure 2. Evolution of the anthropometric measurements between groups and pre-post-test. %MG: body fat percentage; %MM: muscle mass percentage.

The results of the %MM shown in Figure 2 were also not significantly affected after the intervention, with respect to the factor Group $F_{(1-108)} = 0.61$, $p = 0.438$, with respect to the factor Momentum $F_{(1-108)} = 0.08$, $p = 0.777$ and with respect to the interaction (Group × Momentum) $F_{(1-108)} = 0.01$, $p = 0.933$.

3.2. Results of the Strength of the Lower Body Musculature (SJ)

In SJ, significant differences were found with respect to the factor Group $F_{(1-108)} = 4.21$, $p = 0.043$, with respect to the factor Momentum $F_{(1-108)} = 5.04$, $p = 0.027$ and with respect to the interaction (Group × Momentum) $F_{(1-108)} = 4.11$, $p = 0.045$. With a medium effect size and percentage improvement of 21.28% in jump height (Table 3). SJ's results can be observed more graphically in Figure 3.

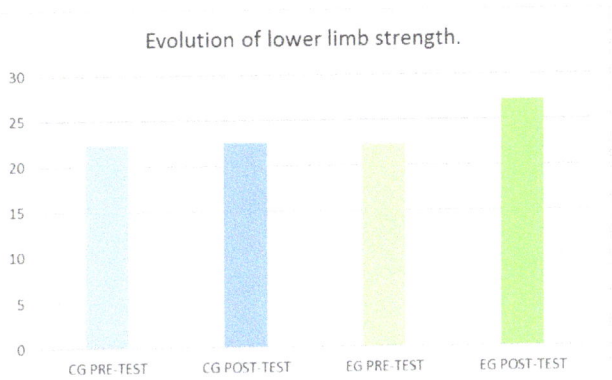

Figure 3. Evolution of lower limb strength between groups and pre-post-test.

3.3. Results of the Capacity to Control Balance (EQUI)

In EQUI, as detailed in Table 3, significant differences were found for the factor Group $F_{(1-108)} = 1.48$, $p = 0.222$, for the factor Momentum $F_{(1-108)} = 6.86$, $p = 0.010$ and for the interaction (Group × Momentum) $F_{(1-108)} = 7.43$, $p = 0.008$, with a large effect size and a percentage of improvement of 59%. These results can be observed more graphically in Figure 4.

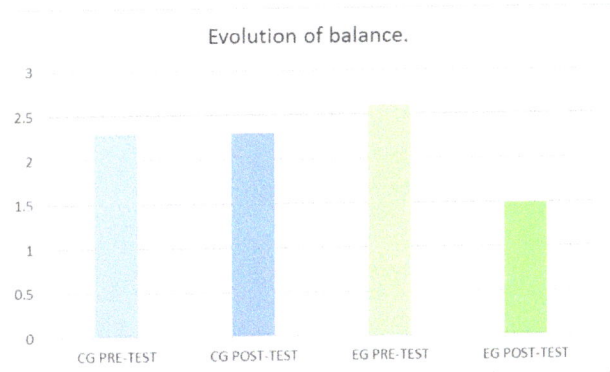

Figure 4. Evolution of the capacity to control balance between groups and pre-post-test.

3.4. Results of the Quality of Life (QoL)

The results obtained for pSF-12, shown in Figure 5, indicate that it was not significantly affected after the intervention, with respect to the factor Group $F_{(1-108)} = 0.59$, $p = 0.654$, with respect to the factor Momentum $F_{(1-108)} = 0.59$, $p = 0.654$ and with respect to the interaction (Group × Momentum) $F_{(1-108)} = 0.03$, $p = 0.862$ (Table 3).

The results obtained for fSF-12, shown in Figure 5, indicate that it was not significantly affected after the intervention, with respect to the factor Group $F_{(1-108)} = 0.64$, $p = 0.424$, with respect to the factor Momentum $F_{(1-108)} = 0.02$, $p = 0.899$ and with respect to the interaction (Group × Momentum) $F_{(1-108)} = 0.00$, $p = 0.958$ (Table 3).

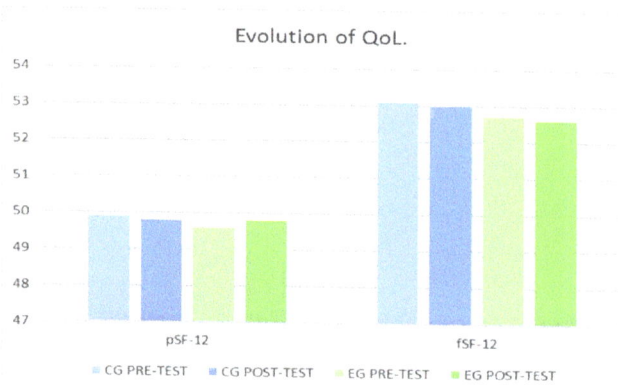

Figure 5. Evolution of the two dimensions of QoL between groups and pre-post-test.

4. Discussion

The aim of this study was to test if the proposed eccentric training protocol improves body composition, lower body strength, balance and quality of life in a healthy adult population. The results suggest a positive effect on the parameters analysed, highlighting the differences obtained in the jumping and balance tests obtained in the EG.

For the other variables, %MG, %MM and SF-12 (fSF-12 and pSF-12), no significant differences were obtained for the sample analysed.

In reference to anthropometric variables such as %GM and %MM, no significant improvements were achieved in accordance with the findings shown in other studies [15,22] which stated that improvements in weight and BMI were achieved with moderate intensity training, although in their case with a study of a much longer duration and conducted with subjects suffering from obesity with an average BMI of 38 points, which by WHO classification is considered class II obesity, and a stair descent protocol with obese women with a BMI of 26.2 and a %MG of 36.4%, respectively; our subjects had an average BMI of 24.9, being at the upper limit of what this organisation considers normal values and a similar %MG with an average score of 25.5%.

Motalebi et al. [11] and Gordon et al. [27] report in their work that eccentric strength training increases strength levels, in this case of the lower body musculature. As in our case, using the SJ, we measured jump height, which is an indirect measure of the strength of the lower body musculature. In the study of Gordon et al. [27], they proposed an eccentric strength training protocol compared to a traditional leg press of two sessions per week for four weeks, and they said that these levels improved. In their case, they observed improvements both at two and four weeks, that is, with four and eight sessions; in our case, the results were evaluated after twelve training sessions, obtaining an improvement of 21.28%.

Regarding the results obtained on balance, they support the hypothesis that an eccentric training programme using gliding discs would improve balance, as they showed a significant improvement after the intervention. We agree with the results obtained in other studies [11,28], which state that strength work improves the capacity to control balance, as well as being relatively simple and safe. On the other hand, in the training proposed in their research, strength work was achieved using whole-body vibration platforms, Bosus and elastic bands, respectively, instead of the gliding discs used in our protocol, as well as lasting for a shorter time (six weeks) and using a sample of female athletes with chronic ankle instability in the case of Chang et al. [28] and lasting longer and using a smaller sample size in the EG in the case of Motalebi et al. [11].

These findings are also consistent with those shown in the work of Olson et al. [1], who found significant improvements in the capacity to control balance in older people with a home training programme.

Regarding the results of the quality of life obtained by the SF-12 survey, we started from values similar to the average of the Spanish population for this age group, both in the physical and psychosocial dimensions [29]. These values were not significantly improved after the application of the training protocol.

These results are consistent with the findings of an extensive systematic literature review and meta-analysis, which analysed 37 articles and concluded that there is a high correlation between strength and balance [12]. This is similar to our work, since both the parameters of lower body strength measured by means of the SJ jump and the ability to control balance were significantly improved after the intervention (21.28 and 59%, respectively), so we can affirm that the eccentric training protocol using gliding discs proposed in this study serves to increase the strength of the musculature of the lower body and to improve the ability to control balance in healthy middle-aged subjects.

A limitation of our study is the diversity in the age of the participants, as well as not stratifying the results by age and gender due to the small number of participants. Another limitation is the restrained number of participants. In terms of future research, it would be interesting to use a much larger sample or to conduct research by age range and gender. It would also be interesting to do a long-term follow-up to see if the risk of falls was reduced. However, as far as we know, this is the first study in which gliding discs have been used for this purpose, and it is important to integrate new technologies in training for fall prevention.

5. Conclusions

The implementation of this eccentric training programme using gliding discs, of 12 sessions of 45′ duration, produced an increase in lower body strength and improved the ability to control balance, which may reduce the probability of falls in a healthy adult population. On the other hand, no improvements in body composition or quality of life were obtained. It should be noted that this type of training can be performed both in gyms and at home without the use of a large amount of equipment, with the consequent socioeconomic benefit in terms of time and money.

Author Contributions: Conceptualization, J.L.-B. and P.H.-L.; methodology, J.L.-B., P.H.-L., J.L.G.-S. and V.R.-P.; software, J.L.G.-S. and V.R.-P.; formal analysis, J.L.-B., P.H.-L., J.L.G.-S. and V.R.-P.; investigation, J.L.-B. and P.H.-L.; writing—original draft preparation, J.L.-B. and P.H.-L.; writing—review and editing, J.L.-B., P.H.-L., J.L.G.-S. and V.R.-P. All authors have read and agreed to the published version of the manuscript.

Funding: This research received no external funding.

Institutional Review Board Statement: The study was conducted according to the guidelines of the Declaration of Helsinki and approved by the Ethics Committee of Facultad de Ciencias de la Educación y de Deportes de la Universidade de Vigo protocol code 04-0721.

Informed Consent Statement: Informed consent was obtained from all subjects involved in the study.

Data Availability Statement: The datasets generated during and analysed during the current study are available from the aim author or the corresponding author on reasonable request.

Acknowledgments: We thank the participants for their contribution.

Conflicts of Interest: The authors declare no conflict of interest.

References

1. Olson, S.L.; Chen, S.-S.; Wang, C.-Y. Effect of a Home Exercise Program on Dynamic Balance in Elderly with a History of Falls. *J. Aging Phys. Act.* **2011**, *19*, 291–305. [CrossRef]
2. Graafmans, W.; Ooms, M.; Hofstee, H.; Bezemer, P.; Bouter, L.M.; Lips, P. Falls in the Elderly: A Prospective Study of Risk Factors and Risk Profiles. *Am. J. Epidemiol.* **1996**, *143*, 1129–1136. [CrossRef]
3. Alamgir, H.; Muazzam, S.; Nasrullah, M. Unintentional Falls Mortality among Elderly in the United States: Time for Action. *Injury* **2012**, *43*, 2065–2071. [CrossRef] [PubMed]

4. Chen, M.; Tang, Q.; Xu, S.; Leng, P.; Pan, Z. Design and Evaluation of an Augmented Reality-Based Exergame System to Reduce Fall Risk in the Elderly. *Int. J. Environ. Res. Public Health* **2020**, *17*, 7208. [CrossRef] [PubMed]
5. Cho, K.H.; Bok, S.K.; Kim, Y.-J.; Hwang, S.L. Effect of Lower Limb Strength on Falls and Balance of the Elderly. *Ann. Rehabil. Med.* **2012**, *36*, 386. [CrossRef] [PubMed]
6. Díaz, L.B.; Casuso-Holgado, M.J.; Labajos-Manzanares, M.T.; Barón-López, F.J.; Pinero-Pinto, E.; Romero-Galisteo, R.P.; Moreno-Morales, N. Analysis of Fall Risk Factors in an Aging Population Living in Long-Term Care Institutions in Spain: A Retrospective Cohort Study. *Int. J. Environ. Res. Public Health* **2020**, *17*, 7234. [CrossRef] [PubMed]
7. Campbell, A.J.; Borrie, M.J.; Spears, G.F. Risk Factors for Falls in a Community-Based Prospective Study of People 70 Years and Older. *J. Gerontol.* **1989**, *44*, M112–M117. [CrossRef] [PubMed]
8. Tinetti, M.E.; Speechley, M.; Ginter, S.F. Risk Factors for Falls among Elderly Persons Living in the Community. *N. Engl. J. Med.* **1988**, *319*, 1701–1707. [CrossRef]
9. Mora, M.; Villalobos, D.; Araya, G.; Ozols, A. Perspectiva Subjetiva de La Calidad de Vida Del Adulto Mayor, Diferencias Ligadas al Género Ya La Práctica de La Actividad Físico Recreativa. *MHSALUD Rev. En Cienc. Del Mov. Hum. Y Salud* **2004**, *1*, 1–11. [CrossRef]
10. Loecker, C.; Schmaderer, M.; Zimmerman, L. Frailty in Young and Middle-Aged Adults: An Integrative Review. *J. Frailty Aging* **2021**, *10*, 327–333. [CrossRef]
11. Motalebi, S.A.; Cheong, L.S.; Iranagh, J.A.; Mohammadi, F. Effect of Low-Cost Resistance Training on Lower-Limb Strength and Balance in Institutionalized Seniors. *Exp. Aging Res.* **2018**, *44*, 48–61. [CrossRef] [PubMed]
12. Muehlbauer, T.; Gollhofer, A.; Granacher, U. Associations between Measures of Balance and Lower-Extremity Muscle Strength/Power in Healthy Individuals across the Lifespan: A Systematic Review and Meta-Analysis. *Sports Med.* **2015**, *45*, 1671–1692. [CrossRef] [PubMed]
13. Benford, J.; Hughes, J.; Waldron, M.; Theis, N. Concentric versus Eccentric Training: Effect on Muscle Strength, Regional Morphology, and Architecture. *Transl. Sports Med.* **2021**, *4*, 46–55. [CrossRef]
14. Büker, N.; Şavkin, R.; Süzer, A.; Akkaya, N. Effect of Eccentric and Concentric Squat Exercise on Quadriceps Thickness and Lower Extremity Performance in Healthy Young Males. *Acta Gymnica* **2021**, *51*. [CrossRef]
15. Chen, T.C.; Hsieh, C.-C.; Tseng, K.-W.; Ho, C.-C.; Nosaka, K. Effects of Descending Stair Walking on Health and Fitness of Elderly Obese Women. *Med. Sci. Sports Exerc.* **2017**, *49*, 1614–1622. [CrossRef]
16. Chen, T.C.-C.; Tseng, W.-C.; Huang, G.-L.; Chen, H.-L.; Tseng, K.-W.; Nosaka, K. Superior Effects of Eccentric to Concentric Knee Extensor Resistance Training on Physical Fitness, Insulin Sensitivity and Lipid Profiles of Elderly Men. *Front. Physiol.* **2017**, *8*, 209. [CrossRef]
17. Gremeaux, V.; Duclay, J.; Deley, G.; Philipp, J.; Laroche, D.; Pousson, M.; Casillas, J. Does Eccentric Endurance Training Improve Walking Capacity in Patients with Coronary Artery Disease? A Randomized Controlled Pilot Study. *Clin. Rehabil.* **2010**, *24*, 590–599. [CrossRef]
18. Wilke, J.; Alfredson, H. Eccentric Training: The Key for a Stronger, More Resilient Athlete? In *Oncology Massage*; Handspring Publishing Limited: Pencaitland, UK, 2021.
19. Lukman, G. *Osnovne Pilates Vaje z Drsniki*; Handspring Publishing Limited: Pencaitland, UK, 2018.
20. Prieto, J.A.; Valle, M.D.; Nistal, P.; Méndez, D.; Barcala-Furelos, R.; Abelairas-Gómez, C. Relevancia de Un Programa de Equilibrio En La Calidad de Vida Relacionada Con La Salud de Mujeres Adultas Mayores Obesas. *Nutr. Hosp.* **2015**, *32*, 2800–2807. [CrossRef] [PubMed]
21. Sylejmani, B.; Myrtaj, N.; Maliqi, A.; Gontarev, S.; Georgiev, G.; Kalac, R. Physical Fitness in Children and Adolescents in Rural and Urban Areas. *J. Hum. Sport Exerc.* **2019**, *14*, 866–875. [CrossRef]
22. Gatterer, H.; Haacke, S.; Burtscher, M.; Faulhaber, M.; Melmer, A.; Ebenbichler, C.; Strohl, K.P.; Högel, J.; Netzer, N.C. Normobaric Intermittent Hypoxia over 8 Months Does Not Reduce Body Weight and Metabolic Risk Factors-a Randomized, Single Blind, Placebo-Controlled Study in Normobaric Hypoxia and Normobaric Sham Hypoxia. *Obes. Facts* **2015**, *8*, 200–209. [CrossRef] [PubMed]
23. Bosco, C.; Viitasalo, J.; Komi, P.; Luhtanen, P. Combined Effect of Elastic Energy and Myoelectrical Potentiation during Stretch-shortening Cycle Exercise. *Acta Physiol. Scand.* **1982**, *114*, 557–565. [CrossRef] [PubMed]
24. Jenkinson, C.; Layte, R. Development and Testing of the UK SF-12. *J. Health Serv. Res. Policy* **1997**, *2*, 14–18. [CrossRef] [PubMed]
25. Leirós-Rodríguez, R.; Romo-Pérez, V.; García-Soidán, J.L. Validity and Reliability of a Tool for Accelerometric Assessment of Static Balance in Women. *Eur. J. Physiother.* **2017**, *19*, 243–248. [CrossRef]
26. Cohen, J. *Statistical Power Analysis for the Behavioural Sciences*, 2nd ed.; Lawrence Earlbaum: Hillsdale, NJ, USA, 1988.
27. Gordon, J.P.; Thompson, B.J.; Crane, J.S.; Bressel, E.; Wagner, D.R. Effects of Isokinetic Eccentric versus Traditional Lower Body Resistance Training on Muscle Function: Examining a Multiple-Joint Short-Term Training Model. *Appl. Physiol. Nutr. Metab.* **2019**, *44*, 118–126. [CrossRef] [PubMed]
28. Chang, W.; Chen, S.; Tsou, Y. Effects of Whole-Body Vibration and Balance Training on Female Athletes with Chronic Ankle Instability. *J. Clin. Med.* **2021**, *10*, 2380. [CrossRef]
29. Vilagut, G.; Valderas, J.M.; Ferrer, M.; Garin, O.; López-García, E.; Alonso, J. Interpretación de Los Cuestionarios de Salud SF-36 y SF-12 En España: Componentes Físico y Mental. *Med. Clínica* **2008**, *130*, 726–735. [CrossRef]

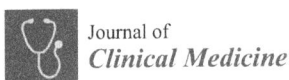

Article

Trunk Alignment in Physically Active Young Males with Low Back Pain

Magdalena Plandowska [1,*], Agnieszka Kędra [1], Przemysław Kędra [1] and Dariusz Czaprowski [2,3]

1 Faculty of Physical Education and Health, Jozef Pilsudski University of Physical Education in Warsaw, 21-500 Biala Podlaska, Poland; agnieszka.kedra@awf.edu.pl (A.K.); przemyslaw.kedra@awf.edu.pl (P.K.)
2 Department of Health Sciences, University College in Olsztyn, 10-283 Olsztyn, Poland; dariusz.czaprowski@interia.pl
3 Center of Body Posture, Bydgoska 33, 10-243 Olsztyn, Poland
* Correspondence: magdalena.plandowska@awf.edu.pl

Abstract: Background: Systematic physical activity has become an essential part of the guidelines for the prevention and treatment of low back pain (LBP). The aim of this study was to assess differences in trunk alignment parameters with regard to the level of physical activity in groups of individuals with and without LBP. Methods: 43 participants with LBP and 37 healthy persons were recruited. Participants were divided into two subgroups: (1) students with a moderate level of physical activity (MPA); (2) students with a high level of physical activity (HPA). An original questionnaire was used to assess the prevalence of LBP. The spinal posture was measured using the Formetric 4D rasterstereographic system. Results: There were no significant differences between groups for any of the parameters assessed: trunk imbalance, trunk inclination, trunk torsion, pelvic tilt, pelvic inclination, pelvic torsion, kyphotic angle and lordotic angle. Conclusions: There are no differences in trunk alignment parameters in the sagittal, frontal and transversal planes between physically active males with and without LBP. Therefore, it can be assumed that physical activity may reduce the risk of the deterioration of trunk alignment in males with LBP younger than 25 years.

Keywords: low back pain; physical activity; trunk alignment; rasterstereographic system; young males

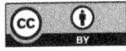

1. Introduction

The ability to maintain an upright posture is fundamental to normal activities of daily living. The normal curvatures of the spine in the sagittal plane (cervical lordosis, thoracic kyphosis and lumbar lordosis) are balanced with each other in normal upright posture [1], while abnormal curvatures of the spine (sagittal imbalance) cause increased muscular effort and energy expenditure, causing pain, fatigue, and disability [2]. It has been reported in many disorders, especially low back pain (LBP). The studies suggest that people with LBP often have disturbances in the motor control of deep trunk muscles [3–7].

There is a lack of literature that analyses and compares the difference in spinal posture in the LBP population with healthy counterparts considering the level of physical activity. The recent Lancet low back pain series recommended exercises [8]. Physical activity is effective in the prevention and treatment of LBP [9]. Physical activity is significant to improving functional activity, influences bone modeling, helps to strengthen the muscles and prevents a reduction in postural stability [10,11]. This is very important for all people, especially individuals with LBP. On the other hand, a high level of physical activity might increase the risk of LBP prevalence. Heneweer et al. [12] described the association between physical activity and LBP as a U-shaped curve—inactivity and over-activity are harmful to the health of the spine.

The influence of a low level of physical activity on body posture is known, while the potential impact of a high level of physical activity in people with LBP has received less attention to date. Therefore, the aim of this study was to assess differences in trunk alignment parameters with regard to the level of physical activity in groups of individuals with and without LBP.

2. Materials and Methods

2.1. Participants

Eighty university students of a Bachelor course in Physical Education participated in this cross-sectional study, including 43 individuals with a history of LBP and 37 healthy persons without LBP. Based on the sample size ($n = 80$), a power analysis was set at 0.75. The inclusion criteria for the LBP group were as follows: (a) male; (b) age between 20 and 23 years; (c) experiencing LBP for the last year; (d) reporting an average low back pain intensity of 4 or greater as measured by the Visual Analogue Scale (VAS; 4–10). Participants were excluded from the study if they: (a) were experiencing very rare pain; (b) had any neurological, cardiovascular, rheumatic or vestibular disorders; (c) had conditions that could interfere with the measure of the Formetric Diers such as back tattoos or prostheses; (d) were experiencing low back pain at the time of the examination. Healthy individuals had no history of LBP within the last year. The demographic characteristics of the participants are presented in Table 1.

Table 1. Characteristics of study population ($n = 80$).

Characteristics	LBP $n = 43$ Mean (SD)	Healthy $n = 37$ Mean (SD)
Age (years)	21.2 (0.8)	21.4 (0.9)
Weight (kg)	81.2 (9.1)	79.8 (9.6)
Height (cm)	183.2 (7.7)	181.1 (5.4)
BMI (kg/m^2)	24.6 (3.5)	24.0 (2.6)

Participants were divided into two subgroups, i.e., (1) students with a moderate level of physical activity (MPA) and (2) students with a high level of physical activity (HPA). The inclusion criteria in the MPA group were as follows: (a) attending physical education classes included in the curriculum; (b) taking up leisure-time physical activity no more than once per week and no longer than 60 min. The inclusion criteria in the HPA group were as follows: (a) attending physical education classes included in the curriculum; (b) training a minimum of 90 min per day—5 times per week; (c) training experience—a minimum of 3 years. The HPA group included students who trained handball or volleyball.

All the participants gave their written informed consent. The study was conducted in accordance with the Declaration of Helsinki, and the research was accepted by the Senate Scientific Research Ethics Commission.

2.2. Questionnaire

A questionnaire was used to assess the prevalence of LBP [13]. The first page of the questionnaire included an explanation of the study purpose, instructions and questions on age, body mass and body height.

The next page of the questionnaire included questions related to:

(a) training (sport)—sports discipline, number of training days per week, number of training hours per day;

(b) experiencing LBP within the last year (12 months). Individuals who responded positively ("yes") to question "Have you experienced low back pain for the last year (12 months)?" answered the question in the second part. Individuals who responded negatively ("no") to this question were asked not to answer the remaining questions.

The second part of the questionnaire included questions on the frequency and intensity of LBP, the types of situation in which LBP occurred or increased.

The Visual Analogue Scale (VAS) was used to assess average pain intensity. Participants were asked to rate their maximal pain intensity from the last year on a 10 cm line.

The centimetres marked by the participants were measured and classified according to the following key: 0—no pain, 1–3—mild pain, 4–6—moderate pain and 7–10—severe pain [14].

In this study, we defined LBP as the pain localized below the costal margin and the inferior gluteal folds without sciatica, with an average pain intensity of 4 or greater (moderate or severe pain), as measured by the Visual Analogue Scale (VAS).

Information about musculoskeletal disorders was also obtained from systematic medical examinations conducted by a sports doctor.

2.3. Spine Shape Evaluation

The spinal posture was measured using the Formetric 4D rasterstereographic system (DIERS, International GmbH, Schlangenbad, Germany). It is a valid and reliable method used for three-dimensional analysis of the spine [15,16].

Prior to the study, each participant was given detailed information on the testing procedures and research methodology.

It was assumed that the participants experiencing low back pain at the time of the examination would adopt a non-habitual body posture which may be accompanied by an unnatural positioning of body parts. Therefore, the participants were asked whether they felt pain at the time of taking the measurement. None of the participants reported pain when they were tested.

Participants removed all clothing except for a pair of shorts. The subject's back was exposed from the beginning of the intergluteal fissure to the occiput. Subjects were placed barefoot in a comfortable standing position, with their knees extended and their arms resting naturally alongside their hips. To standardize the subjects' positioning, a horizontal line was drawn on the floor to provide a reference for their heels. Participants were positioned 2 m from the Formetric 4D projection and camera unit. The unit projected stripes of light on the surface of the participant's back. In accordance with the recommendations of Guidetti et al. [17], no reflective markers were positioned on participants.

Each scan was completed in the DIERS data collection and processing software. During each scan, 12 images were recorded over the 6 s (2 Hz). Each scan was processed as per the manufacturer's instructions. On each of the collected images, the software automatically indicated the location of the left (DL) and right (DR) sacral dimples associated with the posterior superior iliac spine and the location of the vertebral prominens (VP). The middle point between the dimples (DM) was determined from the location of DL and DR.

The test was performed by the same examiner. Participants were examined individually. They were supplied with the same instructions before the test.

The following trunk alignment parameters were analysed:

Trunk and pelvic parameters: trunk imbalance VP-DM [mm], trunk inclination VP-DM [mm], trunk torsion [°], pelvic tilt DL-DR [mm], pelvic inclination DL-DR [°] (dimples), pelvic torsion DL-DR [°];

Spinal curve angles: kyphotic angle VP-ITL [°], lordotic angle ITL-DM [°] (Table 2, Figure 1).

All the tests were performed during morning hours in the laboratory room at the Regional Centre for Research and Development.

2.4. Statistical Analysis

The parameters were described using basic descriptive statistics measurements, i.e., percentage for qualitative variables, mean and standard deviation for quantitative variables. Descriptive statistics were calculated separately for both LBP and healthy groups. The chi-square test was used for categorical variables (the prevalence and frequency of LBP with regard to the level of physical activity). The Shapiro–Wilk test was used to check the compliance of the results with normal distribution. The data were analysed using a two-factor ANOVA. The between-subject factors were group (LBP and healthy) and the level of physical activity (MPA and HPA). Statistical significance was set at $p < 0.05$. The collected material was organised and analysed using Statistica 13.3 calculation software.

Table 2. Trunk alignment parameters and their description.

Trunk Alignment Parameters	Description
Trunk imbalance VP-DM [mm]	The lateral deviation of VP from DM
Trunk inclination VP-DM [mm]	A difference in height between VP and DM, based on a vertical plane
Trunk torsion [°]	The torsion of the surface normals of DM and VP
Pelvic tilt DL-DR [mm]	The difference in height of the DL and DR
Pelvic inclination DL-DR [°] (dimples)	The mean torsion of the DL and DR surface normals
Pelvic torsion DL-DR [°]	The torsion of the surface normals on DL and DR
Kyphotic angle VP-ITL [°]	The angle between VP and the thoracic-lumbar inflection point ITL
Lordotic angle ITL-DM [°]	The angle between the surface tangents of the thoracic-lumbar inflection point ITL and the lower lumbar-sacral inflection point ILS

VP—vertebra prominens; DM—midpoint between the left and right sacral dimples; DL—left sacral dimple; DR—right sacral dimple; ITL—thoracic-lumbar inflection point.

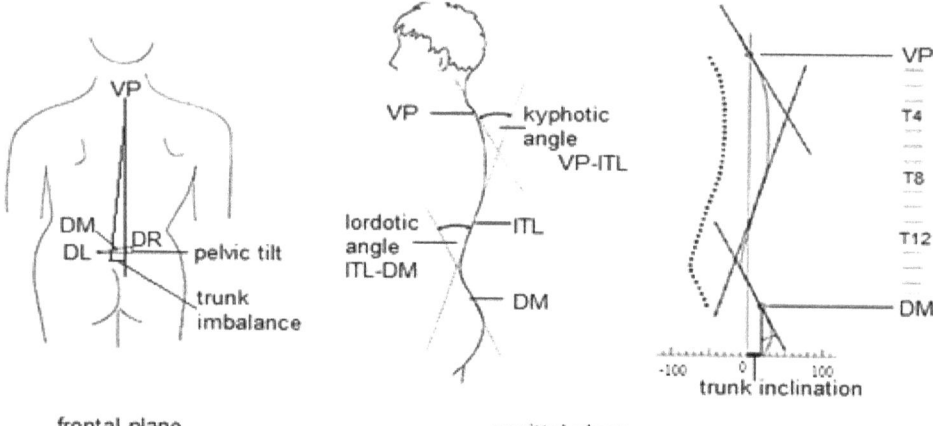

Figure 1. Trunk alignment parameters, measured with Diers Formetric. Abbreviations: VP—vertebra prominens; DM—midpoint between the left and right sacral dimples; DL—left sacral dimple; DR—right sacral dimple; ITL—thoracic-lumbar inflection point.

3. Results

LBP was common among participants with a HPA than among their peers with a MPA (59.1% vs. 47.2%, respectively). The difference was not significant ($p = 0.29$) (Table 3).

Table 3. The prevalence of LBP.

				MPA $n = 36$	HPA $n = 44$	p Value
LBP	$n = 43$	n (%)		17 (47.2)	26 (59.1)	0.29
Healthy	$n = 37$	n (%)		19 (52.8)	18 (40.9)	

LBP—low back pain; MPA—moderate level of physical activity; HPA—high level of physical activity. Statistical significance was set at $p < 0.05$.

The largest group was those who experienced LBP a few times a year (3–6/year) (60.5%). Participants with HPA declared frequent or constant pain more often than their peers with MPA (42.3% vs. 35.3%, respectively). The difference was not statistically significant ($p = 0.64$). The analysis of LBP intensity showed that 62.8% of the participants declared moderate pain. Nearly 40% of the participants limited their physical activity when the pain was very intensive. In 46.5% of participants, LBP intensified during physical activity, more often among the participants with HPA than among students with MPA (57.7% vs. 29.4%, respectively) (Table 4).

Table 4. The frequency and intensity of LBP, the influence of LBP on the undertaken PA.

		All $n = 43$	MPA $n = 17$	HPA $n = 26$	p Value
LBP frequency					
LBP a few times a year (3–6/year)	n (%)	26 (60.5)	11 (64.7)	15 (57.7)	0.64
Frequent or constant LBP (more than 1–2 months)	n (%)	17 (39.5)	6 (35.3)	11 (42.3)	
LBP intensity					
Moderate	n (%)	27 (62.8)	10 (58.8)	17 (65.4)	0.66
Severe	n (%)	16 (37.2)	7 (41.2)	9 (34.6)	
The influence of LBP on the undertaken PA					
No influence	n (%)	25 (58.1)	10 (58.8)	15 (57.7)	0.94
I limit the amount of PA when the pain is very intensive.	n (%)	16 (37.2)	7 (41.2)	11 (42.3)	
A higher intensity of LBP during physical exercises					
No	n (%)	23 (53.5)	12 (70.6)	11 (42.3)	0.06
Yes	n (%)	20 (46.5)	5 (29.4)	15 (57.7)	

LBP—low back pain; PA—physical activity; MPA—moderate level of physical activity; HPA—high level of physical activity. Statistical significance was set at $p < 0.05$.

The analysis of trunk alignment revealed no differences in trunk alignment parameters in the sagittal, frontal and transversal planes between active participants with and without LBP regardless of the level of physical activity (Tables 5 and 6).

Table 5. Means and standard deviations for trunk alignment parameters.

		MPA M (SD)	HPA M (SD)	All M (SD)
Trunk and pelvic parameters				
Trunk inclination VP-DM [mm]	LBP	18.4 (15.4)	24.0 (13.8)	21.8 (14.5)
	Healthy	12.9 (10.2)	18.9 (16.7)	15.8 (13.9)
Trunk imbalance VP-DM [mm]	LBP	10.1 (5.8)	9.4 (8.1)	9.7 (7.2)
	Healthy	8.3 (7.1)	7.1 (5.0)	7.7 (6.1)
Trunk torsion [°]	LBP	3.4 (2.6)	4.2 (3.0)	3.9 (2.9)
	Healthy	3.5 (2.2)	3.5 (2.9)	3.5 (2.5)
Pelvic tilt DL-DR [mm]	LBP	4.4 (4.1)	4.7 (3.9)	4.6 (3.9)
	Healthy	4.3 (3.0)	4.0 (1.8)	4.1 (2.4)
Pelvic inclination (dimples) [°]	LBP	16.7 (5.1)	18.4 (4.1)	17.8 (4.6)
	Healthy	17.2 (4.9)	18.4 (4.0)	17.8 (4.4)
Pelvic torsion DL-DR [°]	LBP	2.9 (2.0)	2.3 (1.7)	2.6 (1.8)
	Healthy	2.6 (1.6)	2.5 (1.4)	2.5 (1.5)

Table 5. Cont.

		MPA	HPA	All
		M (SD)	M (SD)	M (SD)
Spinal curve angles				
Kyphotic angle VP-ITL [°]	LBP	43.5 (8.7)	45.3 (7.2)	44.6 (7.8)
	Healthy	44.4 (6.8)	45.2 (6.5)	44.8 (6.6)
Lordotic angle ITL-DM [°]	LBP	31.3 (6.7)	30.6 (6.2)	30.9 (6.3)
	Healthy	31.3 (7.1)	31.0 (6.9)	31.1 (6.9)

LBP—low back pain; M—mean; SD—standard deviation; PA—physical activity; MPA—moderate level of physical activity; HPA—high level of physical activity; VP—vertebra prominens; DM—midpoint between the left and right sacral dimples; DL—left sacral dimple; DR—right sacral dimple; ITL—thoracic-lumbar inflection point.

Table 6. Summary of analysis of variance for trunk alignment parameters.

	Group	Level of PA	Group × Level of PA
Trunk and pelvic parameters			
Trunk inclination VP-DM [mm]	$F = 2.769$ $p = 0.100$	$F = 3.275$ $p = 0.074$	$F = 0.006$ $p = 0.939$
Trunk imbalance VP-DM [mm]	$F = 1.897$ $p = 0.172$	$F = 0.351$ $p = 0.555$	$F = 0.032$ $p = 0.857$
Trunk torsion [°]	$F = 0.270$ $p = 0.604$	$F = 0.481$ $p = 0.489$	$F = 0.518$ $p = 0.473$
Pelvic tilt DL-DR [mm]	$F = 0.310$ $p = 0.579$	$F = 0.000$ $p = 0.994$	$F = 0.122$ $p = 0.727$
Pelvic inclination (dimples) [°]	$F = 0.052$ $p = 0.819$	$F = 1.936$ $p = 0.168$	$F = 0.073$ $p = 0.787$
Pelvic torsion DL-DR [°]	$F = 0.071$ $p = 0.789$	$F = 0.745$ $p = 0.390$	$F = 0.438$ $p = 0.509$
Spinal curve angles			
Kyphotic angle VP-ITL [°]	$F = 0.057$ $p = 0.811$	$F = 0.638$ $p = 0.427$	$F = 0.073$ $p = 0.787$
Lordotic angle ITL-DM [°]	$F = 0.010$ $p = 0.921$	$F = 0.111$ $p = 0.739$	$F = 0.020$ $p = 0.888$

PA—physical activity; VP—vertebra prominens; DM—midpoint between the left and right sacral dimples; DL—left sacral dimple; DR—right sacral dimple; ITL—thoracic-lumbar inflection point. Group: LBP vs. Healthy; Level of PA: MPA vs. HPA. Statistical significance was set at $p < 0.05$.

4. Discussion

The aim of this study was to assess differences in trunk alignment with regard to the level of physical activity in groups of individuals with and without LBP. Our results revealed that no differences were found in trunk alignment parameters in active males with LBP compared with healthy individuals. Similar findings were reported in other studies [18,19]. A systematic review by Laird et al. [18] showed that people with LBP display no difference in their lordosis angle and pelvic tilt angle in standing. A study conducted by Tatsumi et al. [20] indicates that participants with LBP have a large anteversion of the pelvic angle. Authors suggested that large lumbar lordosis is not associated with LBP. Other studies showed that participants with LBP are characterized by a loss of lumbar lordosis and an increase of pelvic tilt [21–24]. A systematic review and meta-analysis demonstrate a strong relationship between LBP and decreased lumbar lordotic curvature [24]. Moreover, Barrey et al. [22,23] showed that participants with chronic LBP and lumbar degenerative disease are characterized by sagittal imbalance. Our study did not observe a significant difference in pelvic asymmetry parameters between participants with and without LBP. Other studies showed that pelvic asymmetry is unlikely to be associated with the prevalence of LBP [25,26].

Studies based on the analysis of the relation between physical activity and LBP reported that a moderate level of physical activity is associated with lower prevalence of LBP [9,27]. Another study found that there is strong evidence that a heavy physical workload is a risk factor for back pain [28]. LBP is common in the athletic population [29]. Although it is well known that physical activity can reduce risk for musculoskeletal diseases by improving muscle strength, bone metabolism and functional health [10,11], there is a lack of literature that analyses and compares the difference in spinal posture in the LBP population considering the level of physical activity. Therefore, the aim of this study was to assess differences in trunk alignment parameters with regard to the level of physical activity in groups of individuals with and without LBP. The results of our study showed that there are no significant differences in trunk alignment parameters in the sagittal, frontal and transversal planes between active males with and without LBP, regardless of the level of physical activity. Despite the fact that a high level of physical activity might increase the risk of LBP prevalence, this study showed that physical activity may reduce the risk of the deterioration of trunk alignment in males with LBP younger than 25 years. Our findings are consistent with recommendations from LBP management. Prevention and treatment guidelines recommend staying active and continuing with normal activities. Exercise can be utilised as a central component of treatment. Recommended physical treatments include a graduated activity or exercise programme that targets the improvement of function and prevention of worsening disability [8]. Exercise is of great importance to improve functional ability and health-related quality of life in patients with LBP. Being active is associated with less pain, including LBP, and injury, as long as the rate of increase in activity is managed appropriately and other important factors are also taken into account (e.g., sleep, mood, relationships) [30].

4.1. Limitations

The present study is limited by its cross-sectional design; therefore, causality cannot be inferred. The characterization of pain was not our aim; therefore, the detailed characterization of pain has been omitted. Another limitation was a small number of study participants. The research was planned with all students in the 1st, 2nd and 3rd year of PE on a day of testing. The target group was smaller due to the fact that this was during the COVID-19 pandemic. Moreover, different sports were considered together. It is worth continuing the observation with a larger athlete sample size to verify the observed results, with a view to identifying differences between sports.

4.2. Study Strenghts

According to the authors' knowledge, it is the first study to compare differences in trunk alignment parameters taking into account different levels of physical activity (MPA and HPA). The spinal posture was measured using a valid and reliable method used for three-dimensional analysis of the spine (the Formetric 4D rasterstereographic system, DIERS) [15,16]. However, the study showed that reliability of trunk imbalance and pelvic torsion is lower than the overall excellent reliability of sagittal plane parameters [16]. Prevalence of LBP was measured using a reliable questionnaire, and the Kappa coefficient value for all the analysed variables was equal to or higher than 0.93 [13].

5. Conclusions

There are no differences in trunk alignment in the sagittal, frontal and transversal planes between physically active males with and without LBP, regardless of the level of physical activity. Therefore, it can be assumed that physical activity may reduce the risk of the deterioration of trunk alignment in males with LBP younger than 25 years.

Supplementary Materials: The following supporting information can be downloaded at: https://www.mdpi.com/article/10.3390/jcm11144206/s1, supplementary file: Dataset.

Author Contributions: Conceptualization, M.P. and A.K.; methodology, M.P. and A.K.; formal analysis, M.P. and A.K.; writing—original draft preparation, M.P., A.K. and P.K.; writing—review and editing, M.P., A.K., P.K. and D.C.; supervision, D.C. All authors have read and agreed to the published version of the manuscript.

Funding: This research received no external funding.

Institutional Review Board Statement: The study was conducted in accordance with the Declaration of Helsinki, and the research was accepted by the Senate Scientific Research Ethics Commission.

Informed Consent Statement: Informed consent was obtained from all subjects involved in the study.

Data Availability Statement: Data are contained within the article or Supplementary Materials.

Conflicts of Interest: The authors declare no conflict of interest.

References

1. Le Huec, J.C.; Thompson, W.; Mohsinaly, Y.; Barrey, C.; Faundez, A. Sagittal balance of the spine. *Eur. Spine J.* **2019**, *28*, 1889–1905. [CrossRef]
2. Hiyama, A.; Katoh, H.; Sakai, D.; Sato, M.; Tanaka, M.; Nukaga, T. Correlation analysis of sagittal alignment and skeletal muscle mass in patients with spinal degenerative disease. *Sci. Rep.* **2018**, *8*, 15492. [CrossRef] [PubMed]
3. Hodges, P.W. Changes in motor planning of feedforward postural responses of the trunk muscles in low back pain. *Exp. Brain Res.* **2001**, *14*, 261–266. [CrossRef] [PubMed]
4. Macdonald, D.A.; Moseley, G.L.; Hodges, P.W. People with recurrent low back pain respond differently to trunk loading despite remission from symptoms. *Spine* **2010**, *35*, 818–824. [CrossRef] [PubMed]
5. Cholewicki, J.; Greene, H.S.; Polzhofer, G.K.; Galloway, M.T.; Shah, R.A.; Radebold, A. Neuromuscular function in athletes following recovery from a recent acute low back injury. *J. Orthop. Sports Phys. Ther.* **2002**, *32*, 568–575. [CrossRef] [PubMed]
6. Brumagne, S.; Cordo, P.; Lysens, R.; Verschueren, S.; Swinnen, S. The role of paraspinal muscle spindles in lumbosacral position sense in individuals with and without low back pain. *Spine* **2000**, *25*, 989–994. [CrossRef]
7. Tong, M.; Mousavi, S.J.; Kiers, H.; Ferreira, P.; Refshauge, K.M.; van Dieen, J.H. Is there a relationship between lumbar proprioception and low back pain? A systematic review with meta-analysis. *Arch. Phys. Med. Rehabil.* **2017**, *98*, 120–136. [CrossRef]
8. Foster, N.E.; Anema, J.R.; Cherkin, D.; Chou, R.; Cohen, S.P.; Gross, D.P.; Ferreira, P.H.; Fritz, J.M.; Koes, B.W.; Peul, W.; et al. Lancet Low Back Pain Series Working Group. Prevention and treatment of low back pain: Evidence; challenges; and promising directions. *Lancet* **2018**, *9*, 2368–2383. [CrossRef]
9. Alzahrani, H.; Mackey, M.; Stamatakis, E.; Zadro, J.R.; Shirley, D. The association between physical activity and low back pain: A systematic review and meta-analysis of observational studies. *Sci. Rep.* **2019**, *9*, 8244. [CrossRef]
10. Długołęcka, B.; Jówko, E.; Czeczelewski, J.; Cieśliński, I.; Klusiewicz, A. Bone mineral status of young men with different levels of physical activity. *Pol. J. Sport Tour.* **2019**, *26*, 8–13. [CrossRef]
11. Alsufiany, M.B.; Lohman, E.B.; Daher, N.S.; Gang, G.R.; Shallan, A.I.; Jaber, H.M. Non-specific chronic low back pain and physical activity: A comparison of postural control and hip muscle isometric strength: A cross-sectional study. *Medicine* **2020**, *99*, e18544. [CrossRef] [PubMed]
12. Heneweer, H.; Vanhees, L.; Picavet, H.S. Physical activity and low back pain: A U-shaped relation? *Pain* **2009**, *1431*, 21–25. [CrossRef] [PubMed]
13. Kędra, A.; Kolwicz-Gańko, A.; Kędra, P.; Bochenek, A.; Czaprowski, D. Back pain in physically inactive students compared to physical education students with a high and average level of physical activity studying in Poland. *BMC Musculoskelet. Disord.* **2017**, *18*, 501. [CrossRef] [PubMed]
14. McCaffery, M.; Beebe, A. *Pain: Clinical Manual for Nursing Practice*; C.V. Mosby Company: St Louis, MO, USA, 1989.
15. Degenhardt, B.F.; Starks, Z.; Bhatia, S. Reliability of the DIERS Formetric 4D Spine Shape Parameters in Adults without Postural Deformities. *Biomed. Res. Int.* **2020**, *13*, 1796247. [CrossRef]
16. Schroeder, J.; Reer, R.; Braumann, K.M. Video raster stereography back shape reconstruction: A reliability study for sagittal, frontal, and transversal plane parameters. *Eur. Spine J.* **2015**, *24*, 262–269. [CrossRef]
17. Guidetti, L.; Bonavolontà, V.; Tito, A.; Reis, V.M.; Gallotta, M.C.; Baldari, C. Intra- and interday reliability of spine rasterstereography. *Biomed. Res. Int.* **2013**, *2013*, 745480. [CrossRef]
18. Laird, R.A.; Gilbert, J.; Kent, P.; Keating, J.L. Comparing lumbo-pelvic kinematics in people with and without back pain: A systematic review and meta-analysis. *BMC Musculoskelet. Disord.* **2014**, *15*, 229. [CrossRef]
19. Laird, R.A.; Kent, P.; Keating, J.L. How consistent are lordosis; Range of movement and lumbo-pelvic rhythm in people with and without back pain? *BMC Musculoskelet. Disord.* **2016**, *17*, 403. [CrossRef]

20. Tatsumi, M.; Mkoba, E.M.; Suzuki, Y.; Kajiwara, Y.; Zeidan, H.; Harada, K.; Bitoh, T.; Nishida, Y.; Nakai, K.; Shimoura, K.; et al. Risk factors of low back pain and the relationship with sagittal vertebral alignment in Tanzania. *BMC Musculoskelet. Disord.* **2019**, *20*, 584. [CrossRef]
21. Korovessis, P.G.; Dimas, A.; Iliopoulos, P.; Lambiris, E. Correlative analysis of lateral vertebral radiographic variables and medical outcomes study short-form health survey: A comparative study in asymptomatic volunteers versus patients with low back pain. *J. Spinal Disord. Tech.* **2002**, *15*, 384–390. [CrossRef]
22. Barrey, C.; Jund, J.; Noseda, O.; Roussouly, P. Sagittal balance of the pelvis-spine complex and lumbar degenerative diseases. A comparative study about 85 cases. *Eur. Spine J.* **2007**, *16*, 1459–1467. [CrossRef] [PubMed]
23. Barrey, C.; Jund, J.; Perrin, G.; Roussouly, P. Spinopelvic alignment of patients with degenerative spondylolisthesis. *Neurosurgery* **2007**, *6*, 981–986; discussion 986. [CrossRef]
24. Chun, S.W.; Lim, C.Y.; Kim, K.; Hwang, J.; Chung, S.G. The relationships between low back pain and lumbar lordosis: A systematic review and meta-analysis. *Spine J.* **2017**, *17*, 1180–1191. [CrossRef]
25. Levangie, P.K. The association between static pelvic asymmetry and low back pain. *Spine* **1999**, *24*, 1234–1242. [CrossRef] [PubMed]
26. Yu, Q.; Huang, H.; Zhang, Z.; Hu, X.; Li, W.; Li, L.; Chen, M.; Liang, Z.; Ambrose Lo, W.L.; Wang, C. The association between pelvic asymmetry and non-specific chronic low back pain as assessed by the global postural system. *BMC Musculoskelet. Disord.* **2020**, *21*, 596. [CrossRef]
27. Shiri, R.; Falah-Hassani, K. Does leisure time physical activity protect against low back pain? Systematic review and meta-analysis of 36 prospective cohort studies. *Br. J. Sports Med.* **2017**, *51*, 1410–1418. [CrossRef] [PubMed]
28. Heneweer, H.; Staes, F.; Aufdemkampe, G.; van Rijn, M.; Vanhees, L. Physical activity and low back pain: A systematic review of recent literature. *Eur. Spine J.* **2011**, *20*, 826–845. [CrossRef]
29. Farahbakhsh, F.; Rostami, M.; Noormohammadpour, P.; Mehraki Zade, A.; Hassanmirazaei, B.; Faghih Jouibari, M.; Kordi, R.; Kennedy, D.J. Prevalence of low back pain among athletes: A systematic review. *J. Back Musculoskelet. Rehabil.* **2018**, *31*, 901–916. [CrossRef]
30. Gabbett, T.J. The training—Injury prevention paradox: Should athletes be training smarter and harder? *Br. J. Sports Med.* **2016**, *50*, 273–280. [CrossRef]

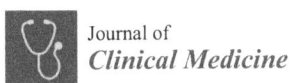

Article

Effectiveness of Warm-Up Exercises with Tissue Flossing in Increasing Muscle Strength

Anna Hadamus [1,*], Tomasz Jankowski [2,3], Karolina Wiaderna [1,2], Aneta Bugalska [1], Wojciech Marszałek [4], Michalina Błażkiewicz [5] and Dariusz Białoszewski [1]

1. Department of Rehabilitation, Faculty of Dental Medicine, Medical University of Warsaw, 02-091 Warsaw, Poland
2. Students Scientific Society for Physiotherapy, Department of Rehabilitation, Faculty of Dental Medicne, Medical University of Warsaw, 02-091 Warsaw, Poland
3. "Fizjopunkt Orlik" Rehabilitation Clinic, 04-041 Warsaw, Poland
4. Institute of Sport Sciences, The Jerzy Kukuczka Academy of Physical Education, 40-065 Katowice, Poland
5. Faculty of Rehabilitation, The Józef Piłsudski University of Physical Education in Warsaw, 00-809 Warsaw, Poland
* Correspondence: anna.hadamus@wum.edu.pl

Abstract: Tissue flossing is an increasingly popular method in physiotherapy and sports. There is a belief that tissue flossing can improve range of motion and muscle strength, shorten muscle recovery time, and reduce the risk of injury. The aim of this study was to analyse the effectiveness of tissue flossing for immediately improving muscle strength in recreational athletes when it is performed during warm-up. All participants were randomly assigned to either an experimental group ($n = 36$) or a control group ($n = 34$) using a random number generator. The experimental group ($n = 36$) performed an intervention comprising exercises with muscle tissue flossing and exercises without flossing. The control group ($n = 30$) performed the same protocol without a floss band. Muscle strength was measured for knee flexion end extension at three speeds (60, 120, and 180 °/s) 3 times. Analysed parameters include peak torque, work, and power related to body weight, flexors–extensors ratio, and time to peak torque. There were no significant changes in the muscle strength parameters from before to after the warm-up in either group ($p > 0.05$). Significantly lower values of peak torque, work, and power were observed in the experimental group during the warm-up with the floss band applied to muscles ($p < 0.05$). No clinically significant changes in time to peak torque or flexors–extensors ratio were observed. A single application of flossing does not improve muscle strength or power and can even reduce individuals' maximum muscle strength capabilities.

Keywords: tissue flossing; floss band; vascular occlusion; muscle strength; muscle endurance; warm-up

1. Introduction

The idea of enhancing strength training via the restriction (occlusion) of blood flow dates back to the mid-1960s in Japan, where it is known as KAATSU. The KAATSU method was developed by Yoshiaki Sato. The occlusive effect in KAATSU training is achieved with narrow elastic tourniquets placed around limbs near joints. Elsewhere, occlusion training refers to blood flow restriction training (BFRT) or low-load blood flow restriction (LL-BFR). For the BFRT technique, wider bands or pressure cuffs are tightened manually or pneumatically so that the inflow of arterial blood is not blocked but venous outflow from the area is blocked [1]. Ongoing and published studies have shown that BFRT is useful in strength training, indicating that this method may stimulate muscle hypertrophy to the same level as high-load resistance training and may be an effective means for increasing muscle strength and muscle mass, even in highly trained individuals. Numerous publications have demonstrated the effectiveness of BFR resistance training at loads of less

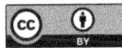

than 50% of a single maximum repetition, although the underlying processes have yet to be fully explained [2–6]. Despite these numerous reports of the effectiveness of this type of training, negative effects have also been indicated. Adverse effects have included blood clot formation, muscle cell damage, and abnormal blood pressure exercise responses or neural responses (such as numbness in the leg or arm). In light of these adverse effects, caution is advised for individuals with cardiovascular disease in particular [6,7].

Along with tourniquets and cuffs, floss bands are also used for exerting external pressure on tissues. Flossing has been popularised as VooDoo Flossing by Starrett and Cordoza [8]. They pointed out numerous advantages of flossing-mediated pressure, including improvements in joint mobilisation, joint range of motion, the mobility of connective tissue, and the quality of muscle contractions and pain relief. Once the brace removal occurs, there is an abrupt increase in perfusion to the joint and tissues, aiding in the renewal of damaged muscle and joint structures [9]. Elastic floss bands may also reduce joint or muscle oedema; compression forces compel the excess fluid into the lymphatic system, which then helps the body excrete the fluid, which may be useful in relieving delayed-onset muscle soreness (DOMS) [8,10]. However, some studies have suggested that floss bands do not reduce DOMS [11].

Tissue flossing is considered to be a method that is moderately effective in increasing patients' range of motion [12] and can be applied by the patient independently without continuous support from a physiotherapist. Flossing has also been shown to be useful for athletes, for example, during warm-up, to rapidly increase a joint's mobility before performing activities requiring maximum effort, such as those in training or competitions [1,13]. On the other hand, our previous study has shown no advantage in comparison to the warm-up procedure without a floss band in increasing trunk flexion measured by sit and reach test [14]. Moreover, only a few studies have assessed the effect of soft tissue flossing on muscle strength parameters, which are very important for performance during training.

There are several factors, that increase the risk of injury, including non-modifiable factors like age, anatomical knee structure, congenital ligaments laxity, and previous injuries, as well as modifiable factors like environment, technique, body weight, muscle laxity, and muscle strength [15–18]. The relationship between injury rate and muscle strength is visible, especially in the knee joint, which transfers high forces and is stabilized both by ligaments and muscles. Insufficiency of the knee flexors and extensor strength can cause dynamic knee valgus being one of the main knee injury risk factors [15,19,20]. Other researchers showed a relationship between muscle strength and the hamstring strain injury risk [16], meniscus damage progression [21], or re-injury following ACL reconstruction [22,23]. Muscle activation exercises are performed during warm-up to increase the possibility to generate high muscle strength during the main exercise sessions or competitions, and therefore to reduce the risk of injury [24,25]. Some other supporting techniques, like tissue flossing, can be applied additionally to enhance the warm-up effects. There are only a few studies concerning the influence of tissue flossing on muscle strength [13,26–28], but the results are inconclusive. The present study investigated the strength parameters of thigh muscles, as they determine lower limb function in many sports and can be a factor in predicting the risk of injury [16,29,30].

The aim of the study was to assess the effect of flossing during the pre-exercise warm-up on selected strength parameters of the knee flexors and extensors. Based on previous studies, it was hypothesized an increase in muscle strength, work and power parameters. Moreover, the time to achieve peak torque was expected to shorten.

2. Materials and Methods

2.1. Participants

The study enrolled 70 recreational athletes (47 women and 23 men) aged 18–29 years, participating in regular physical exercise sessions 3–4 times per week, min. 30 min each. All participants were randomly assigned to either an experimental group ($N = 36$) or a control group ($N = 34$) using the random number generator in Microsoft Excel. An interview to determine whether individuals met the following exclusion criteria: current musculoskeletal complaints, a history of lower limb surgery or injury within the preceding year, cardiac, vascular, or respiratory disorders, blood coagulation disorders, pregnancy, and cancer (at present or within the five years before the study). All participants were informed about the potential risks associated with the tests, especially the tissue flossing procedure, and agreed to participate in the study.

Four participants from the control group did not complete the experiment due to musculoskeletal complaints that occurred during the isokinetic measurement. Therefore, the control group included finally 30 athletes. The characteristics of the participants that completed the study protocol are in Table 1.

Table 1. Characteristics of the participants (mean ± SD).

Group	Gender	Age (Years)	Body Mass (kg)	Body Height (cm)	Body Mass Index BMI (kg/m^2)
Experimental group (n = 36)	21 females 15 males	21.0 ± 2.1	68.8 ± 12.9	171.8 ± 10.9	23.2 ± 2.9
Control group (n = 30)	24 females 6 males	21.8 ± 2.2	65.9 ± 12.9	170.2 ± 8.2	22.6 ± 2.9

2.2. Ethical Approval

The study protocol was approved by the Bioethics Committee of the Medical University of Warsaw (no. KB/217/2020). The work was carried out in accordance with the Declaration of Helsinki.

2.3. Measurements

Leg dominance was defined using the revised version of the Waterloo Footedness Questionnaire (WFQ-R) [31]. Muscle strength in the dominant leg only was then measured with the Humac Norm system (CSMi Inc., Stoughton, MA, USA) under isokinetic conditions for knee flexion and extension (concentric/concentric) in an open kinetic chain at the following speeds, following relevant standards [32]: 60 degrees per second (5 repetitions), 120 degrees per second (7 repetitions) and 180 degrees per second (10 repetitions). Before each series, the participants performed two trial repetitions followed by a 5-s break. Between each series, the participants rested for 20 s.

The following parameters were measured separately for the flexors (Flx) and extensors (Ext): peak torque (PT) [Nm], work per repetition (WR) [Nm], mean power (MP) [W], and time to peak torque (TPT) [s]. All torque values included gravity correction. Peak torque, work per repetition and mean power values are then related to body weight (BW) in kilograms. For each parameter flexors-extensor ratio was calculated as follows:

$$Rat_{FlxExt} = \frac{x_{Flx}}{x_{Ext}},$$

where x_{Flx} is the value of the parameter for flexors, and x_{Ext} is the value of the parameter for extensors.

2.4. Procedures

At the beginning, each participant was tested with WFQ-R. Then, participants performed an 8 min initial warm-up, consisting of slow running (300 m), high knee skips (300 m), 10 squats, skipping for 30 s, and a cycloergometer for 2 min with ca. 30% resistance. All participants were familiar with performed exercises.

2.4.1. Experimental Group

After initial warm-up the experimental group performed the first isokinetic measurement, followed by a 1 min break. Then, a plum (strong) Flossband (Sanctband, WAGUS GmbH, Germany) was applied to the participant's muscles during this time. The band was always applied by the same physiotherapist (T.J.) who was highly experienced in performing this technique. The band was applied to the tight muscles of the dominant leg, starting from the epicondyles level along the course of the tight muscles proximally while maintaining 50% tension and with 50% overlap of the previous part of the band (Figure 1) [33–35]. This procedure lasted about 1 min. Immediately after, a participant performed the second isokinetic measurement, which was followed by a 30-s break. The floss band was removed during this time. The warm-up was continued then for the next 5 min, including medium-speed running (200 m), a cycloergometer for 2 min with ca. 60% resistance, and a trampoline jumps for 1 min. Then, the third isokinetic measurement was performed.

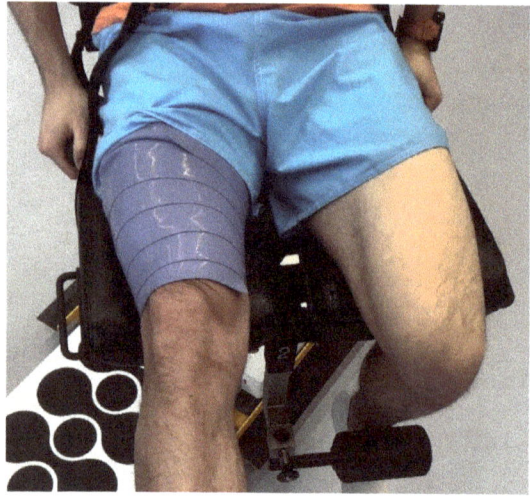

Figure 1. Application of a floss band on tight muscles.

2.4.2. Control Group

Participants assigned to the control group started after initial warm-up with the first isokinetic measurement, followed by a 2 min break. Immediately after, a participant performed the second isokinetic measurement, which was followed by a 30-s break. The warm-up was continued then for the next 5 min, including medium-speed running (200 m), a cycloergometer for 2 min with ca. 60% resistance, and a trampoline jumps for 1 min. Then, the third isokinetic measurement was performed. The same time intervals were kept in the control group as in the experimental group.

2.5. Statistical Analysis

Statistical analysis was performed using PQStat 2021 software v. 1.8.2.238 (PQStat Software, Poznań, Poland). Shapiro–Wilk test showed that the variables have non-normal distribution. Because of this and small group sizes, non-parametric test (Friedmann's ANOVA with post hoc Dunn–Bonferroni test) was used to analyse differences between three measurements (1—before floss band application; 2—with floss band applied on muscles in the experimental group, 3—at the end of a warm-up) within the groups. The results were considered statistically significant for $p < 0.05$.

The effect size was estimated using Cohen's d. Cohen's d was counted for combinations between measurements 1, 2 and 3, as follows:

$$d = \frac{m_a - m_b}{SDpool}; \quad SDpool = \sqrt{\frac{SD_a^2 + SD_b^2}{2}}$$

where: m_a, m_a—means from measurement a and b, respectively; SD_a and SD_b—standard deviations from measurements a and b, respectively (a, b = 1, 2, 3 and a ≠ b). The ranges of effect size for Cohen's d was as follows: d ≤ 0.5—small, 0.5 < d ≤ 0.8—medium; d > 0.8—large [36].

3. Results

3.1. Peak Torque per Body Weight

In the experimental group, PT per BW values both in extensors and flexors were significantly lower in the second measurement at all three speeds ($p < 0.05$), but they returned to the baseline in the third measurement. Flexors' peak torque per BW was slightly higher in the third measurement. In the control group, no significant changes were observed between all three measurements at all speeds, but a detailed analysis of the values showed a slight increase in generated PT per BW, both for extensors and flexors (Figure 2).

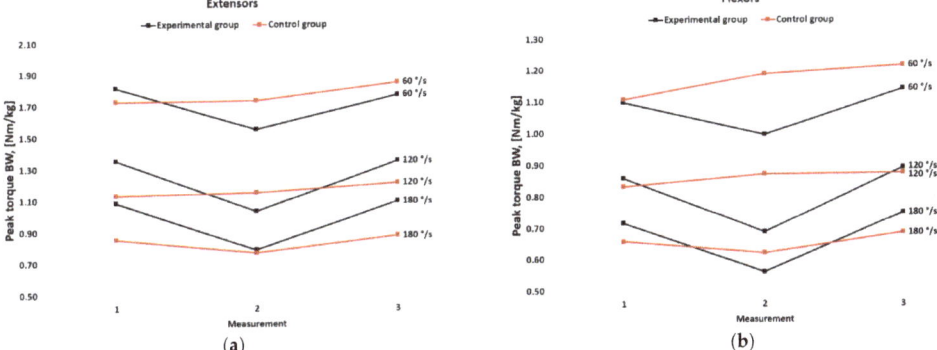

Figure 2. Mean of peak torque per body weight in the experimental and the control group for (**a**) extensors and (**b**) flexors.

3.2. Work per Repetition per Body Weight

WR values related to BW decreased significantly in the second measurement and then increased in the third measurement ($p < 0.05$) in the experimental group. There were no significant differences between measurements no. 1 and 3. No statistically significant differences were observed in the control group, although a slight increase was observed (Figure 3).

3.3. Mean Power per Body Weight

In the experimental group, MP per BW significantly decreased in measurement no. 2 and then returned to the baseline in measurement no. 3 ($p < 0.05$). No differences were shown in the control group (Figure 4)

3.4. Time to Peak Torque

In the experimental group, TPT in the extensors lowered significantly between the first and the second measurement ($p < 0.05$) and remained at this level at the third measurement in all three speeds (Figure 4a). Similar changes were observed in the TPT in the flexors only in the measurement in 60 °/s (Figure 4b). In the control group, no significant changes were observed in all speeds (Figure 5).

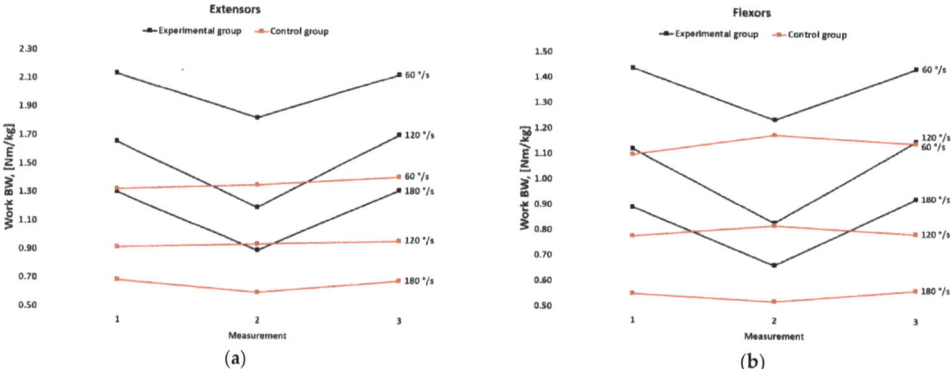

Figure 3. Mean of work per repetition per body weight in the experimental and the control group for (**a**) extensors and (**b**) flexors.

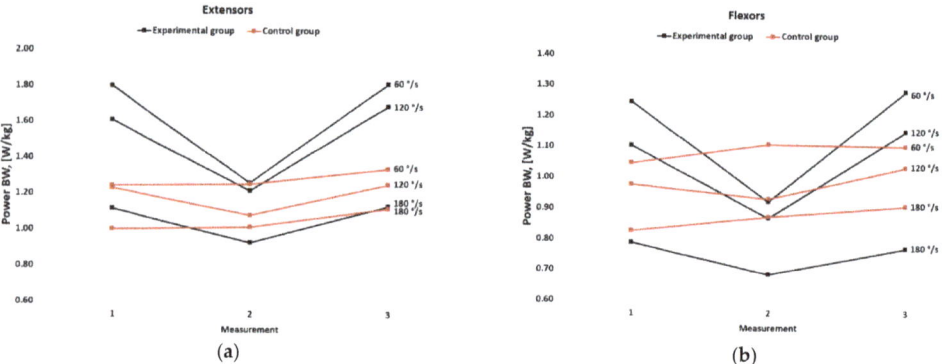

Figure 4. Mean power per body weight in the experimental and the control group for (**a**) extensors and (**b**) flexors.

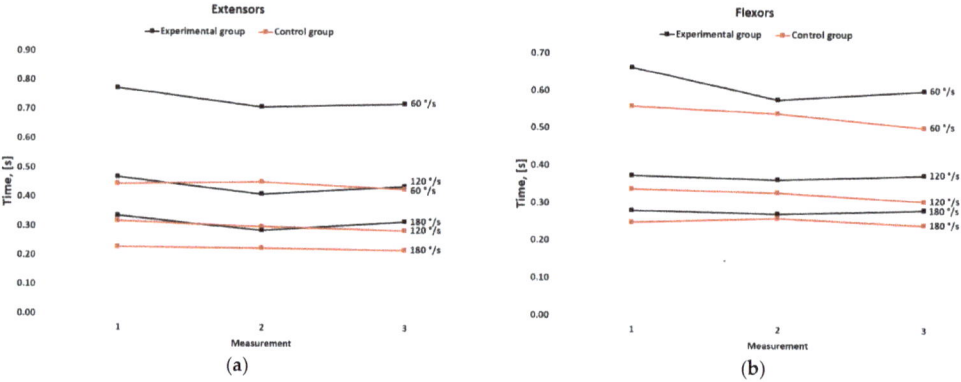

Figure 5. Mean of time to peak torque in the experimental and the control group for (**a**) extensors and (**b**) flexors.

3.5. Flexors–Extensors Ratio

In general, flexors to extensors ratio values calculated for all measured parameters showed no significant differences among all three measurements. There were some significant differences observed in the post hoc Dunn–Bonferroni test in the experimental group for time to PT ratio in 180°/s between measurements no. 1 and 2 and in the control group for PT ratio in 60°/s between measurements no. 1 and 2, WR ratio in 60°/s between measurements no. 2 and 3, WR ratio in 180°/s between measurement no. 1 and 2, and MP ratio in 180°/s between measurement no. 1 and 2. Nevertheless, all parameters showed no differences in the flexors–extensors ratio between the first and the third measurements.

All detailed values of the calculated parameters are in Appendix A, including measurements in 60°/s (Table A1), 120°/s (Table A2), and 180°/s (Table A3).

4. Discussion

The objective of this study was to assess the effectiveness of flossing applied during a warm-up in improving the strength and time parameters of the knee flexors and extensors. It was shown that floss band application during exercises does not improve generated peak torque, power, or work immediately after the warm-up. Furthermore, muscle strength parameters were significantly lower during exercising with a floss band than without it. A slight increase in muscle strength in the control group suggests, that the same set of exercises without flossing is even more effective in improving muscle strength parameters than with floss band application. There were some changes observed in the time to peak-torque and flexors–extensors ratio, but they seem to be clinically irrelevant.

Among the current literature, few studies on floss bands can be directly compared with the present investigation. Most published works have analysed Starett's and Cordoza's [8] original assumptions and examined the effectiveness of tissue flossing in improving range of motion, overall joint performance, and tissue flexibility [8,14]. Studies have predominantly been carried out on athletes and in the setting of post-injury rehabilitation for sports. Most of the protocols involved several repeated flossing sessions combined with sports practice sessions, and the outcomes are inconsistent [1,12,13,26,37]. Such outcomes are also reported after a single session of floss band intervention [13,26–28,35,38,39].

Chang et al. [38] reported a significant increase in quadriceps peak torque per BW and a decrease in hamstrings peak torque per BW immediately after single floss band application. Intervention with a floss band was at some points different from the intervention in the present study, as it included walking knee lift, side squat, and lunge and lasted 3 min. In the present study, participants performed high-intensity exercises in an open kinetic chain (isokinetic measurement), which also lasted about 3 min, but the intensity and biomechanics of muscle contraction were different. Although Chang et al. [38] did not calculate a flexors–extensors ratio, it seems that the direction of this ratio changed in their study from above 1 before, to less than 1 immediately after flossing and coming to baseline in 20 min after exercises. Such a result was not confirmed in the present study and by other researchers, as the flexors–extensors ratio is expected to be close to 0.60 when tested with a speed of 60°/s [22]. It is worth noting that in the cited paper, the torque generated by the hamstring muscles before and 20 min after the intervention remained unchanged. In contrast, the quadriceps torque increased. In addition, in both cases, the hamstring torque is almost twice as high as that achieved for the quadriceps muscle. This makes the presented results significantly different from those recorded in our work.

Vogrin et al. [34] assessed nineteen recreational athletes in three different conditions (high floss band pressure, low floss band pressure, and control). They reported small to medium benefits associated with flossing application compared to controls regarding maximum voluntary contraction in isometric conditions for knee extensors (421.37 Nm before and 445.94 Nm after flossing with low pressure; 418.47 Nm before and 429.16 Nm after flossing with high pressure) and unclear to small benefits for flexors (215.82 Nm before and 220.26 Nm after flossing; 203.33 Nm before and 211.07 Nm after flossing with high pressure). A slight increase in the muscle torque obtained for flexors seems to be comparable with the results presented above, while those for extensors seem to be better than those achieved in the present study, although they did not refer to body weight. Konrad et al. [27] reported a slight increase in maximal isometric knee extension (from

293.10 Nm to 309.56 Nm), while Kaneda et al. [35] confirmed these results for isometric knee flexion (63.8 to 66.3% of body weight). However, Konrad et al. [27] reported no group effect. Both studies were performed on relatively small study groups (16 and 17 recreational male athletes, respectively) and the increase in muscle strength was comparable with those reported for flexors peak torque per body weight in the present study, although we noticed non-significant changes. Kaneda et al. [35] measured also maximal eccentric knee flexion and extension torque. They reported an average increase of almost 30% BW for knee extension and 10% BW for knee flexion after flossing application [35]. The methodology of this study was in some points different from the above-cited studies: 70 athletes were assessed and divided into two groups, included also female participants. Additionally, concentric peak torque in isokinetic conditions was measured instead of isometric or isokinetic eccentric peak torque. Therefore, direct comparison between the results of these studies is limited.

The present study was based on a large study population of recreational athletes. It is similar in this respect to the publications of Driller et al., who assessed the effect of tissue flossing on the ankle joint and the ability to jump and run [13,26,28]. The results were positive, as the authors stated that flossing can contribute to the prevention of injuries by improving joint mobility and that it can be used during warm-up among both recreational athletes and elite rugby union athletes. The first of these studies showed a significant improvement in height (from 23 to 27 cm) and velocity (from 1.88 to 2.03 m/s) in a single-leg vertical jump test immediately following the application of a flossing band, possibly indicating improved muscle strength and power [13]. These findings, however, were not confirmed in another study, where the persistence of the effects of flossing was assessed using a counter-movement jump (CMJ) test [28]. There were no significant time and intervention interaction effects in the CMJ test results for either the study or control group, but there were small benefits associated with flossing 30 min after application. In addition, there were no differences between the study and control groups in the CMJ test results in a similar study involving elite rugby union athletes [26].

The positive influence of warm-up visible in the control group in the present study was confirmed by Paravlic et al. [40] in their study assessing tensiomyography (TMG) parameters and the CMJ test. At the same time, they reported negative alterations in all TMG parameters and reduced CMJ test results immediately after flossing, which corresponds with the results of the present study. This can suggest that ischemic preconditioning can reduce athletic performance [41,42], which can increase the risk of an injury, especially during competition.

The most noticeable finding in the present study was a marked decrease in the values of the strength parameters investigated in the isokinetic study when the floss band was applied. Blacker et al. [43] showed that knee isokinetic measurements taken within one day have high reproducibility. The results obtained by a control group in the present study, confirm this. Therefore, the effect we observed could be due to a sense of discomfort or pain caused by pressure on the muscles from the tight band, direct contact of the taut rubber with the skin or an additional reduction in comfort as the subjects sat in the chair of the dynamometer with the floss band. While such sensations are subjective experiences, they may affect one's motivation to perform a task at maximum effort. This observation should be considered in future studies on this topic.

A decrease in muscle strength with flossing is considered a sign that this technique should not be used in exercises that require muscle strength and power. In this regard, the work generated by muscles after a floss band was applied can be compared to that after static stretching, which has an undesirable effect on muscles during warm-up, reducing the generated muscle strength by 3% to 9%. Different authors have reported that dynamic stretching can improve muscle strength by as much as 9% or cause a slight decrease by 4%, and some authors have found no effect on the force generated [44,45]. The findings of the present study indicate that tissue flossing ranks between static and dynamic stretching concerning its effect on strength parameters. The application of a floss band resulted in decreases in most parameters tested, but on the third measurement, after the floss band had been removed, the parameters returned to baseline or near-baseline values. On one hand, this may be a sign that the effects of flossing have a short duration or do not influence muscle strength directly after use. On the other hand, a slight increase in strength parameters in the control group suggests, that the influence of tissue flossing on muscles is not positive when analysed directly after exercises with a floss band. Therefore, there is no rationale for using soft tissue flossing during warm-up to improve muscle strength parameters before the main exercise session or competition.

Although an innovative approach to assessing the effectiveness of flossing was applied, the present study has some limitations. The floss-band stretch force was not quantified [34,46] and the blood flow restriction is also not quantifiable [47]. Possible differences in band application were minimized by involving only one, highly experienced physiotherapist in this task. The study protocol also did not include fatigue parameters, especially from high-speed tests. Calculating the fatigue ratio for different strength and time variables could give additional information about the influence of tissue flossing on muscle physiology. This study, due to its design, was not blinded to participants or investigators.

In future studies, it would be worthful to analyse, how tissue flossing application applied during warm-up influences results achieved in the main session or during competition. It is warranted to consider different pressure levels, intensity, and duration of warm-up exercises, as well as the type of sports activities to draw reliable conclusions.

5. Conclusions

Based on the above-described results and their comparison to the literature, it can be concluded that a single session of muscle flossing does not improve muscle strength or power and may even decrease maximum muscle strength. It is therefore not recommended for use during warm-up. Additional research is warranted to determine the effects of flossing on other muscle-related indices, such as muscle excitability, endurance or contraction velocity.

Author Contributions: Conceptualization, A.H. and T.J.; Data curation, A.H., T.J., K.W. and A.B.; Formal analysis, A.H. and W.M.; Funding acquisition, M.B. and D.B.; Investigation, T.J., K.W. and A.B.; Methodology, A.H., T.J. and D.B.; Project administration, A.H.; Resources, A.H., T.J., K.W. and W.M.; Supervision, A.H. and D.B.; Visualization, W.M.; Writing—original draft, A.H.; Writing—review and editing, A.H. and M.B.. All authors have read and agreed to the published version of the manuscript.

Funding: This research was funded from the statutory funds of the Medical University of Warsaw (grant no. 2F1/N/22), statutory funds of the Jerzy Kukuczka Academy of Physical Education, and by the Ministry of Science and Higher Education in the year 2020–2022 under Research Group no. 3 at the Józef Piłsudski University of Physical Education in Warsaw "Motor system diagnostics in selected dysfunctions as a basis for planning the rehabilitation process".

Institutional Review Board Statement: The study was conducted in accordance with the Declaration of Helsinki, and approved by the Bioethics Committee of the Medical University of Warsaw (no. KB/217/2020, approval date 22 July 2020).

Informed Consent Statement: Informed consent was obtained from all subjects involved in the study.

Data Availability Statement: The measurement data used to support the findings of this study are available from the corresponding author upon request.

Conflicts of Interest: The authors declare no conflict of interest. The funders had no role in the design of the study; in the collection, analyses, or interpretation of data; in the writing of the manuscript, or in the decision to publish the results.

Appendix A

Table A1. Results of the measurement in the 60 °/s test for the experimental and the control group, where: s—means small, m—medium and l—large effect size calculated by Cohen's d.

Group	Parameter	Measurement 1	p-Value 1–2	Measurement 2	p-Value 2–3	Measurement 3	p-Value 1–3
Experimental group	Ext peak torque BW [Nm/kg]	Me 1.75 IQR 1.49–2.06	<0.001 m	Me 1.51 IQR 1.28–1.81	0.017 s	Me 1.70 IQR 1.39–2.03	0.949 s
	Flx peak torque BW [Nm/kg]	Me 1.09 IQR 0.89–1.25	0.007 s	Me 0.97 IQR 0.88–1.12	0.002 m	Me 1.12 IQR 0.98–1.30	>0.999 s
	Peak torque flx-ext ratio	Me 0.60 IQR 0.55–0.68	0.065 s	Me 0.65 IQR 0.61–0.73	>0.999 s	Me 0.66 IQR 0.56–0.74	0.335 s
	Ext work BW [Nm/kg]	Me 2.09 IQR 1.82–2.43	<0.001 s	Me 1.76 IQR 1.43–2.23	<0.001 s	Me 2.02 IQR 1.66–2.58	>0.999 s
	Flx work BW [Nm/kg]	Me 1.43 IQR 1.19–1.69	<0.001 s	Me 1.16 IQR 0.98–1.42	0.001 s	Me 1.40 IQR 1.21–1.69	>0.999 s
	Work flx-ext ratio	Me 0.68 IQR 0.60–0.76	>0.999 s	Me 0.71 IQR 0.62–0.80	>0.999 s	Me 0.67 IQR 0.58–0.78	>0.999 s
	Ext power BW [W/kg]	Me 1.08 IQR 0.95–1.32	0.010 m	Me 0.86 IQR 0.74–1.16	0.007 m	Me 1.08 IQR 0.90–1.39	>0.999 s
	Flx power BW [W/kg]	Me 0.79 IQR 0.64–0.91	0.004 m	Me 0.67 IQR 0.62–0.78	0.003 s	Me 0.77 IQR 0.66–0.91	>0.999 s
	Power flx-ext ratio	Me 0.70 IQR 0.63–0.82	>0.999 s	Me 0.76 IQR 0.65–0.85	>0.999 s	Me 0.72 IQR 0.59–0.80	>0.999 s
	Ext time to peak torque [s]	Me 0.77 IQR 0.615–0.895	0.047 s	Me 0.69 IQR 0.54–0.81	>0.999 s	Me 0.735 IQR 0.595–0.87	0.422 s
	Flx time to peak torque [s]	Me 0.605 IQR 0.50–0.81	0.231 s	Me 0.545 IQR 0.465–0.65	>0.999 s	Me 0.585 IQR 0.49–0.64	0.867 s
	Time to PT flx-ext ratio	Me 0.86 IQR 0.72–1.00	>0.999 s	Me 0.87 IQR 0.68–1.07	>0.999 s	Me 0.79 IQR 0.69–0.99	>0.999 s
Control group	Ext peak torque BW [Nm/kg]	Me 1.63 IQR 1.13–2.26	0.736 s	Me 1.82 IQR 1.10–2.15	0.244 s	Me 1.90 IQR 1.40–2.24	>0.999 s
	Flx peak torque BW [Nm/kg]	Me 1.13 IQR 0.83–1.43	0.413 s	Me 1.21 IQR 1.01–1.34	>0.999 s	Me 1.25 IQR 0.98–1.46	>0.999 s
	Peak torque flx-ext ratio	Me 0.68 IQR 0.56–0.78	0.024 l	Me 0.68 IQR 0.62–0.81	0.212 s	Me 0.69 IQR 0.54–0.78	>0.999 s
	Ext work BW [Nm/kg]	Me 1.30 IQR 0.80–1.61	>0.999 s	Me 1.27 IQR 1.01–1.64	>0.999 s	Me 1.45 IQR 0.98–1.70	>0.999 s
	Flx work BW [Nm/kg]	Me 1.24 IQR 0.69–1.49	0.212 s	Me 1.21 IQR 0.86–1.43	0.590 s	Me 1.22 IQR 0.86–1.40	>0.999 s
	Work flx-ext ratio	Me 0.90 IQR 0.66–0.98	0.364 s	Me 0.91 IQR 0.81–1.13	0.020 s	Me 0.82 IQR 0.68–1.00	0.735 s
	Ext power BW [W/kg]	Me 0.96 IQR 0.62–1.34	>0.999 s	Me 1.00 IQR 0.62–1.34	0.051 s	Me 1.06 IQR 0.79–1.38	0.117 s
	Flx power BW [W/kg]	Me 0.83 IQR 0.59–1.05	>0.999 s	Me 0.86 IQR 0.77–0.99	>0.999 s	Me 0.95 IQR 0.73–1.10	0.504 s
	Power flx-ext ratio	Me 0.91 IQR 0.67–1.00	0.051 s	Me 0.89 IQR 0.63–1.16	0.071 s	Me 0.83 IQR 0.68–1.00	>0.999 s
	Ext time to peak torque [s]	Me 0.42 IQR 0.34–0.50	>0.999 s	Me 0.43 IQR 0.35–0.56	>0.999 s	Me 0.445 IQR 0.36–0.49	>0.999 s
	Flx time to peak torque [s]	Me 0.54 IQR 0.48–0.67	>0.999 s	Me 0.55 IQR 0.49–0.61	0.107 s	Me 0.50 IQR 0.43–0.56	0.302 s
	Time to PT flx-ext ratio	Me 1.35 IQR 1.02–1.59	0.198 s	Me 1.21 IQR 0.88–1.50	>0.999 s	Me 1.16 IQR 0.94–1.46	0.567 s

Ext—extensors; Flx—flexors; PT—peak torque; BW—body weight; Me—median; IQR—inter-quartile range; p-values for post hoc Dunn–Bonferroni test.

Table A2. Results of the measurement in the 120 °/s test for the experimental and the control group, where: s—means small, m—medium and l—large effect size calculated by Cohen's d.

	Parameter	Measurement 1	*p*-Value 1–2	Measurement 2	*p*-Value 2–3	Measurement 3	*p*-Value 1–3
Experimental group	Ext peak torque BW [Nm/kg]	Me 1.33 IQR 1.09–1.52	<0.001 m	Me 1.01 IQR 0.77–1.19	<0.001 m	Me 1.28 IQR 1.10–1.61	>0.999 s
	Flx peak torque BW [Nm/kg]	Me 0.85 IQR 0.77–0.95	<0.001 l	Me 0.71 IQR 0.56–0.75	<0.001 l	Me 0.91 IQR 0.79–1.04	>0.999 s
	Peak torque flx-ext ratio	Me 0.67 IQR 0.56–0.75	>0.999 s	Me 0.70 IQR 0.60–0.83	>0.999 s	Me 0.67 IQR 0.59–0.77	>0.999 s
	Ext work BW [Nm/kg]	Me 1.57 IQR 1.37–2.00	<0.001 l	Me 1.16 IQR 0.98–1.42	<0.001 l	Me 1.63 IQR 1.40–1.99	>0.999 s
	Flx work BW [Nm/kg]	Me 1.12 IQR 0.92–1.33	<0.001 l	Me 0.83 IQR 0.69–1.00	<0.001 l	Me 1.13 IQR 0.98–1.34	0.867 s
	Work flx-ext ratio	Me 0.69 IQR 0.60–0.80	>0.999 s	Me 0.71 IQR 0.64–0.84	>0.999 s	Me 0.66 IQR 0.61–0.81	>0.999 s
	Ext power BW [W/kg]	Me 1.45 IQR 1.35–1.91	<0.001 m	Me 1.18 IQR 0.90–1.46	<0.001 l	Me 1.56 IQR 1.32–2.06	>0.999 s
	Flx power BW [W/kg]	Me 1.13 IQR 0.94–1.34	0.002 l	Me 0.84 IQR 0.70–0.99	<0.001 l	Me 1.18 IQR 0.97–1.33	>0.999 s
	Power flx-ext ratio	Me 0.72 IQR 0.63–0.82	>0.999 s	Me 0.73 IQR 0.67–0.88	0.472 s	Me 0.71 IQR 0.62–0.81	>0.999 s
	Ext time to peak torque [s]	Me 0.46 IQR 0.415–0.525	0.003 m	Me 0.405 IQR 0.34–0.46	>0.999 s	Me 0.43 IQR 0.40–0.475	0.020 s
	Flx time to peak torque [s]	Me 0.385 IQR 0.31–0.425	0.262 s	Me 0.37 IQR 0.31–0.40	0.789 s	Me 0.37 IQR 0.335–0.425	>0.999 s
	Time to PT flx-ext ratio	Me 0.80 IQR 0.68–0.93	0.178 s	Me 0.85 IQR 0.76–1.03	>0.999 s	Me 0.85 IQR 0.76–0.99	0.297 s
Control group	Ext peak torque BW [Nm/kg]	Me 1.07 IQR 0.69–1.37	>0.999 s	Me 1.13 IQR 0.83–1.37	0.881 s	Me 1.15 IQR 0.89–1.64	0.263 s
	Flx peak torque BW [Nm/kg]	Me 0.79 IQR 0.60–1.10	>0.999 s	Me 0.89 IQR 0.66–1.07	>0.999 s	Me 0.95 IQR 0.66–1.19	>0.999 s
	Peak torque flx-ext ratio	Me 0.78 IQR 0.59–0.96	>0.999 s	Me 0.80 IQR 0.64–1.00	0.054 s	Me 0.75 IQR 0.57–0.87	0.147 s
	Ext work BW [Nm/kg]	Me 0.79 IQR 0.63–1.25	>0.999 s	Me 0.86 IQR 0.69–1.28	>0.999 s	Me 0.95 IQR 0.98–1.55	>0.999 s
	Flx work BW [Nm/kg]	Me 0.79 IQR 0.54–0.95	>0.999 s	Me 0.83 IQR 0.51–1.10	>0.999 s	Me 0.83 IQR 0.48–1.10	>0.999 s
	Work flx-ext ratio	Me 0.94 IQR 0.65–1.07	0.345 s	Me 0.93 IQR 0.74–1.16	0.054 s	Me 0.82 IQR 0.70–1.05	>0.999 s
	Ext power BW [W/kg]	Me 1.14 IQR 0.88–1.56	>0.999 s	Me 1.23 IQR 0.88–1.58	>0.999 s	Me 1.27 IQR 0.95–1.91	0.567 s
	Flx power BW [W/kg]	Me 1.01 IQR 0.79–1.43	>0.999 s	Me 1.12 IQR 0.79–1.36	>0.999 s	Me 1.20 IQR 0.79–1.34	>0.999 s
	Power flx-ext ratio	Me 0.94 IQR 0.66–1.08	0.263 s	Me 0.95 IQR 0.79–1.21	0.077 s	Me 0.85 IQR 0.73–1.06	>0.999 s
	Ext time to peak torque [s]	Me 0.31 IQR 0.26–0.36	0.637 s	Me 0.30 IQR 0.24–0.34	>0.999 s	Me 0.28 IQR 0.25–0.32	0.567 s
	Flx time to peak torque [s]	Me 0.32 IQR 0.28–0.37	>0.999 s	Me 0.33 IQR 0.27–0.38	0.147 s	Me 0.28 IQR 0.25–0.35	0.504 s
	Time to PT flx-ext ratio	Me 1.02 IQR 0.76–1.36	0.302 s	Me 1.13 IQR 0.95–1.26	0.263 s	Me 1.10 IQR 0.88–1.21	>0.999 s

Ext—extensors; Flx—flexors; PT—peak torque; BW—body weight; Me—median; IQR—inter-quartile range; *p*-values for post hoc Dunn–Bonferroni test.

Table A3. Results of measurement in the 180 °/s test for the experimental and control groups, where: s—means small, m—medium and l—large effect size calculated by Cohen's d.

	Parameter	Measurement 1	p-Value 1–2	Measurement 2	p-Value 2–3	Measurement 3	p-Value 1–3
Experimental group	Ext peak torque BW [Nm/kg]	Me 1.06 IQR 0.88–1.25	<0.001 s	Me 0.74 IQR 0.57–0.92	<0.001 s	Me 1.07 IQR 0.85–1.25	>0.999 s
	Flx peak torque BW [Nm/kg]	Me 0.74 IQR 0.65–0.82	<0.001 s	Me 0.59 IQR 0.47–0.66	<0.001 s	Me 0.74 IQR 0.63–0.88	>0.999 s
	Peak torque flx-ext ratio	Me 0.71 IQR 0.58–0.79	0.585 s	Me 0.71 IQR 0.64–0.80	>0.999 s	Me 0.71 IQR 0.57–0.88	0.526 s
	Ext work BW [Nm/kg]	Me 1.24 IQR 1.01–1.53	<0.001 s	Me 0.83 IQR 0.63–1.06	<0.001 s	Me 1.21 IQR 1.01–1.52	>0.999 s
	Flx work BW [Nm/kg]	Me 0.86 IQR 0.77–1.01	<0.001 s	Me 0.68 IQR 0.51–0.79	<0.001 s	Me 0.91 IQR 0.76–1.06	>0.999 s
	Work flx-ext ratio	Me 0.70 IQR 0.61–0.81	>0.999 s	Me 0.77 IQR 0.62–0.86	>0.999 s	Me 0.73 IQR 0.60–0.86	>0.999 s
	Ext power BW [W/kg]	Me 1.69 IQR 1.39–2.11	<0.001 s	Me 1.19 IQR 0.87–1.52	<0.001 s	Me 1.77 IQR 1.37–2.25	>0.999 s
	Flx power BW [W/kg]	Me 1.26 IQR 1.08–1.44	<0.001 s	Me 0.97 IQR 0.71–1.12	<0.001 s	Me 1.27 IQR 1.04–1.59	>0.999 s
	Power flx-ext ratio	Me 0.72 IQR 0.60–0.81	>0.999 s	Me 0.77 IQR 0.62–0.89	>0.999 s	Me 0.72 IQR 0.60–0.89	>0.999 s
	Ext time to peak torque [s]	Me 0.335 IQR 0.30–0.36	<0.001 s	Me 0.28 IQR 0.255–0.32	0.789 s	Me 0.31 IQR 0.285–0.33	0.020 s
	Flx time to peak torque [s]	Me 0.28 IQR 0.255–0.31	0.648 s	Me 0.27 IQR 0.235–0.31	>0.999 s	Me 0.27 IQR 0.245–0.30	>0.999 s
	Time to PT flx-ext ratio	Me 0.82 IQR 0.73–0.95	0.029 m	Me 0.92 IQR 0.80–1.10	0.789 s	Me 0.87 IQR 0.75–1.00	0.422 s
Control group	Ext peak torque BW [Nm/kg]	Me 0.83 IQR 0.63–1.07	>0.999 s	Me 0.72 IQR 0.57–0.98	0.125 s	Me 0.83 IQR 0.66–1.13	0.567 s
	Flx peak torque BW [Nm/kg]	Me 0.63 IQR 0.48–0.89	>0.999 s	Me 0.69 IQR 0.36–0.83	>0.999 s	Me 0.74 IQR 0.45–0.83	>0.999 s
	Peak torque flx-ext ratio	Me 0.80 IQR 0.68–1.00	0.446 s	Me 0.77 IQR 0.67–1.00	0.567 s	Me 0.77 IQR 0.64–1.00	>0.999 s
	Ext work BW [Nm/kg]	Me 0.65 IQR 0.42–0.89	0.712 s	Me 0.57 IQR 0.42–0.75	0.504 s	Me 0.63 IQR 0.51–0.92	>0.999 s
	Flx work BW [Nm/kg]	Me 0.53 IQR 0.39–0.72	>0.999 s	Me 0.57 IQR 0.27–0.77	>0.999 s	Me 0.59 IQR 0.33–0.80	>0.999 s
	Work flx-ext ratio	Me 0.83 IQR 0.68–1.00	0.031 s	Me 0.91 IQR 0.70–1.11	0.147 s	Me 0.78 IQR 0.61–1.00	>0.999 s
	Ext power BW [W/kg]	Me 1.22 IQR 0.81–1.63	>0.999 s	Me 1.08 IQR 0.77–1.30	0.198 s	Me 1.22 IQR 0.88–1.74	0.567 s
	Flx power BW [W/kg]	Me 0.96 IQR 0.68–1.27	>0.999 s	Me 0.95 IQR 0.53–1.34	>0.999 s	Me 1.06 IQR 0.68–1.43	>0.999 s
	Power flx-ext ratio	Me 0.84 IQR 0.67–0.96	0.012 s	Me 0.92 IQR 0.71–1.15	0.446 s	Me 0.81 IQR 0.65–1.03	0.446 s
	Ext time to peak torque [s]	Me 0.23 IQR 0.19–0.27	>0.999 s	Me 0.22 IQR 0.18–0.26	>0.999 s	Me 0.23 IQR 0.17–0.25	>0.999 s
	Flx time to peak torque [s]	Me 0.225 IQR 0.20–0.28	>0.999 s	Me 0.25 IQR 0.21–0.28	0.125 s	Me 0.22 IQR 0.20–0.26	0.263 s
	Time to PT flx-ext ratio	Me 1.05 IQR 0.95–1.22	0.881 s	Me 1.13 IQR 0.89–1.50	0.393 s	Me 0.98 IQR 0.83–1.40	>0.999 s

Ext—extersors; Flx—flexors; PT—peak torque; BW—body weight; Me—median; IQR—inter-quartile range; p-values for post hoc Dunn–Bonferroni test.

References

1. Ross, S.; Kandassamy, G. The effects of 'Tack and Floss' active joint mobilisation on ankle dorsiflexion range of motion using Voodoo Floss Bands. *J. Phys. Ther.* 2017; in press.
2. Cook, C.J.; Kilduff, L.P.; Beaven, C.M. Improving strength and power in trained athletes with 3 weeks of occlusion training. *Int. J. Sports Physiol. Perform.* 2014, 9, 166–172. [CrossRef]
3. Schoenfeld, B.J. The mechanisms of muscle hypertrophy and their application to resistance training. *J. Strength Cond. Res.* 2010, 24, 2857–2872. [CrossRef] [PubMed]
4. Pearson, S.J.; Hussain, S.R. A review on the mechanisms of blood-flow restriction resistance training-induced muscle hypertrophy. *Sports Med.* 2015, 45, 187–200. [CrossRef] [PubMed]
5. Lowery, R.P.; Joy, J.M.; Loenneke, J.P.; de Souza, E.O.; Machado, M.; Dudeck, J.E.; Wilson, J.M. Practical blood flow restriction training increases muscle hypertrophy during a periodized resistance training programme. *Clin. Physiol. Funct. Imaging* 2014, 34, 317–321. [CrossRef] [PubMed]
6. Spranger, M.D.; Krishnan, A.C.; Levy, P.D.; O'Leary, D.S.; Smith, S.A. Blood flow restriction training and the exercise pressor reflex: A call for concern. *Am. J. Physiol. Heart Circ. Physiol.* 2015, 309, H1440–H1452. [CrossRef]
7. Vanwye, W.R.; Weatherholt, A.M.; Mikesky, A.E. Blood Flow Restriction Training: Implementation into Clinical Practice. *Int. J. Exerc. Sci.* 2017, 10, 649–654.
8. Starrett, K.; Cordoza, G. *Becoming a Supple Leopard. The Ultimate Guide to Resolving Pain, Preventing Injury, and Optimizing Athletic Performance*; Victory Belt Publishing Inc: Las Vegas, NV, USA, 2015.
9. Borda, J.; Selhorst, M. The use of compression tack and flossing along with lacrosse ball massage to treat chronic Achilles tendinopathy in an adolescent athlete: A case report. *J. Man. Manip. Ther.* 2017, 25, 57–61. [CrossRef]
10. Prill, R.; Schulz, R.; Michel, S. Tissue flossing: A new short-term compression therapy for reducing exercise-induced delayed-onset muscle soreness. A randomized, controlled and double-blind pilot crossover trial. *J. Sports Med. Phys. Fit.* 2019, 59, 861–867. [CrossRef]
11. Gorny, V.; Stöggl, T. Tissue flossing as a recovery tool for the lower extremity after strength endurance intervals. *Sportverletz. Sportschaden* 2018, 32, 55–60. [CrossRef]
12. Kielur, D.S.; Powden, C.J. Changes of Ankle Dorsiflexion Using Compression Tissue Flossing: A Systematic Review and Meta-Analysis. *J. Sport Rehabilitation* 2020, 30, 306–314. [CrossRef]
13. Driller, M.W.; Overmayer, R.G. The effects of tissue flossing on ankle range of motion and jump performance. *Phys. Ther. Sport* 2017, 25, 20–24. [CrossRef] [PubMed]
14. Hadamus, A.; Kowalska, M.; Kędra, M.; Wiaderna, K.; Białoszewski, D. Effect of hamstring tissue flossing during warm-up on sit and reach performance. *J. Sports Med. Phys. Fit.* 2022, 62, 51–55. [CrossRef] [PubMed]
15. Dauty, M.; Crenn, V.; Louguet, B.; Grondin, J.; Menu, P.; Fouasson-Chailloux, A. Anatomical and Neuromuscular Factors Associated to Non-Contact Anterior Cruciate Ligament Injury. *J. Clin. Med.* 2022, 11, 1402. [CrossRef] [PubMed]
16. Green, B.; Bourne, M.N.; van Dyk, N.; Pizzari, T. Recalibrating the risk of hamstring strain injury (HSI): A 2020 systematic review and meta-analysis of risk factors for index and recurrent hamstring strain injury in sport. *Br. J. Sports Med.* 2020, 54, 1081–1088. [CrossRef] [PubMed]
17. Edouard, P.; Pollock, N.; Guex, K.; Kelly, S.; Prince, C.; Navarro, L.; Branco, P.; Depiesse, F.; Gremeaux, V.; Hollander, K. Hamstring Muscle Injuries and Hamstring Specific Training in Elite Athletics (Track and Field) Athletes. *Int. J. Environ. Res. Public Health* 2022, 19, 10992. [CrossRef]
18. Hietamo, J.; Rantala, A.; Parkkari, J.; Leppanen, M.; Rossi, M.; Heinonen, A.; Steffen, K.; Kannus, P.; Mattila, V.; Pasanen, K. Injury History and Perceived Knee Function as Risk Factors for Knee Injury in Youth Team-Sports Athletes. *Sports Health* 2022, 19417381211065443. [CrossRef]
19. Giustino, V.; Messina, G.; Patti, A.; Padua, E.; Zangla, D.; Drid, P.; Battaglia, G.; Palma, A.; Bianco, A. Effects of a Postural Exercise Program on Vertical Jump Height in Young Female Volleyball Players with Knee Valgus. *Int. J. Environ. Res. Public Health* 2022, 19, 3953. [CrossRef]
20. Collings, T.J.; Diamond, L.E.; Barrett, R.S.; Timmins, R.G.; Hickey, J.T.; Du Moulin, W.S.; Williams, M.D.; Beerworth, K.A.; Bourne, M.N. Strength and Biomechanical Risk Factors for Noncontact ACL Injury in Elite Female Footballers: A Prospective Study. *Med. Sci. Sports Exerc.* 2022, 54, 1242–1251. [CrossRef]
21. Li, M.; Nie, Y.; Li, K.; Zeng, Y.; Wu, Y.; Liu, Y.; Wu, L.; Shen, B. Effect of Extensor Muscle Strength on Meniscus Damage Progression in Subjects Without Radiologic Knee Osteoarthritis: Data From the Osteoarthritis Initiative. *Am. J. Phys. Med. Rehabil.* 2022, 101, 836–842. [CrossRef]
22. Rivera-Brown, A.M.; Frontera, W.R.; Fontánez, R.; Micheo, W.F. Evidence for isokinetic and functional testing in return to sport decisions following ACL surgery. *PM&R* 2022, 14, 678–690. [CrossRef]
23. Bodkin, S.G.; Hertel, J.; Diduch, D.R.; Saliba, S.A.; Novicoff, W.M.; Brockmeier, S.F.; Miller, M.D.; Gwathmey, F.W.; Werner, B.C.; Hart, J.M. Predicting ACL Reinjury from Return to Activity Assessments at 6-months Post-Surgery: A Prospective Cohort Study. *J. Athl. Train.* 2021, 57, 325–333. [CrossRef] [PubMed]
24. Fiorilli, G.; Quinzi, F.; Buonsenso, A.; Di Martino, G.; Centorbi, M.; Giombini, A.; Calcagno, G.; di Cagno, A. Does Warm-up Type Matter? A Comparison between Traditional and Functional Inertial Warm-up in Young Soccer Players. *J. Funct. Morphol. Kinesiol.* 2020, 5, 84. [CrossRef] [PubMed]

25. Patti, A.; Giustino, V.; Hirose, N.; Messina, G.; Cataldi, S.; Grigoli, G.; Marchese, A.; Mulè, G.; Drid, P.; Palma, A.; et al. Effects of an experimental short-time high-intensity warm-up on explosive muscle strength performance in soccer players: A pilot study. *Front. Physiol.* **2022**, *13*, 1644. [CrossRef] [PubMed]
26. Mills, B.; Mayo, B.; Tavares, F.; Driller, M. The Effect of Tissue Flossing on Ankle Range of Motion, Jump, and Sprint Performance in Elite Rugby Union Athletes. *J. Sport Rehabil.* **2020**, *29*, 282–286. [CrossRef]
27. Konrad, A.; Bernsteiner, D.; Budini, F.; Reiner, M.M.; Glashüttner, C.; Berger, C.; Tilp, M. Tissue flossing of the thigh increases isometric strength acutely but has no effects on flexibility or jump height. *Eur. J. Sport Sci.* **2021**, *21*, 1648–1658. [CrossRef]
28. Driller, M.; Mackay, K.; Mills, B.; Tavares, F. Tissue flossing on ankle range of motion, jump and sprint performance: A follow-up study. *Phys. Ther. Sport* **2017**, *28*, 29–33. [CrossRef]
29. Rouis, M.; Coudrat, L.; Jaafar, H.; Filliard, J.R.; Vandewalle, H.; Barthelemy, Y.; Driss, T. Assessment of isokinetic knee strength in elite young female basketball players: Correlation with vertical jump. *J. Sports Med. Phys. Fit.* **2015**, *55*, 1502–1508.
30. Vieira, A.; Alex, S.; Martorelli, A.; Brown, L.E.; Moreira, R.; Bottaro, M. Lower-extremity isokinetic strength ratios of elite springboard and platform diving athletes. *Physician Sportsmed.* **2017**, *45*, 87–91. [CrossRef]
31. Schneiders, A.G.; Sullivan, S.J.; O'Malley, K.J.; Clarke, S.V.; Knappstein, S.A.; Taylor, L.J. A valid and reliable clinical determination of footedness. *PM&R* **2010**, *2*, 835–841. [CrossRef]
32. Davies, G.J. *A Compendium of Isokinetics in Clinical Usage and Rehabilitation Techniques*; S&S Publishers: Onalaska, WI, USA, 1992.
33. Pavlů, D.; Pánek, D.; Kuncová, E.; Thung, J.S. Effect of Blood Circulation in the Upper Limb after Flossing Strategy. *Appl. Sci.* **2021**, *11*, 1634. [CrossRef]
34. Vogrin, M.; Kalc, M.; Ličen, T. Acute Effects of Tissue Flossing Around the Upper Thigh on Neuromuscular Performance: A Study Using Different Degrees of Wrapping Pressure. *J. Sport Rehabil.* **2020**, *30*, 601–608. [CrossRef] [PubMed]
35. Kaneda, H.; Takahira, N.; Tsuda, K.; Tozaki, K.; Kudo, S.; Takahashi, Y.; Sasaki, S.; Kenmoku, T. Effects of Tissue Flossing and Dynamic Stretching on Hamstring Muscles Function. *J. Sports Sci. Med.* **2020**, *19*, 681–689. [PubMed]
36. Cohen, J. *Statistical Power Analysis for the Behavioral Sciences*; Routledge: New York, NY, USA, 1988.
37. Kiefer, B.N.; Lemarr, K.E.; Enriquez, C.C.; Tivener, K.A.; Todd, D. A pilot study: Perceptual effects of the voodoo floss band on glenohumeral flexibility. *Int. J. Athl. Ther. Train.* **2017**, *22*, 29–33. [CrossRef]
38. Chang, N.-J.; Hung, W.-C.; Lee, C.-L.; Chang, W.-D.; Wu, B.-H. Effects of a Single Session of Floss Band Intervention on Flexibility of Thigh, Knee Joint Proprioception, Muscle Force Output, and Dynamic Balance in Young Adults. *Appl. Sci.* **2021**, *11*, 12052. [CrossRef]
39. Wu, S.Y.; Tsai, Y.H.; Wang, Y.T.; Chang, W.D.; Lee, C.L.; Kuo, C.A.; Chang, N.J. Acute Effects of Tissue Flossing Coupled with Functional Movements on Knee Range of Motion, Static Balance, in Single-Leg Hop Distance, and Landing Stabilization Performance in Female College Students. *Int. J. Environ. Res. Public Health* **2022**, *19*, 1427. [CrossRef]
40. Paravlic, A.H.; Segula, J.; Drole, K.; Hadzic, V.; Pajek, M.; Vodicar, J. Tissue Flossing Around the Thigh Does Not Provide Acute Enhancement of Neuromuscular Function. *Front. Physiol.* **2022**, *13*, 702. [CrossRef]
41. Salvador, A.F.; De Aguiar, R.A.; Lisbôa, F.D.; Pereira, K.L.; Cruz, R.S.; Caputo, F. Ischemic Preconditioning and Exercise Performance: A Systematic Review and Meta-Analysis. *Int. J. Sports Physiol. Perform.* **2016**, *11*, 4–14. [CrossRef]
42. Husmann, F.; Mittlmeier, T.; Bruhn, S.; Zschorlich, V.; Behrens, M. Impact of Blood Flow Restriction Exercise on Muscle Fatigue Development and Recovery. *Med. Sci. Sports Exerc.* **2018**, *50*, 436–446. [CrossRef]
43. Blacker, S.D.; Fallowfield, J.L.; Bilzon, J.L.J.; Willems, M.E.T. Within-day and between-days reproducibility of isokinetic parameters of knee, trunk and shoulder movements. *Isokinet. Exerc. Sci.* **2010**, *18*, 45–55. [CrossRef]
44. Yamaguchi, T.; Ishii, K. Effects of static stretching for 30 seconds and dynamic stretching on leg extension power. *J. Strength Cond. Res.* **2005**, *19*, 677–683. [CrossRef]
45. McHugh, M.P.; Cosgrave, C.H. To stretch or not to stretch: The role of stretching in injury prevention and performance. *Scand. J. Med. Sci. Sports* **2010**, *20*, 169–181. [CrossRef] [PubMed]
46. Cheatham, S.W.; Baker, R. Quantification of the Rockfloss® Floss Band Stretch Force at Different Elongation Lengths. *J. Sport Rehabil.* **2020**, *29*, 377–380. [CrossRef] [PubMed]
47. Lee, Y.; Choi, J. A Study to Identify the Optimum Forearm Floss Band Intensity in 29 Young Adults Performing Blood Flow Restriction Training. *Med Sci. Monit.* **2022**, *28*, e935771. [CrossRef] [PubMed]

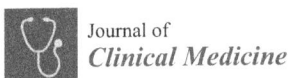

Article

Efficacy of Acupuncture on Quality of Life, Functional Performance, Dyspnea, and Pulmonary Function in Patients with Chronic Obstructive Pulmonary Disease: Protocol for a Randomized Clinical Trial

Renato Fleury Cardoso [1], Ana Cristina Rodrigues Lacerda [1,2], Vanessa Pereira Lima [2], Lucas Fróis Fernandes de Oliveira [2], Sofia Fróis Fernandes de Oliveira [2], Rafaela Paula Araújo [2], Cecylia Leiber Fernandes e Castro [2], Flávia Pereira da Silva [2], Lizânia Vieira de Paiva [3], Lia Dietrich [4], Pedro Henrique Scheidt Figueiredo [2], Henrique Silveira Costa [2], Mario Bernardo-Filho [5], Danúbia da Cunha de Sá-Caputo [5], Vanessa Amaral Mendonça [1,2] and Redha Taiar [6,*]

[1] Postgraduate Program in Health Sciences (PPGCS), Federal University of Jequitinhonha and Mucuri Valleys (UFVJM), Diamantina 39803-371, Brazil; cardoso.renato@ufvjm.edu.br (R.F.C.); lacerda.acr@ufvjm.edu.br (A.C.R.L.); vaafisio@hotmail.com (V.A.M.)

[2] Physiotherapy Department, Federal University of Jequitinhonha and Mucuri Valleys, Diamantina 39803-371, Brazil; vanessa.lima@ufvjm.edu.br (V.P.L.); lucaasfrois@hotmail.com (L.F.F.d.O.); sofiafroisf@hotmail.com (S.F.F.d.O.); rafaela.araujo@ufvjm.edu.br (R.P.A.); cecylialeiber@hotmail.com (C.L.F.e.C.); flavia.silva@ufvjm.edu.br (F.P.d.S.); pedro.figueiredo@ufvjm.edu.br (P.H.S.F.); henriquesilveira@yahoo.com.br (H.S.C.)

[3] Postgraduate Program in Health, Society and Environment (PPGSASA), Federal University of Jequitinhonha and Mucuri Valleys (UFVJM), Diamantina 39803-371, Brazil; lizania.paiva@ufvjm.edu.br

[4] Dentistry Department, Federal University of Jequitinhonha and Mucuri Valleys, Diamantina 39803-371, Brazil; lia.dietrich@ufvjm.edu.br

[5] Laboratory of Mechanical Vibrations and Integrative Practices, State University of Rio de Janeiro, Rio de Janeiro 20550-013, Brazil; bernardofilhom@gmail.com (M.B.-F.); dradanubia@gmail.com (D.d.C.d.S.-C.)

[6] MATériaux et Ingénierie Mécanique (MATIM), Université de Reims Champagne-Ardenne, 51100 Reims, France

* Correspondence: redha.taiar@univ-reims.fr

Abstract: Chronic obstructive pulmonary disease (COPD) is a respiratory disease characterized by the presence of chronic airflow obstruction. Previous studies have evaluated the effect of acupuncture treatment (AT) in patients with COPD. Nevertheless, these studies show a great deal of heterogeneity in treatment protocols, having sample sizes that are too small to estimate and clarify effect size and heterogeneity in patients' baseline. The aim of this study is to evaluate the effectiveness of acupuncture on quality of life, functional performance, dyspnea, and pulmonary function in patients with COPD. As such, patients will go through the following three phases: Phase I–pretreatment: period of subject selection and inclusion in the protocol, with an interview and performance of exams and tests as follows: Mini-Cog, dual-energy X-ray absorptiometry, spirometry, the Patient-Generated Index, Saint George's Respiratory Questionnaire, the six-minute walk test, the London Chest Activity of Daily Living, and the COPD Assessment Test. Phase II–8 weeks of treatment, with AT 3 times a week, with two parallel groups: Group I–with 50 subjects–AT according to the recommended technical standards; Group II–with 50 subjects–Control, without acupuncture. Phase III–Continuation of AT for 8 weeks, maintaining the subjects in the previously allocated groups and following the same methodology.

Keywords: chronic obstructive pulmonary disease; COPD; acupuncture; acupuncture therapy; acupuncture treatment; quality of life; health-related quality of life

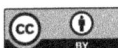

1. Introduction

Chronic obstructive pulmonary disease (COPD) is a preventable and treatable respiratory disease characterized by the presence of chronic airflow obstruction that is not fully reversible [1] and by the presence of systemic oxidative stress and inflammation biomarkers [2,3]. Studies on the prevalence of COPD suggest that around a quarter (1/4) of adults aged 40 years and older have moderate airflow obstruction [4].

Although COPD compromises the lungs, it also has significant systemic consequences [1,4–6]. COPD patients often adopt a sedentary lifestyle that can precipitate the onset of muscle deconditioning through inactivity and a cycle of clinical deterioration [1,7–9], negatively impacting the quality of life of patients with COPD [1,10]. Thus, although these patients maintain activities of daily living (ADL) related to self-care, mobility, food, and personal hygiene, their ADLs are considered to be of lesser intensity when compared to healthy individuals [11]. The same is true for physical activity as COPD patients often maintain lower levels of physical activity, according to international guidelines for maintaining physical health [7,8].

The concept of quality of life (QoL) refers to objective and, to a greater extent, subjective indicators of happiness and satisfaction [12]. According to the World Health Organization, QoL is defined as "an individual's perception of their position in life in the context of the culture and value system in which they live, and in relation to their goals, expectations, standards, and concerns" [13]. In this sense, the administration of questionnaires to assess the HRQoL of patients with COPD has been widely used, generating reliable, valid, and reproducible evidence [14,15].

The complementary role of acupuncture in alleviating the symptoms of various diseases has become increasingly relevant [16]. It is currently accepted that the stimulation of acupuncture points causes the release of neurotransmitters in the central nervous system, in addition to other substances responsible for the responses promoting analgesia, restoration of organic functions, and immune modulation. The World Health Organization recommends acupuncture to its member states, having produced several publications on its efficacy and safety, training of professionals, research methods, and evaluation of the therapeutic results of complementary and traditional medicines [17,18]. In addition, the consensus of the National Institutes of Health of the United States endorsed the indication of acupuncture, alone or as an adjunct, in several chronic conditions including COPD [19]. Additionally, a portion of COPD patients do not respond significantly to pulmonary rehabilitation, and therefore require alternative forms of intervention [20].

Previous studies have evaluated the effect of acupuncture treatment (AT) on COPD patients [21,22], but recent systematic reviews demonstrate great heterogeneity in treatment protocols, including different types and numbers of points of acupuncture, treatment regimens, treatment durations, inappropriate sample size to estimate and clarify effect size, and heterogeneity in the main outcomes of patients evaluated at baseline and in treatments received, demonstrating low methodological quality [23,24]. In addition, there are also studies that evaluate the additive effect [21] and studies that compare AT with certain other interventions [25], leaving a gap regarding the isolated effect of AT. This study hypothesizes that AT will result in an improvement in the quality of life (primary outcome) of patients with COPD, in addition to an improvement in functional performance and pulmonary function, promoting a reduction in the impact of the disease on the lives of such patients.

2. Materials and Methods

2.1. Design

The study will be a two-arm, parallel-group, prospective, computer-randomized, controlled, evaluator-blind design lasting for 16 weeks (two eight-week intervention periods). The study was registered on the www.ensaiosclinicos.gov.br (accessed on 23 May 2022) (REBEC) website. The protocol has been developed according to the SPIRIT guidelines [26] and described according to the CONSORT statements [27]. The acupuncture protocol will follow the recommendations of the Standards for Reporting Interventions in Clinical Trials of Acupuncture (STRICTA), a formal extension of CONSORT. STRICTA was designed to improve the integrity and transparency of reporting interventions in clinical trials of acupuncture so that such trials can be more accurately interpreted and easily replicated [28]. Furthermore, the intervention will be reported according to the Model for Intervention Description and Replication (TIDieR) checklist and guide [29].

2.2. Patients

Patients with a clinical diagnosis of COPD who meet the inclusion criteria will be recruited from the waiting list of the Federal University of the Jequitinhonha and Mucuri Valleys (UFVJM) Physiotherapy school clinic, as well as in doctors' offices and hospitals and through pamphlets and advertisements on local radio.

Patients will be aware that they will be randomized into one of two groups. Group I will receive AT and Group II will be without AT–we chose a control group without any intervention in order to analyze the isolated effect of AT. At the end of the project, if the results are favorable, patients in the control group will be offered the possibility of receiving AT.

The sample size was estimated using the GPower® program (Franz Faul, Universitat Kiel, Kiel, Germany), version 3.1.9.2. For this, a priori analysis was used, considering the t-test for comparisons between groups, for the quality-of-life variable evaluated by the Saint George Respiratory Questionnaire (SGRQ)-Total score [22]. Thus, considering an effect size of 0.59 [22], power of 0.80%, and alpha error of 5%, the sample size was estimated at 50 patients for each group, totaling 100 patients. These calculations assumed a 20% loss in the worst-case scenario.

2.3. Randomization

Randomization will be generated by a website (https://www.randomizer.org/ (accessed on 23 May 2022)) and performed by a researcher not involved in the recruitment, treatment, or evaluation of patients. This investigator will be instructed not to disclose the scheduled intervention to the other investigators until the completion of the study. Since randomization will occur after the initial evaluation, it is characterized as a blind distribution. The sequence will be generated in blocks of four patients in random order. The allocation will be hidden in numerical sequence, in opaque sealed envelopes.

2.4. Eligibility

2.4.1. Inclusion Criteria

I. Clinical diagnosis of COPD according to GOLD [1].
II. Ability to offer written authorization or nominate a person to read the Statement of Free and Informed Consent, giving the research patient's agreement.
III. Patients over 65 years of age with preserved cognitive function according to the Mini-Cog, that is, those who scored at least 3 to 5 points [30].
IV. Absence of exacerbation and stability of drug treatment in the last month.
V. A 3-month absence from participation in a pulmonary rehabilitation program.

2.4.2. Exclusion Criteria

I. Patient with a previous medical diagnosis of a disease that affects cognitive function and inhibits understanding of the questionnaires.
II. Patients unable to perform any of the assessments.
III. Previous acupuncture therapy.
IV. Being, or having been, in a rehabilitation group in the last 3 months before starting the protocol.
V. Patients who present an exacerbation of the clinical condition during the collection period will be excluded.

2.5. Intervention

The tests and questionnaires applied after phases II and III will be carried out within 48 h after the last session.

The period for carrying out this protocol will be from 2022 to 2025. Figure 1 presents the flow chart of the full study protocol.

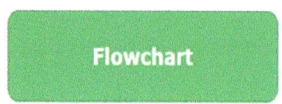

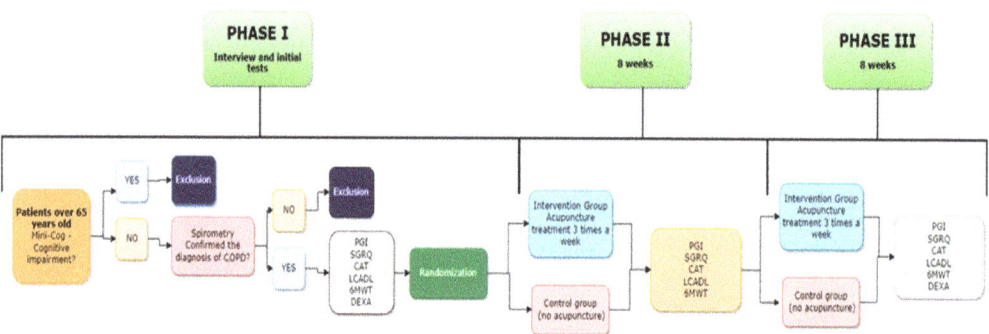

Figure 1. Flow of participants throughout in all stages of the research.

Acupuncture

Acupuncture needles made of stainless steel, 0.25 mm gauge and 3 cm long, approved by the Brazilian National Health Surveillance Agency (ANVISA) will be used.

The description of the technique and methodology follows the principles suggested by the Standards for Reporting Interventions in Clinical Trials of Acupuncture (STRICTA) [28], described below:

(a) the Traditional Chinese Medicine needling style will be used, based on the literature in the area and clinical consensus.
(b) treatment reasoning will be based on Chinese acupuncture literature, consensual methods, and literary references.
(c) the selection of needling points will not change throughout the treatment.
(d) the needling will be manual.

After the insertion of needles, manipulation will be carried out with adequate stimulus to obtain Dé Qi (acupuncture sensation) at determined and preestablished points for all patients.

The procedure for each session will be as follows:

Patients in the supine position will have the needles removed 30 min after the last needle is inserted.

The following acupoints will be used:

- Zusanli-stomach 36 (ST36 bilateral).
- Xuehai-spleen 10 (SP10 bilateral)
- Qihai-Ren Mai 6 (RM6 or CV6).
- Danzhong–Ren Mai 17 (RM17 or CV17).
- Chize-lung 5 (LU5 bilateral).
- Lieque-lung 7 (LU7 bilateral).

A total of 10 needles will be used per session.

After a thorough evaluation (Hsieh and colleagues, 2020) of the acupoints used in prior randomized clinical trial studies for COPD therapy, the points were chosen. Furthermore, sites were chosen that allows the patient to remain supine during treatment without changing positions [31].

The order of puncture will follow the traditional concept of needling. Because the problem (COPD) is at the top (lungs), the puncturing starts from the bottom. Thus, the order of puncture will follow the sequence: ST36, SP10, RM6, RM17, LU5, and LU7.

2.6. Outcome Measures

The primary outcome (quality of life) will be assessed using the SGRQ and PGI questionnaires. Secondary outcomes will be evaluated using DEXA, Spirometry, 6MWT, LCADL, and CAT.

2.6.1. Questionnaires, Scales and Tests

Mini-Cog

The Mini-Cog will be applied only in the first phase of the experiment, as an inclusion criterion for patients over 65 years of age. The test consists of a three-word memorization task and a clock drawing task. The individual must be able to remember the three words after making the drawing, scoring 1 point for each word they remember and 2 points for correctly drawing the clock [30,32].

The Mini-Cog has a total score of 5 points. Results ranging from 3 to 5 points are considered normal [32].

Double Energy X-ray Absorptiometry (DEXA)

Total body mass, fat mass, lean mass, bone mineral density, and height will be evaluated using dual-energy radiological absorbance (DEXA) (Lunar Radiation Corporation, Madison, WI, USA, DPX model). Fat mass and lean mass will be evaluated by total body analysis and by body segment (upper, lower and trunk). For this analysis, patients will be positioned in the scanning area of the equipment so that the sagittal line marked on the equipment passes under the center of certain anatomical points such as the skull, spine, pelvis, and lower limbs. Patients will be evaluated wearing light clothes, without the use of any metal object that could interfere with the measurements.

DEXA will be used to characterize the sample and to assess changes in the subjects' body composition. Therefore, it will be evaluated in Phase I and at the end of Phase III.

Spirometry

Spirometry is the measurement of the air that enters and leaves the lungs [33,34]. Spirometry is a test that enables the diagnosis and quantification of ventilatory disorders. It will be used to assess the individual's pulmonary function and characterize the studied sample according to the GOLD criteria [1].

Spirometry will be performed using the MIR Spirometer, Model Minispir, manufactured by MIR Medical International Research (Rome, Italy), with the individual sitting with trunk support, with arms along the body and wearing a nose clip. The subject will be asked to place the mouthpiece above the tongue and close the mouth tightly around it; at the researcher's command, the individual will make a deep inspiration until total lung capacity (TLC) has been reached, followed by a "fast and prolonged" forced expiration, until the examiner's end signal, when the patient will make another maximum inspiration with the mouthpiece still in the mouth. At least three measurements will be performed, three of which are acceptable and two reproducible, for evaluation; the best values will be recorded according to the 1st Brazilian Consensus on Spirometry. The test will analyze forced vital capacity (FVC); forced expiratory volume in the first second (FEV1); forced expiratory flows at 25%, 75%, and 25–75% of the FVC curve; peak expiratory flow (PEF); the relationship between FEV1 and FVC (FEV1/FVC); and inspiratory capacity (IC), which is the amount of air that can be inhaled from resting expiratory level to TLC. These parameters will be expressed in absolute values and percentage of the predicted value, according to the GOLD reference values [1].

The spirometer will be calibrated each day before the tests. Calibration will involve measuring the output of the spirometer and the sensitivity of the recording device or generating a software correction factor, and it will therefore involve tuning the equipment for performance within certain limits. For this purpose, a 3 L syringe supplied by the manufacturer will be used along with the equipment.

Spirometry will be applied in Phase I to confirm the diagnosis according to GOLD and characterize the sample, and at the end of Phase II and Phase III to evaluate the response to the acupuncture intervention.

Patient-Generated Index (PGI)

The PGI is completed in three steps: (1) Patients identify the five most important areas of their life affected by the disease, in this case, chronic obstructive pulmonary disease; (2) patients rate how much each area was affected by COPD using a scale of 0 to 6, where 0 is the worst imaginable and 6 is exactly how they would like it to be; (3) patients now imagine they have 10 "tokens" to spend on improving selected areas and allocate these tokens to areas according to their priority. An overall index is then calculated by multiplying the ratings for each area in Step 2 by the proportion of tokens given to that area in Step 3, which are then added to produce an index where higher scores indicate higher QoL [14].

It is worth mentioning that for the PGI there is a minimum detectable difference of 10.8 [14].

The PGI will be used to assess QoL, which will be analyzed in Phase I and at the ends of Phase II and Phase III.

Saint George's Respiratory Questionnaire (SGRQ)

The SGRQ addresses aspects related to three domains: symptoms, activity, and psychosocial impacts that respiratory disease inflicts on the patient. Each domain has a maximum possible score; the points for each answer are added up and the total is referred to as a percentage of the maximum. A total score is calculated from 0 (no health impairment) to 100 (maximum health impairment). In addition to the total score, there is also a score for each domain of symptoms, activity, and impact, which are also scored from 0 to 100. Values above 10% reflect an altered QOL in that domain. Changes equal to or greater than 4% after an intervention, in any domain or the total number of points, indicate a significant change in the patients' QoL [35].

The SGRQ will be used to assess QoL, which will be analyzed in Phase I and at the ends of Phase II and Phase III.

London Chest Activity of Daily Living (LCADL)

The London Chest Activity of Daily Living (LCADL) scale has four domains (personal care, household activities, physical activities, and leisure activities), with 15 questions in total, to assess the limitations to ADLs in patients with COPD [36]. Each question in the domains receives a score from 0 to 5, indicated by the patient, with the highest value representing the maximum inability to perform ADL due to dyspnea. The total score can range from 0 to 75 points, and the higher the value, the greater the limitation in ADL. The scale also has question 16, which refers to a specification of ADL impairment due to dyspnea, in any situation, and the patient must answer this question by ticking one of the three alternatives: "a lot", "little", or "not at all" [37].

The LCADL will be used to assess ADLs, which will be analyzed in Phase I and at the ends of Phase II and Phase III.

Six-Minute Walk Test (6MWT)

To evaluate functional performance, the 6MWT will also be applied according to the recommendations of the American Thoracic Society [38]. The test will be performed in a

30 m corridor, on a flat surface on which the subjects will be instructed to walk as fast as possible, without running, for six minutes. The subject will be allowed to rest during the test and resume walking as soon as they are able. During the walk, the examiner will give verbal stimuli every minute, always using the same tone of voice and the standardized phrase: "you are doing very well". The subject will be instructed to interrupt the test if he presents pain in the lower limbs, tachycardia, dizziness, or any other symptom of discomfort. Immediately before and after the test, systemic blood pressure (BP), heart rate (HR), oxygen saturation (SpO2), and level of dyspnea and lower limb fatigue (Borg scale) will be measured. Two tests will be performed with an interval of 30 min between them, and the test in which the patient has walked the longest distance will be used for analysis. If the difference in the distance walked between the two tests is greater than 10%, a third test will be performed [38,39]. It is noteworthy that a mean increase of 30 m in 6MWT covered distance after pulmonary rehabilitation in COPD patients indicates a minimal clinically important increase [39,40].

The 6MWT will be used to evaluate functional performance; therefore, it will be evaluated in Phase I and at the ends of Phase II and Phase III.

COPD Assessment Test (CAT)

The CAT is composed of eight items, called cough, phlegm, chest tightness, shortness of breath, limitations in household activities, confidence in leaving home, sleep, and energy. For each item, the patient chooses only one answer option, the score of which varies from zero to five. At the end of the test, all response scores are added up, and the clinical impact of COPD is evaluated according to the stratification score of the CAT development and validation study [41]. The results vary according to the range of scores obtained, being classified for clinical impact as follows: 6–10 points, mild; 11–20, moderate; 21–30, severe; and 31–40, very severe [42].

The CAT will be used to assess the impact of COPD on patients' lives, which will be analyzed in Phase I and at the ends of Phase II and Phase III.

2.7. Ethics

Each patient will receive information about the purpose and structure of the research and written consent will be required through the Free and Informed Consent Form (ICF) to participate in the study. Patients may opt out of the study at any time before or during implementation of the protocol.

The project has been approved by the Ethics and Research Committee of the Federal University of Jequitinhonha and Mucuri Valleys (reference number 5.274.273).

2.8. Analyses

Statistical analysis will be performed following the intention-to-treat principle. Data will be analyzed using the SPSS Statistics statistical package (v.22.0; IBM Corp, Armonk, NY, USA). The normality of the data will be verified using the Kolmogorov-Smirnov test and the homoscedasticity of the data through the Levene test. The parametric data will be expressed as mean and standard deviation. In the case of nonparametric data, the median and its upper and lower limits will be expressed. The data will be analyzed using generalized linear mixed-effects models for repeated measures with post hoc Bonferroni analysis for correction. For all tests, an alpha of 5% will be adopted. Effect sizes will be interpreted based on their minimal clinically important differences (MCIDs).

Treatment of Lost Data (Missing Data)

Missing data will be classified as missed and nonrandom (PNA) when dropouts are due to a lack of efficacy and adverse effects and as missed completely by chance (PCA) when a loss to follow-up does not depend on observed or unobserved measures (e.g., patient moves to another city for non-health reasons). We are planning to perform mixed-effects models for repeated measures (repeated-measures ANOVA) to deal with missing data due to PCA and use single imputation methods (such as best- or worst-case imputation, i.e., assigning the worst possible value of the result for dropouts for a negative reason–treatment failure and the best possible value for positive dropouts (cures)) when considering the absence a PNA. We are planning sensitivity analyses to assess whether the methods used to deal with missing data produce any important differences in the results [43].

3. Discussion

Previous studies on acupuncture for the treatment of COPD demonstrate that acupuncture can result in important clinical improvements in quality of life and dyspnea [21,44]. However, existing studies provide insufficient evidence due to methodological limitations, including poor study design, inadequate control groups, and variations in AT. A systematic review on the topic published in 2018 showed that the methodological quality of the included studies was generally low. For example, most of the included studies were at high risk of performance bias. In addition, most analyses of the data in the meta-analysis indicated heterogeneity across studies. Finally, there were several forms of intervention adjunct to acupuncture, which makes it difficult to assess the effectiveness of acupuncture alone [45].

Therefore, more rigorously designed studies are needed to elucidate the efficacy of acupuncture therapy for the treatment of patients with COPD and its response in regard to HRQoL (primary outcome). Moreover, there is also a need to analyze functional performance limited by dyspnea in ADLs, the impact of COPD on patients' lives, and these patients' pulmonary function (secondary outcomes). We therefore propose a randomized clinical trial with the evaluators blinded in addition to blinding the researcher to patient allocation. The data will be coded in a nonidentifiable way and will not contain any information that could indicate bias regarding patient allocation. The study will have a 16-week follow-up, with reapplication of tests and questionnaires at 8 weeks, enabling assessment of the responses in the short and long term, which, according to our previous review, has not yet been performed. In addition, our control group will not undergo any intervention, thereby providing analysis of the isolated effect of acupuncture on patients with COPD.

Control procedures involving invasive or noninvasive sham needling techniques can be therapeutically active, evoking localized neurophysiological and/or immune and circulatory responses [46–49]. There are also variations in assumptions about the accuracy needed for point location, as some acupuncturists and researchers consider acupuncture points areas of reactivity rather than action points. These assumptions affect the integrity of sham acupuncture as an appropriate control [28].

The PEDro (Physiotherapy Evidence Database) provides easy access to high-quality clinical research by physical therapists around the world, enabling the application of evidence in practice and effective teaching. All randomized clinical trials indexed in the PEDro are classified and can receive a maximum score of 10 points, according to their quality through the PEDro scale. This classification enables readers to identify relevant and valid studies to guide them in clinical practice [50].

A bibliographic survey using the PEDro database shows only one study that evaluated the effect of AT on the quality of life of patients with COPD with a score of 8; the other studies had scores of 5 or less, that is, were of low methodological quality according to the database. Although Feng's 2016 study obtained a score of 8 in terms of methodological quality, gaps remain regarding the isolated effects of acupuncture, as the study used a sham group as a comparator [22]. The use of sham acupuncture using the application of the needle at points other than those of oriental medicine or the use of seeds in place of the needle or even the use of a placebo needle can generate interpretation bias considering the mechanical effects and the pressure exerted on the biological tissue. Given the consideration that sham acupuncture can be as effective as traditional acupuncture [46–49], there remains a gap regarding the isolated effects of acupuncture. Furthermore, in addition to HRQoL, secondary outcomes such as functional performance, functional limitations, dyspnea in activities of daily living, and the impact of the disease on life are crucial for the global understanding of the effectiveness of acupuncture in patients with COPD. Therefore, conducting the present study is justified in terms of relevance and practical potential for application.

Our work predicts a score of 8 on the PEDro scale as we plan to specify eligibility criteria, randomly assign patients, and use veiled subject allocation by a researcher designated exclusively for this role during research planning, performed using a computer program; we will have well-defined inclusion and exclusion criteria ensuring similar groups with regard to the most important prognostic indicators at baseline; and there will be blinding of the evaluators who will measure the outcomes. Furthermore, we will aim to ensure patient adherence, ensuring that measurements of at least one key outcome will be obtained in more than 85% of subjects initially distributed among the groups, using weekly telephone calls made to patients in the control group; data will be analyzed by intent to treat; we will describe the results of intergroup statistical comparisons in at least one key result; and we will describe measures of precision as measures of variability for at least one key outcome. We will lose in points that do not apply to studies with acupuncture, i.e., blinding of subjects and blinding of the therapist who will apply the therapy. In addition, we will follow up for a total of 16 weeks by reapplying the tests and questionnaires at 8 weeks, which will enable assessment of the responses in the short and long term, which, according to our previous review, has not yet been undertaken.

Author Contributions: Conceptualization, R.F.C., A.C.R.L., V.P.L. and V.A.M.; formal analysis, R.F.C., A.C.R.L. and V.P.L.; methodology, R.F.C., A.C.R.L., V.P.L., V.A.M., L.V.d.P. and L.D.; funding acquisition, A.C.R.L. and V.P.L.; project administration, R.F.C., A.C.R.L. and V.P.L.; resources, R.F.C., A.C.R.L., V.P.L., V.A.M., L.F.F.d.O., S.F.F.d.O., R.P.A., C.L.F.e.C., F.P.d.S.; supervision, A.C.R.L., V.P.L.; validation, R.F.C., A.C.R.L., V.P.L., L.F.F.d.O., S.F.F.d.O., R.P.A., C.L.F.e.C. and F.P.d.S.; writing—original draft, R.F.C., A.C.R.L., V.P.L., V.A.M., L.V.d.P. and L.D.; writing—review and editing, R.F.C., A.C.R.L., V.P.L., L.F.F.d.O., S.F.F.d.O., R.P.A., C.L.F.e.C., F.P.d.S., P.H.S.F., H.S.C., M.B.-F., D.d.C.d.S.-C. and R.T. All authors have read and agreed to the published version of the manuscript.

Funding: This research received no external funding.

Institutional Review Board Statement: The study will be conducted according to the guidelines of the Declaration of Helsinki and was approved by the Institutional Ethics and Research Committee of Federal University of Jequitinhonha and Mucuri Valleys (protocol code 5.274.2738 on 1 February 2022)

Informed Consent Statement: Informed consent will be obtained from all subjects involved in the study.

Data Availability Statement: The data presented in this study are available on request from the corresponding author. The data are not publicly available due to the privacy guarantee of the data collected individually.

Acknowledgments: We thank the volunteers, authors, and collaborators. Data collections: Federal University of Jequitinhonha and Mucuri Valleys.

Conflicts of Interest: The authors declare no conflict of interest.

References

1. Global Initiative for Chronic Obstructive Lung Disease. *Global Strategy for Prevention, Diagnosis and Management of COPD*; Global Initiative for Chronic Obstructive Lung Disease: Fontana, WI, USA, 2022; p. 177.
2. Sin, D.D.; Anthonisen, N.R.; Soriano, J.B.; Agusti, A.G. Mortality in COPD: Role of comorbidities. *Eur. Respir. J.* **2006**, *28*, 1245–1257. [CrossRef] [PubMed]
3. da Silva Lage, V.K.; de Paula, F.A.; Dos Santos, J.M.; Costa, H.S.; da Silva, G.P.; Lima, L.P.; Santos, J.N.V.; de Almeida, H.C.; Figueiredo, P.H.S.; Bernardo-Filho, M.; et al. Are oxidative stress biomarkers and respiratory muscles strength associated with COPD-related sarcopenia in older adults? *Exp. Geront.* **2021**, *157*, 111630. [CrossRef]
4. Decramer, M.; Janssens, W.; Miravitlles, M. Chronic obstructive pulmonary disease. *Lancet* **2012**, *379*, 1341–1351. [CrossRef]

5. Arrieiro, A.N.; Soares, L.A.; Prates, A.C.N.; Figueiredo, P.H.S.; Costa, H.S.; Simão, A.P.; Neves, C.D.C.; dos Santos, J.M.; Santos, L.M.D.M.; Avelar, N.C.P.; et al. Inflammation Biomarkers Are Independent Contributors to Functional Performance in Chronic Conditions: An Exploratory Study. *Int. J. Med. Sci. Health Res.* **2021**, *5*, 30–37. [CrossRef]
6. De-Miguel-Diez, J.; Jimenez-Garcia, R.; Hernandez-Barrera, V.; De-Miguel-Yanes, J.M.; Carabantes-Alarcon, D.; Lopez-De-Andres, A. Assessing the Impact of Gender and COPD on the Incidence and Mortality of Hospital-Acquired Pneumonia. A Retrospective Cohort Study Using the Spanish National Discharge Database (2016–2019). *J. Clin. Med.* **2021**, *10*, 5453. [CrossRef]
7. Man, W.; Donaldson, A.V.; Maddocks, M.; Martolini, D.; Polkey, M. Muscle function in COPD: A complex interplay. *Int. J. Chronic Obstr. Pulm. Dis.* **2012**, *7*, 523–535. [CrossRef] [PubMed]
8. Pimenta, S.; Silva, C.G.; Flora, S.; Hipólito, N.; Burtin, C.; Oliveira, A.; Morais, N.; Brites-Pereira, M.; Carreira, B.P.; Januário, F.; et al. What Motivates Patients with COPD to Be Physically Active? A Cross-Sectional Study. *J. Clin. Med.* **2021**, *10*, 5631. [CrossRef]
9. Lage, V.K.D.S.; da Silva, G.P.; Lacerda, A.C.R.; de Paula, F.A.; Lima, L.P.; Santos, J.N.V.; de Almeida, H.C.; Pinto, A.G.F.; Figueiredo, P.H.S.; Costa, H.S.; et al. Functional tests associated with sarcopenia in moderate chronic obstructive pulmonary disease. *Expert Rev. Respir. Med.* **2020**, *15*, 569–576. [CrossRef]
10. Sanchez-Ramirez, D.C. Impact of Pulmonary Rehabilitation Services in Patients with Different Lung Diseases. *J. Clin. Med.* **2022**, *11*, 407. [CrossRef]
11. Regueiro, E.M.G.; Di Lorenzo, V.A.P.; Parizotto, A.P.D.D.; Negrini, F.; Sampaio, L.M.M. Analysis of metabolic and ventilatory demand during the execution of daily life activities in individuals with chronic obstructive pulmonary disease. *Rev. Lat. Am. Enfermagem.* **2006**, *14*, 41–47. [CrossRef]
12. Guyatt, G.H.; Feeny, D.H.; Patrick, D.L. Measuring health-related quality of life. *Ann. Intern. Med.* **1993**, *118*, 622–629. [CrossRef] [PubMed]
13. WHOQOL Group. The World Health Organization Quality of Life assessment (WHOQOL): Position paper from the World Health Organization. *Soc. Sci. Med.* **1995**, *41*, 1403–1409. [CrossRef]
14. Cardoso, R.F.; Ruta, D.; De Oliveira, T.M.; Costa, M.C.B.; Fonseca, A.A.; Figueiredo, P.H.S.; Bastone, A.D.C.; De Alcântara, M.A.; Lacerda, A.C.R.; Lima, V.P. Portuguese translation and validation of the Patient Generated Index instrument for patients with Chronic Obstructive Pulmonary Disease: Individualized quality of life assessment. *J. Bras. Pneumol.* **2020**, *46*, e20190272. [CrossRef] [PubMed]
15. Li, J.-S. Guidelines for Chinese medicine rehabilitation of chronic obstructive pulmonary disease. *World J. Tradit. Chin. Med.* **2020**, *6*, 295. [CrossRef]
16. Suzuki, M.; Yokoyama, Y.; Yamazaki, H. Research into Acupuncture for Respiratory Disease in Japan: A Systematic Review. *Acupunct. Med.* **2009**, *27*, 54–60. [CrossRef] [PubMed]
17. World Health Organization. *Benchmarks for the Practice of Acupuncture*; World Health Organization: Geneva, Switzerland, 2020.
18. World Health Organization. *WHO Global Report on Traditional and Complementary Medicine 2019*; World Health Organization: Geneva, Switzerland, 2019.
19. Ministério da Saúde, Secretaria de Atenção à Saúde, Departamento de Atenção Básica. *Política Nacional de Práticas Integrativas e Complementares No SUS*; Ministério da Saúde, Secretaria de Atenção à Saúde, Departamento de Atenção Básica: Rio de Janeiro, Brazil, 2015.
20. Souto-Miranda, S.; Mendes, M.A.; Cravo, J.; Andrade, L.; Spruit, M.A.; Marques, A. Functional Status Following Pulmonary Rehabilitation: Responders and Non-Responders. *J. Clin. Med.* **2022**, *11*, 518. [CrossRef] [PubMed]
21. Deering, B.M.; Fullen, B.; Egan, C.; McCormack, N.; Kelly, E.; Pender, M.; Costello, R.W. Acupuncture as an Adjunct to Pulmonary Rehabilitation. *J. Cardiopulm. Rehabil. Prev.* **2011**, *31*, 392–399. [CrossRef]
22. Feng, J.; Wang, X.; Li, X.; Zhao, D.; Xu, J. Acupuncture for chronic obstructive pulmonary disease (COPD). *Medicine* **2016**, *95*, e4879. [CrossRef]
23. Fernández-Jané, C.; Vilaró, J.; Fei, Y.; Wang, C.; Liu, J.; Huang, N.; Xia, R.; Tian, X.; Hu, R.-X.; Yu, M.; et al. Filiform needle acupuncture for copd: A systematic review and meta-analysis. *Complement. Ther. Med.* **2019**, *47*, 102182. [CrossRef]
24. Hsieh, P.-C.; Yang, M.-C.; Wu, Y.-K.; Chen, H.-Y.; Tzeng, I.-S.; Hsu, P.-S.; Lee, C.-T.; Chen, C.-L.; Lan, C.-C. Acupuncture therapy improves health-related quality of life in patients with chronic obstructive pulmonary disease: A systematic review and meta-analysis. *Complement. Ther. Clin. Pract.* **2019**, *35*, 208–218. [CrossRef]
25. Xie, Y.; Li, J.-S.; Yu, X.-Q.; Li, S.-Y.; Zhang, N.-Z.; Li, Z.-G.; Shao, S.-J.; Guo, L.-X.; Zhu, L.; Zhang, Y.-J. Effectiveness of Bufei Yishen Granule combined with acupoint sticking therapy on quality of life in patients with stable chronic obstructive pulmonary disease. *Chin. J. Integr. Med.* **2013**, *19*, 260–268. [CrossRef] [PubMed]
26. Chan, A.-W.; Tetzlaff, J.M.; Gøtzsche, P.C.; Altman, D.G.; Mann, H.; Berlin, J.A.; Dickersin, K.; Hróbjartsson, A.; Schulz, K.F.; Parulekar, W.R.; et al. SPIRIT 2013 explanation and elaboration: Guidance for protocols of clinical trials. *BMJ* **2013**, *346*, e7586. [CrossRef] [PubMed]
27. Eldridge, S.M.; Chan, C.L.; Campbell, M.J.; Bond, C.M.; Hopewell, S.; Thabane, L.; Lancaster, G.A. CONSORT 2010 statement: Extension to randomised pilot and feasibility trials. *BMJ* **2016**, *355*, i5239. [CrossRef] [PubMed]
28. MacPherson, H.; Altman, D.G.; Hammerschlag, R.; Youping, L.; Taixiang, W.; White, A.; Moher, D.; on behalf of the STRICTA Revision Group. Revised STandards for Reporting Interventions in Clinical Trials of Acupuncture (STRICTA): Extending the CONSORT Statement. *PLoS Med.* **2010**, *7*, e1000261. [CrossRef] [PubMed]

29. Hoffmann, T.C.; Glasziou, P.P.; Boutron, I.; Milne, R.; Perera, R.; Moher, D.; Altman, D.G.; Barbour, V.; Macdonald, H.; Johnston, M.; et al. Better reporting of interventions: Template for intervention description and replication (TIDieR) checklist and guide. *BMJ* **2014**, *348*, g1687. [CrossRef] [PubMed]
30. Filho, S.T.R.; Lourenço, R.A. The performance of the Mini-Cog in a sample of low educational level elderly. *Dement. Neuropsychol.* **2009**, *3*, 81–87. [CrossRef]
31. Hsieh, P.-C.; Cheng, C.-F.; Wu, C.-W.; Tzeng, I.-S.; Kuo, C.-Y.; Hsu, P.-S.; Lee, C.-T.; Yu, M.-C.; Lan, C.-C. Combination of Acupoints in Treating Patients with Chronic Obstructive Pulmonary Disease: An Apriori Algorithm-Based Association Rule Analysis. *Evid. Based Complement. Altern. Med.* **2020**, *2020*, 8165296. [CrossRef]
32. Borson, S.; Scanlan, J.M.; Chen, P.; Ganguli, M. The Mini-Cog as a Screen for Dementia: Validation in a Population-Based Sample. *J. Am. Geriatr. Soc.* **2003**, *51*, 1451–1454. [CrossRef]
33. Pereira, C.A.D.C.; Sato, T.; Rodrigues, S.C. Novos valores de referência para espirometria forçada em brasileiros adultos de raça branca. *J. Bras. Pneumol.* **2007**, *33*, 397–406. [CrossRef]
34. Sociedade Brasileira de Pneumologia e Tisiologia. II Consenso Brasileiro sobre Doença Pulmonar Obstrutiva Crônica—DPOC. *J. Bras. Pneumol.* **2004**, *30*, 1–52.
35. De Sousa, T.C.; Jardim, J.R.; Jones, P.W. Validação do Questionário do Hospital Saint George na Doença Respiratória (SGRQ) em pacientes portadores de doença pulmonar obstrutiva crônica no Brasil. *J. Pneumol.* **2000**, *26*, 119–128. [CrossRef]
36. Carpes, M.F.; Mayer, A.F.; Simon, K.M.; Jardim, J.R.; Garrod, R. Versão brasileira da escala London Chest Activity of Daily Living para uso em pacientes com doença pulmonar obstrutiva crônica. *J. Bras. Pneumol.* **2012**, *34*, 128–139. [CrossRef] [PubMed]
37. Muller, J.P.; Gonçalves, P.A.G.; da Fontoura, F.F.; Mattiello, R.; Florian, J. Aplicabilidade da escala London Chest Activity of Daily Living em pacientes em lista de espera para transplante de pulmão. *J. Bras. Pneumol.* **2013**, *39*, 92–97. [CrossRef] [PubMed]
38. Crapo, R.O.; Casaburi, R.; Coates, A.L.; Enright, P.L.; MacIntyre, N.R.; McKay, R.T.; Johnson, D.; Wanger, J.S.; Zeballos, R.J.; Bittner, V.; et al. ATS statement: Guidelines for the six-minute walk test. *Am. J. Respir. Crit. Care Med.* **2002**, *166*, 111–117. [CrossRef]
39. Holland, A.E.; Spruit, M.A.; Troosters, T.; Puhan, M.A.; Pepin, V.; Saey, D.; McCormack, M.C.; Carlin, B.W.; Sciurba, F.C.; Pitta, F.; et al. An official European Respiratory Society/American Thoracic Society technical standard: Field walking tests in chronic respiratory disease. *Eur. Respir. J.* **2014**, *44*, 1428–1446. [CrossRef] [PubMed]
40. Neves, C.D.; Lage, V.K.; Lima, L.P.; Matos, M.A.; Vieira, L.; Teixeira, A.L.; Figueiredo, P.H.; Costa, H.S.; Lacerda, A.C.R.; Mendonça, V.A. Inflammatory and oxidative biomarkers as determinants of functional capacity in patients with COPD assessed by 6-min walk test-derived outcomes. *Exp. Gerontol.* **2021**, *152*, 111456. [CrossRef]
41. Jones, P.W.; Harding, G.; Berry, P.; Wiklund, I.; Chen, W.H.; Kline Leidy, N. Development and first validation of the COPD Assessment Test. *Eur. Respir. J.* **2009**, *34*, 648–654. [CrossRef]
42. Silva, G.P.F.D.; Morano, M.T.A.P.; Viana, C.M.S.; Magalhães, C.B.D.A.; Pereira, E.D.B. Validação do Teste de Avaliação da DPOC em português para uso no Brasil. *J. Bras. Pneumol.* **2013**, *39*, 402–408. [CrossRef]
43. Committee for Medicinal Products for Human Use (CHMP). Guideline on missing data in confirmatory clinical trials. *Lond. Eur. Med. Agency* **2010**, *44*, 1–12.
44. Lewith, G.T.; Prescott, P.; Davis, C.L. Can a standardized acupuncture technique palliate disabling breathlessness: A single-blind, placebo-controlled crossover study. *Chest* **2004**, *125*, 1783–1790. [CrossRef]
45. Wang, J.; Li, J.; Yu, X.; Xie, Y. Acupuncture Therapy for Functional Effects and Quality of Life in COPD Patients: A Systematic Review and Meta-Analysis. *Biomed. Res. Int.* **2018**, *2018*, 3026726. [CrossRef] [PubMed]
46. Chae, Y. The Dilemma of Placebo Needles in Acupuncture Research. *Acupunct. Med.* **2017**, *35*, 383–384. [CrossRef] [PubMed]
47. Chae, Y.; Lee, Y.S.; Enck, P. How placebo needles differ from placebo pills? *Front. Psychiatry* **2018**, *9*, 243. [CrossRef] [PubMed]
48. Moffet, H.H. Sham acupuncture may be as efficacious as true acupuncture: A systematic review of clinical trials. *J. Altern. Complement. Med.* **2009**, *15*, 213–216. [CrossRef]
49. Zhang, C.S.; Tan, H.Y.; Zhang, G.S.; Zhang, A.L.; Xue, C.C.; Xie, Y.M. Placebo devices as effective control methods in acupuncture clinical trials: A systematic review. *PLoS ONE* **2015**, *10*, e0140825. [CrossRef]
50. Shiwa, S.R.; Costa, L.O.P.; Moser, A.D.D.L.; Aguiar, I.D.C.; Oliveira, L.V.F.D. PEDro: A base de dados de evidências em fisioterapia. *Fisioter. Em. Mov.* **2011**, *24*, 523–533. [CrossRef]

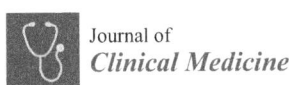

Article

Approach to Knee Arthropathy through 180-Degree Immersive VR Movement Visualization in Adult Patients with Severe Hemophilia: A Pilot Study

Roberto Ucero-Lozano [1], Raúl Pérez-Llanes [2], José Antonio López-Pina [3] and Rubén Cuesta-Barriuso [4,*]

1. Department of Physiotherapy, European University of Madrid, 28670 Madrid, Spain
2. Department of Physiotherapy, Catholic University San Antonio-UCAM, 30107 Murcia, Spain
3. Department of Basic Phycology and Methodology, University of Murcia, 30100 Murcia, Spain
4. Department of Surgery and Medical-Surgical Specialties, University of Oviedo, 33006 Oviedo, Spain
* Correspondence: cuestaruben@uniovi.es; Tel.: +34-985103386

Abstract: (1) Background: Hemarthrosis is a typical clinical manifestation in patients with hemophilia. Its recurrence causes hemophilic arthropathy, characterized by chronic joint pain. Watching movement recorded from a first-person perspective and immersively can be effective in the management of chronic pain. The objective of this study was to evaluate the effectiveness of an immersive virtual reality intervention in improving the pain intensity, joint condition, muscle strength and range of motion in patients with hemophilic knee arthropathy. (2) Methods: Thirteen patients with hemophilic knee arthropathy were recruited. The patients wore virtual reality glasses and watched a flexion–extension movement of the knee on an immersive 180° video, recorded from a first-person perspective over a 28-day period. The primary variable was the pain intensity (visual analog scale). The secondary variables were the joint status (Hemophilia Joint Health Score), quadriceps and hamstring strength (dynamometry), and range of motion (goniometry). (3) Results: After the intervention period, statistically significant differences were observed in the intensity of the joint pain (Standard error [SE] = 19.31; 95% interval confidence [95%CI] = −1.05; −0.26), joint condition (SE = 18.68; 95%CI = −1.16; −0.52) and quadriceps strength (SE = 35.00; 95%CI = 2.53; 17.47). We found that 38.46% and 23.07% of the patients exhibited an improvement in their quadriceps muscle strength and joint condition above the minimum detectable change for both variables (8.21% and 1.79%, respectively). (4) Conclusions: One hundred and eighty degree immersive VR motion visualization can improve the intensity of joint pain in patients with hemophilic knee arthropathy. An intervention using immersive virtual reality can be an effective complementary approach to improve the joint condition and quadriceps strength in these patients.

Keywords: hemophilia; knee; virtual reality exposure therapy; joint pain; physiotherapy

1. Introduction

Hemophilia is a rare disease linked to the X chromosome. It affects 1:10,000 live births. From the pathophysiological point of view, it is characterized by the absence or deficiency of any of the clotting factors. In hemophilia A, clotting factor VIII is missing, while in hemophilia B, the deficiency is related to factor IX [1]. This hematological pathology is characterized by the development of bleeding, mainly in the musculoskeletal system. Intraarticular bleeding (hemarthrosis) is the most common sign, mainly affecting the elbows, ankles, and knees [2].

The recurrence of bleeding events in the same joint causes progressive joint degeneration from an early age [3]; this is known as hemophilic arthropathy [4]. Such arthropathy is characterized by chronic proliferative synovial hypertrophy and osteochondral changes [5]. Joint pain associated with the development of arthropathy can start in childhood. Up to 20% of these patients report chronic pain [6], affecting their perceived quality of life [7].

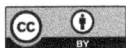

The gold standard in the treatment of hemophilia for the prevention of hemarthrosis and hemophilic arthropathy is the prophylactic administration of blood clotting concentrates [8] or, more recently, bispecific monoclonal antibodies [9]. Although prophylactic treatment is now widely used, it is scarcely available to patients residing in developing countries. Similarly, most patients now in their adulthood did not have access to such prophylactic treatment during childhood and adolescence [10], thus presenting in advanced degenerative joint damage.

From a neurobiological point of view, pain is a warning system that serves to protect us from potential damage [11]. This system, which receives information from external receptors, also evaluates the relevance of such information in relation to previous information, beliefs, experiences, etc. In the same way, it triggers physiological and behavioral responses [12]. All these responses are influenced by the environment, the tissues, and the evaluation generated by our brain based on all the information, beliefs, emotions, and sensations [12]. This constant assessment of experiences and memories can result in painful responses [13] or may down-modulate the nociceptive information [14].

The therapeutic approach, in connection with pain modulation from the cerebral response and not from peripheral information, has developed a hands-off model in the treatment of pain and, especially, chronic pain [15]. Therapies such as motor imagery, mirror therapy or motion visualization are based on this approach [16]. These therapies are based on the activation of mirror neurons through the observation of a movement. Watching a movement can cause the same cortical activation as if the movement were actually being performed [14]. However, this activation lacks the nociceptive input that could be generated by performing the movement. This makes the movement less relevant [12].

Similarly, the greater the immersion and the reality perceived by the brain, the greater the effect. Therefore, immersive virtual reality (VR) from a first-person perspective can help the patient to feel part of the immersive experience, being a valid option in the approach to patients with pain [17,18].

The aim of this study was to evaluate the effectiveness of an immersive virtual reality intervention in improving the intensity of joint pain, the joint condition, muscle strength, and the range of motion in adult patients with hemophilic knee arthropathy.

2. Materials and Methods

2.1. Study Design

A prospective, multicenter pilot study was developed in adult patients with hemophilic knee arthropathy. The aim of this pilot study was to evaluate the changes after an immersive virtual reality intervention.

2.2. Patient Recruitment and Selection

Patients with hemophilia were recruited in September 2021 from the Hemophilia Associations of Galicia and Malaga and the Spanish Federation of Hemophilia. The study took place between September 2021 and January 2022.

The inclusion criteria of the study were (i) subjects being over 18 years of age; (ii) with a diagnosis of hemophilia A or B; (iii) with a severe hemophilia phenotype (<1% of FVIII/FIX); (iv) with a medical diagnosis of hemophilic knee arthropathy (and more than 4 points on the Hemophilia Joint Health Score) [19]; (v) patients on prophylactic treatment; and (vi) who signed the informed consent document. Patients excluded from the study were those: (i) who developed hemarthrosis during the study period; (ii) without chronic knee pain for at least one year prior to the study; (iii) having neurological or cognitive alterations that prevented their understanding of the questionnaires and evaluation tests; (iv) amputees, epileptic patients, or those with severe vision problems that made it difficult for them to visualize movement with the mobile application; (v) patients who had developed antibodies to clotting factor concentrates (inhibitors); and (vi) those patients who were receiving other physiotherapy treatment at the time of the study.

2.3. Ethical Considerations

The main researcher informed the patients about the potential risks and benefits of the study. Subsequently, the patients received an information sheet listing all the characteristics of the study. All subjects signed the informed consent document before being included in the study. The study was conducted in accordance with the Declaration of Helsinki. The study was approved by the Clinical Research Ethics Committee of the Virgen de la Arrixaca University Hospital (ID: 2020-2-9-HCUVA). Prior to the recruitment of patients, the research project was registered (www.clinicaltrials.gov; ID: NCT04549402).

2.4. Measurement Instruments

Prior to the experimental phase, the main anthropometric (weight and height) and clinical variables (type of treatment, development of inhibitors, and knee joint condition) of the patients recruited in the study were collected.

Two evaluations were performed: pretreatment (T0) and at the end of the intervention (T1). The primary variable was the intensity of the knee joint pain. The knee joint condition, quadriceps and hamstring muscle strength, and range of motion were the secondary variables. All assessments were performed by the same physiotherapist, with years of experience in the evaluation and treatment of patients with hemophilia, blinded to the study's objectives.

The intensity of the perceived pain was evaluated using the visual analog scale [20]. This scale has shown an excellent intraobserver reliability (intraclass correlation coefficient [ICC]: 0.97) in assessing the intensity of knee pain [21]. This tool assesses the intensity of pain perceived by patients on a 10 cm line. The patients made a mark on the line that represented the average intensity of their usual joint pain suffered during the last week. Scores ranged from 0 (no pain) to 10 (the worst perceived pain) points.

The joint condition was evaluated using the Hemophilia Joint Health Score [19]. This scale, specific for use in patients with hemophilia, evaluates eight items: swelling and the duration of swelling, pain, atrophy and muscle strength, crepitus, and a loss of flexion and extension. This instrument has shown a high intraobserver reliability (Chronbach's $\alpha = 0.88$) in the evaluation of the joint condition in adult patients with hemophilia [5]. The scores, per joint, range from 0 (no joint damage) to 20 points (maximum joint damage).

Muscle strength was measured with a pressure dynamometer (Lafayette Manual Muscle Tester 01165) [22]. Pressure dynamometry has shown high intra-evaluator reliability in adult subjects in knee flexion (CHF: 0.91–0.93) and extension (CHF: 0.82–0.93) movements [23]. The evaluation of quadriceps muscle strength was performed according to the protocol described by Skou et al. [24]. Based on the functional characteristics of these patients, adaptations were made for the evaluation of patients with severe ROM restrictions [2]. With the patient in the supine position and at 75° of hip and knee flexion, the pressure dynamometer was placed perpendicular to the leg, just above the lateral malleolus. The patient was asked to keep the leg in the same position. For the evaluation of hamstring muscle strength, the patient was placed in a prone position and the knee flexed 45°, placing the dynamometer on the back of the leg at the Achilles tendon [25]. For the evaluation of both muscles, the patient was asked to exert two maximum isometric contractions against the dynamometer. These contractions lasted for 5 s, with a 30 s break in between [26]. The mean value of both the measurements was used [27]. The higher the value, the greater the muscle strength. The unit of measurement was Newton.

Knee ROM was assessed with an analog goniometer [28]. This instrument has shown an excellent intraobserver reliability (ICC = 0.91–0.99) in the measurement of mobility in this joint [29]. It was measured in the sagittal plane under no-load pain-free conditions, with the patient in the supine position. The goniometer was positioned with its axis on the joint interline, the reference points being the longitudinal axis of the femur and fibula [30]. The higher the degrees, the greater the range of motion. The unit of measurement is the degree.

Before starting the study, a pilot study was carried out to calculate the evaluator's intraobserver reliability. Reliability in assessing the joint condition, muscle strength, and range of motion was assessed. Six patients with hemophilia, not included in the study, were evaluated on two consecutive days. An excellent intraobserver reliability was obtained in the variables joint status (CHF = 0.982), and the muscle strength in the quadriceps (CHF = 0.903) and hamstrings (CHF = 0.978), and was good for the range of motion in flexion (CHF = 0.790) and extension (CHF = 0.876) movements.

2.5. Intervention

The intervention consisted of immersively visualizing the knee flexion–extension movement. For this purpose, a 180-degree immersive video in a first-person perspective was used. This video was viewed on the patient's smartphone, regardless of the operating system. In order to view the video immersively, the smartphone was coupled to virtual reality glasses (3D virtual reality glasses with remote control; model Q-MAX) [18]. The video was hosted on YouTube® with access from the He-Mirror App®, designed for this study by the research group. After installing the mobile application on the patients' cell phones, the mobile terminal was coupled to the virtual reality glasses. All patients were given the same model VR glasses, so they all underwent the same intervention with the same program and the same VR system. The patients had to be seated in a chair, with their feet relaxed and only resting on their heels. The intervention was performed for 28 consecutive days at home. The patients performed one daily session. Each session was 15 min long, uninterrupted, without any breaks. During each session, patients had to only watch the movement of both knees on the video, without imagining the movement or performing it. As the procedure was performed in a seated no-load and no-movement position, the patients were informed that even in the event of joint bleeding, they could continue with the intervention. The main study researcher regularly followed up on patients via telephone, clarifying possible doubts about the intervention or solving issues that may arise, encouraging the patients to persevere and adhere to the treatment. Figure 1 shows the intervention as performed by one of the patients included in the study.

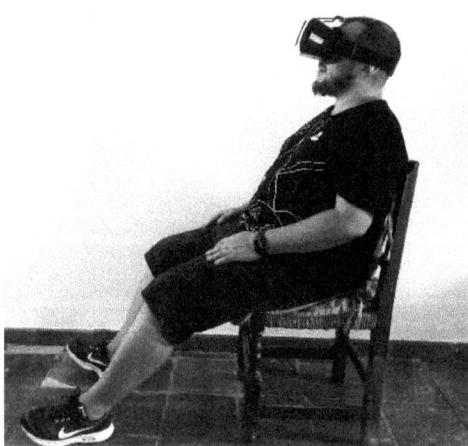

Figure 1. Patient completing the 180° immersive VR motion visualization intervention.

2.6. Sample Size

The sample size was calculated using the statistical package G*Power (version 3.1.9.2; Heinrich-Heine-Universität Düsseldorf, Germany) before recruiting the patients. Assuming a large effect size (d = 0.80), with an alpha level (type I error) of 0.05 and a statistical power of 80% ($1 - \beta = 0.80$), a sample size of 12 patients was estimated. Accounting for potential dropouts during the experimental phase, a total of 13 patients with hemophilia and knee arthropathy were recruited.

2.7. Statistical Analysis

The statistical analysis was performed with the software SPPS, version 21.0 for Windows (IBM Company, Armonk, NY, USA). The descriptive statistics (median and interquartile range) of the patients were calculated at the baseline. The changes between the pre- and post-treatment evaluations were calculated with the non-parametric Wilcoxon test. The minimum detectable change (MDC) was calculated with the standard error of measurement (SEM). The SEM was calculated with the formula: SEM = SDpre $* \sqrt{1-}$ intraclass correlation coefficient (ICC) [31]. Based on the SEM, the MDC was obtained (MDC = Z-score $* \sqrt{2} *$ SEM). The confidence level was set at 95% (Z score = 1.96) [32]. In the same way, the proportion of patients whose change after the intervention exceeded the MDC in the study variables was calculated. In this study, an analysis by intent to treat has been carried out. The selected significance level was 0.025 ($\alpha = 0.05/2$).

3. Results

None of the patients developed knee hemarthrosis during the experimental phase as a result of the intervention. There were no adverse effects resulting from the intervention of this study. The median age of the patients was 37 (IR: 14.5) years with a median body mass index of 26.76 (IR: 6.74) kg/m^2. The majority of patients had a diagnosis of hemophilia A (92.3%). All patients presented a severe hemophilia phenotype (<1% FVIII/FIX) and received prophylactic treatment. Table 1 shows the descriptive characteristics of the patients included in the study.

Table 1. Descriptive characteristics of patients with hemophilia at baseline.

Variables		Median (IR)
Age (years)		37 (14.5)
Weight (kg)		82.5 (21.2)
Height (cm)		173.0 (8.00)
Body Mass Index (kg/m^2)		26.76 (6.74)
		n (%)
Type of hemophilia	A	12 (92.3)
	B	1 (7.7)

IR: interquartile range.

When comparing the changes after the intervention period, statistically significant differences were observed in the variables for the intensity of the joint pain (Standard error [SE] = 19.31; 95% confidence interval [95%CI] = $-1.05; -0.26$; $p < 0.001$), joint condition (SE = 18.68; 95%CI = $-1.16; -0.52$; $p < 0.001$), and quadriceps strength (SE = 35.00; 95%CI = $-1.16; -0.52$; $p < 0.001$). 95% CI = 2.53; 17.47; $p = 0.012$). Table 2 shows the changes after the study period in each variable.

Table 2. Means (standard deviations) and changes evaluated in the different assessments.

Variables	T0	T1	MD (SE)	95%CI	Sig.
Intensity of joint pain (0–10)	1.41 (1.54)	0.75 (1.40)	−0.66 (19.31)	−1.05; −0.26	0.000
Joint health (0–20)	10.77 (3.44)	9.92 (3.07)	−0.84 (18.68)	−1.16; −0.52	0.000
Flexion (degrees)	114.42 (18.29)	115.04 (18.37)	0.61 (22.79)	−0.41; 1.64	0.254
Loss of extension (degrees)	10.31 (13.46)	9.35 (12.32)	−0.96 (15.85)	−1.94; 0.02	0.063
Quadriceps strength (N)	235.02 (77.07)	245.03 (83.25)	10.01 (35.00)	2.53; 17.47	0.012
Hamstring strength (N)	218.06 (37.67)	220.06 (44.32)	1.99 (35.00)	−7.08; 11.08	0.511

Outcome measures at baseline (T0) and after the 4-week period of interventions (T1); MD: means difference; SE: standard error; 95%CI: 95% interval confidence; Sig.: significance.

After the intervention, 38.46% of the patients exhibited an improvement greater than the minimum detectable change (8.21) calculated for quadriceps muscle strength (T0: 235.02; T1: 245.03). Changes in the joint condition (T0: 10.77; T1: 9.92) were greater than the minimum detectable change (1.79) in 23.07% of the patients included in the study. Table 3 shows the calculation of the minimum detectable change and the percentage of patients whose changes exceeded this value.

Table 3. Minimal detectable change of joint status, joint pain, range of motion, and hamstring flexibility evaluated in the different assessments.

Variables	ICC	SEM	MDC (MDCp)
Intensity of joint pain	0.879	0.535	2.027 (7.69)
Joint health	0.985	0.421	1.798 (23.07)
Flexion	0.995	1.293	3.151 (19.23)
Loss of extension	0.991	1.276	3.131 (23.07)
Quadriceps strength	0.987	8.787	8.216 (38.46)
Hamstring strength	0.919	10.721	9.075 (26.92)

ICC: intraclass correlation coefficient; SEM: standard error of measurement; MDC: minimal detectable change; MDCp: proportion of minimal detectable change.

4. Discussion

The aim of this study was to evaluate the changes in the pain intensity, joint condition, range of motion, and muscle strength in patients with hemophilic knee arthropathy after an immersive virtual reality intervention. After the intervention, we found improvements in the perceived pain intensity, joint condition, and quadriceps muscle strength. During the immersive virtual reality intervention, no patient included in the study developed knee hemarthrosis.

Jin et al. [33] noted a significant decrease in pain intensity in patients with total knee arthroplasty after a VR intervention. Byra et al. [34] reported the suitability of using VR in patients with knee and hip osteoarthritis for an effective pain management. Such improvements are due to the multidimensionality of the pain [34]. The illusory effect caused by visualization makes it easier for the brain to evaluate information as something non-aversive, improving downward modulation [12]. These results would be in line with the reduced pain intensity noted in our study.

Adult patients with hemophilia, such as those recruited in this study, have a wide experience of pain from their early childhood as a result of recurring hemarthrosis and arthropathy. It has been described that a change in pain intensity must represent at least two points on the visual analog scale to be clinically relevant [35]. According to our study, the MDC in the pain intensity was 2.027 points and only 7.69% of the subjects experienced changes beyond this value. However, it should be noted that the average intensity of knee pain at the baseline (1.41 points) did not reach two points, so this value should be taken with caution.

Villafañe et al. [36] observed an increase in the knee ROM in patients subject to VR intervention after total arthroplasty. Similarly, Calatayud et al. [37] found changes in the range of shoulder mobility in healthy subjects after a VR exposure with altered visual feedback with regard to the avatar. Changes reported in this study for knee mobility may also be due to the ability to alter statesthesia based on illusory visual inputs [37]. On the other hand, Hsieh et al. [38] found the activation of the same cortical areas after observing a movement or performing it with the hand in healthy subjects. This could cause motion visualization to activate these areas without triggering nociceptive inputs. This non-nociceptive activation may force the brain to reevaluate its available information and modulate the individual's responses to that movement [12]. These responses can be protective, such as reducing the joint range. Although we found no statistically significant differences in the knee range of motion in our study, these results should be taken with caution considering these two aspects: on the one hand, the small sample size, and on the other, the percentage of subjects (23.07%) who achieved an improvement greater than the minimum detectable change (3.131 degrees) in the loss of a knee extension, which is the most limited movement in this population.

Lee et al. [39] reported improvements in the strength of patients with knee osteoarthritis subject to motion visualization. Although a recent study [2] disclosed no immediate changes in strength improvement after a knee flexion–extension movement visualization session in patients with hemophilic arthropathy, the authors noted a large effect size for the activation of the rectus anterior of the quadriceps. The improved strength of the knee muscles predicted with the electromyographic measurement [40] is confirmed by the changes observed in our study regarding the quadriceps strength. However, caution should be exercised pending randomized clinical studies that confirm these changes.

According to the findings of this study, we are optimistic about the suitability of this intervention in the therapeutic approach to patients with hemophilia. Its easy implementation, low cost, and daily home use promotes the democratization of this protocol, making it more accessible.

Limitations of the Study

This pilot study has certain limitations that must be considered. On the one hand, the small sample size limits the generalization of results, although there are a series of changes that must be considered. Multicenter randomized clinical studies with an adequate sample size could confirm the results reported in this study. Another limitation is that in this study, the intake of analgesic drugs was not measured and this may affect the intensity of the pain perceived by these patients. In the same way, changes in the functionality of these patients as a result of the intervention have not been evaluated. The evaluation of variables such as functionality, modifications in muscle contraction, and psychosocial variables would provide more information about this intervention and its usefulness in the approach to patients with hemophilic knee arthropathy.

5. Conclusions

One hundred and eighty degree immersive VR motion visualization can improve the intensity of joint pain in patients with hemophilic knee arthropathy. Conducting daily immersive motion visualization sessions for 4 weeks can improve the joint condition and quadriceps muscle strength in patients with knee arthropathy. Randomized clinical trials with a larger sample size are needed to confirm the changes observed in this pilot study.

Author Contributions: Conceptualization, R.U.-L., J.A.L.-P. and R.C.-B.; methodology, R.U.-L. and R.P.-L.; software, J.A.L.-P.; formal analysis, J.A.L.-P.; investigation, R.U.-L. and R.P.-L.; resources, R.P.-L.; data curation, J.A.L.-P.; writing—original draft preparation, R.U.-L. and R.C.-B.; writing—review and editing, J.A.L.-P. and R.C.-B.; visualization, R.U.-L.; supervision, R.C.-B.; project administration, R.C.-B.; funding acquisition, R.C.-B. All authors have read and agreed to the published version of the manuscript.

Funding: This research was funded by Roche Farma S.A.

Institutional Review Board Statement: The study was conducted in accordance with the Declaration of Helsinki and approved by the Institutional Ethics Committee of Virgen de la Arrixaca University Hospital of Murcia, Spain (protocol code ID: 2020-2-9 HCUVA).

Informed Consent Statement: Informed consent was obtained from all subjects involved in the study. Written informed consent has been obtained from the patients to publish this paper.

Data Availability Statement: The data that support the findings of this study are available on request from the corresponding author. The data are not publicly available due to privacy or ethical restrictions.

Acknowledgments: We would like to thank the patients and participants in this study for taking the time to participate in the assessments and the patient associations for helping with sample recruitment.

Conflicts of Interest: The authors declare no conflict of interest. The funders had no role in the design of the study; in the collection, analyses, or interpretation of data; in the writing of the manuscript; or in the decision to publish the results.

References

1. Pinto, P.; Paredes, A.C.; Almeida, A. Pain Prevalence, Characteristics, and Impact Among People with Hemophilia: Findings from the First Portuguese Survey and Implications for Pain Management. *Pain Med. Malden Mass* **2020**, *21*, 458–471. [CrossRef] [PubMed]
2. Ucero-Lozano, R.; Pérez-Llanes, R.; López-Pina, J.A.; Cuesta-Barriuso, R. One Session Effects of Knee Motion Visualization Using Immersive Virtual Reality in Patients with Hemophilic Arthropathy. *J. Clin. Med.* **2021**, *10*, 4725. [CrossRef] [PubMed]
3. Soucie, J.M.; Cianfrini, C.; Janco, R.L.; Kulkarni, R.; Hambleton, J.; Evatt, B.; Forsyth, A.; Geraghty, S.; Hoots, K.; Abshire, T.; et al. Joint range-of-motion limitations among young males with hemophilia: Prevalence and risk factors. *Blood* **2004**, *103*, 2467–2473. [CrossRef] [PubMed]
4. Manco-Johnson, M.J.; Abshire, T.C.; Shapiro, A.D.; Riske, B.; Hacker, M.R.; Kilcoyne, R.; Ingram, J.D.; Manco-Johnson, M.L.; Funk, S.; Jacobson, L.; et al. Prophylaxis versus Episodic Treatment to Prevent Joint Disease in Boys with Severe Hemophilia. *N. Engl. J. Med.* **2007**, *357*, 535–544. [CrossRef] [PubMed]
5. St-Louis, J.; Abad, A.; Funk, S.; Tilak, M.; Classey, S.; Zourikian, N.; McLaughlin, P.; Lobet, S.; Hernandez, G.; Akins, S.; et al. The Hemophilia Joint Health Score version 2.1 Validation in Adult Patients Study: A multicenter international study. *Res. Pract. Thromb. Haemost.* **2022**, *6*, e12690. [CrossRef]
6. Witkop, M.; Neff, A.; Buckner, T.; Wang, M.; Batt, K.; Kessler, C.M.; Quon, D.; Boggio, L.; Recht, M.; Baumann, K.; et al. Self-reported prevalence, description and management of pain in adults with haemophilia: Methods, demographics and results from the Pain, Functional Impairment, and Quality of life (P-FiQ) study. *Haemophilia* **2017**, *23*, 556–565. [CrossRef]
7. Ucero-Lozano, R.; López-Pina, J.A.; Ortiz-Pérez, A.; Cuesta-Barriuso, R. The relationship between chronic pain and psychosocial aspects in patients with haemophilic arthropathy. A cross-sectional study. *Haemophilia* **2022**, *28*, 176–182. [CrossRef]
8. Oldenburg, J. Optimal treatment strategies for hemophilia: Achievements and limitations of current prophylactic regimens. *Blood* **2015**, *125*, 2038–2044. [CrossRef]
9. Mahlangu, J.; Oldenburg, J.; Paz-Priel, I.; Negrier, C.; Niggli, M.; Mancuso, M.E.; Schmitt, C.; Jiménez-Yuste, V.; Kempton, C.; Dhalluin, C.; et al. Emicizumab Prophylaxis in Patients Who Have Hemophilia A without Inhibitors. *N. Engl. J. Med.* **2018**, *379*, 811–822. [CrossRef]
10. Berg, H.M.V.D.; Fischer, K.; van der Bom, J.G. Comparing outcomes of different treatment regimens for severe haemophilia. *Haemophilia* **2003**, *9*, 27–31. [CrossRef]
11. Butler, D.S. *Explicando el Dolor*; Noigroup Publications: Adelaide, Australia, 2010; ISBN 978-0-9872467-1-4.
12. Jones, M.; Edwards, I.; Gifford, L. Conceptual models for implementing biopsychosocial theory in clinical practice. *Man. Ther.* **2002**, *7*, 2–9. [CrossRef] [PubMed]
13. Apkarian, A.V. Definitions of nociception, pain, and chronic pain with implications regarding science and society. *Neurosci. Lett.* **2019**, *702*, 1–2. [CrossRef] [PubMed]
14. Suso-Martí, L.; León-Hernández, J.V.; La Touche, R.; Paris-Alemany, A.; Cuenca-Martínez, F. Motor Imagery and Action Observation of Specific Neck Therapeutic Exercises Induced Hypoalgesia in Patients with Chronic Neck Pain: A Randomized Single-Blind Placebo Trial. *J. Clin. Med.* **2019**, *8*, 1019. [CrossRef] [PubMed]
15. Girbés, E.L.; Meeus, M.; Baert, I.; Nijs, J. Balancing "hands-on" with "hands-off" physical therapy interventions for the treatment of central sensitization pain in osteoarthritis. *Man. Ther.* **2015**, *20*, 349–352. [CrossRef]
16. Méndez-Rebolledo, G.; Gatica-Rojas, V.; Torres-Cueco, R.; Albornoz-Verdugo, M.; Guzmán-Muñoz, E. Update on the effects of graded motor imagery and mirror therapy on complex regional pain syndrome type 1: A systematic review. *J. Back Musculoskelet. Rehabil.* **2017**, *30*, 441–449. [CrossRef]
17. Yoshimura, M.; Kurumadani, H.; Hirata, J.; Osaka, H.; Senoo, K.; Date, S.; Ueda, A.; Ishii, Y.; Kinoshita, S.; Hanayama, K.; et al. Virtual reality-based action observation facilitates the acquisition of body-powered prosthetic control skills. *J. Neuroeng. Rehabil.* **2020**, *17*, 113. [CrossRef]
18. Choi, J.W.; Kim, B.H.; Huh, S.; Jo, S. Observing Actions Through Immersive Virtual Reality Enhances Motor Imagery Training. *IEEE Trans. Neural Syst. Rehabil. Eng.* **2020**, *28*, 1614–1622. [CrossRef]
19. Hilliard, P.; Funk, S.; Zourikian, N.; Bergstrom, B.-M.; Bradley, C.S.; McLimont, M.; Manco-Johnson, M.; Petrini, P.; Berg, M.V.D.; Feldman, B.M. Hemophilia joint health score reliability study. *Haemophilia* **2006**, *12*, 518–525. [CrossRef]
20. Hawksley, H. Pain assessment using a visual analogue scale. *Prof. Nurse* **2000**, *15*, 593–597.
21. Alghadir, A.H.; Anwer, S.; Iqbal, A.; Iqbal, Z.A. Test–retest reliability, validity, and minimum detectable change of visual analog, numerical rating, and verbal rating scales for measurement of osteoarthritic knee pain. *J. Pain Res.* **2018**, *11*, 851–856. [CrossRef]
22. Pfister, P.B.; De Bruin, E.D.; Sterkele, I.; Maurer, B.; De Bie, R.A.; Knols, R.H. Manual muscle testing and hand-held dynamometry in people with inflammatory myopathy: An intra- and interrater reliability and validity study. *PLoS ONE* **2018**, *13*, e0194531. [CrossRef]
23. Kelln, B.M.; McKeon, P.; Gontkof, L.M.; Hertel, J. Hand-Held Dynamometry: Reliability of Lower Extremity Muscle Testing in Healthy, Physically Active, Young Adults. *J. Sport Rehabil.* **2008**, *17*, 160–170. [CrossRef] [PubMed]

24. Skou, S.T.; Simonsen, O.; Rasmussen, S. Examination of Muscle Strength and Pressure Pain Thresholds in Knee Osteoarthritis: Test-Retest Reliability and Agreement. *J. Geriatr. Phys. Ther.* **2015**, *38*, 141–147. [CrossRef] [PubMed]
25. van der Ploeg, R.J.; Fidler, V.; Oosterhuis, H.J. Hand-held myometry: Reference values. *J. Neurol. Neurosurg. Psychiatry* **1991**, *54*, 244–247. [CrossRef]
26. Andrews, A.W.; Thomas, M.W.; Bohannon, R.W. Normative Values for Isometric Muscle Force Measurements Obtained with Hand-held Dynamometers. *Phys. Ther.* **1996**, *76*, 248–259. [CrossRef]
27. Leffler, A.-S.; Kosek, E.; Lerndal, T.; Nordmark, B.; Hansson, P. Somatosensory perception and function of diffuse noxious inhibitory controls (DNIC) in patients suffering from rheumatoid arthritis. *Eur. J. Pain* **2002**, *6*, 161–176. [CrossRef]
28. Gerhardt, J.; Cocchiarella, L.; Lea, R. *The Practical Guide to Range of Motion Assessment*; American Medical Association: Chicago, IL, USA, 2002.
29. Rothstein, J.M.; Miller, P.J.; Roettger, R.F. Goniometric Reliability in a Clinical Setting. Elbow and Knee Measurements. *Phys. Ther.* **1983**, *63*, 1611–1615. [CrossRef]
30. Pérez-Llanes, R.; Donoso-Úbeda, E.; Meroño-Gallut, J.; Ucero-Lozano, R.; Cuesta-Barriuso, R. Safety and efficacy of a self-induced myofascial release protocol using a foam roller in patients with haemophilic knee arthropathy. *Haemophilia* **2022**, *28*, 326–333. [CrossRef]
31. Schmitt, J.S.; Di Fabio, R.P. Reliable change and minimum important difference (MID) proportions facilitated group responsiveness comparisons using individual threshold criteria. *J. Clin. Epidemiol.* **2004**, *57*, 1008–1018. [CrossRef]
32. De Vet, H.C.; Terwee, C.B.; Ostelo, R.W.; Beckerman, H.; Knol, D.L.; Bouter, L.M. Minimal changes in health status questionnaires: Distinction between minimally detectable change and minimally important change. *Health Qual. Life Outcomes* **2006**, *4*, 54. [CrossRef]
33. Jin, C.; Feng, Y.; Ni, Y.; Shan, Z. Virtual Reality Intervention in Postoperative Rehabilitation after Total Knee Arthroplasty: A Prospective and Randomized Controlled Clinical Trial. *Int. J. Clin. Exp. Med.* **2018**, *11*, 6119–6124.
34. Byra, J.; Czernicki, K. The Effectiveness of Virtual Reality Rehabilitation in Patients with Knee and Hip Osteoarthritis. *J. Clin. Med.* **2020**, *9*, 2639. [CrossRef] [PubMed]
35. Myles, P.S.; Myles, D.B.; Galagher, W.; Boyd, D.; Chew, C.; MacDonald, N.; Dennis, A. Measuring acute postoperative pain using the visual analog scale: The minimal clinically important difference and patient acceptable symptom state. *Br. J. Anaesth.* **2017**, *118*, 424–429. [CrossRef] [PubMed]
36. Villafañe, J.H.; Isgrò, M.; Borsatti, M.; Berjano, P.; Pirali, C.; Negrini, S. Effects of action observation treatment in recovery after total knee replacement: A prospective clinical trial. *Clin. Rehabil.* **2017**, *31*, 361–368. [CrossRef] [PubMed]
37. Bourdin, P.; Martini, M.; Sanchez-Vives, M.V. Altered visual feedback from an embodied avatar unconsciously influences movement amplitude and muscle activity. *Sci. Rep.* **2019**, *9*, 19747. [CrossRef]
38. Hsieh, Y.-W.; Lee, M.-T.; Lin, Y.-H.; Chuang, L.-L.; Chen, C.-C.; Cheng, C.-H. Motor Cortical Activity During Observing a Video of Real Hand Movements versus Computer Graphic Hand Movements: An MEG Study. *Brain Sci.* **2020**, *11*, 6. [CrossRef]
39. Lee, T.-H.; Liu, C.-H.; Chen, P.-C.; Liou, T.-H.; Escorpizo, R.; Chen, H.-C. Effectiveness of mental simulation practices after total knee arthroplasty in patients with knee osteoarthritis: A systematic review and meta-analysis of randomized controlled trials. *PLoS ONE* **2022**, *17*, e0269296. [CrossRef]
40. Chen, J.; Zhang, X.; Gu, L.; Nelson, C. Estimating Muscle Forces and Knee Joint Torque Using Surface Electromyography: A Musculoskeletal Biomechanical Model. *J. Mech. Med. Biol.* **2017**, *17*, 1750069. [CrossRef]

MDPI
St. Alban-Anlage 66
4052 Basel
Switzerland
www.mdpi.com

Journal of Clinical Medicine Editorial Office
E-mail: jcm@mdpi.com
www.mdpi.com/journal/jcm

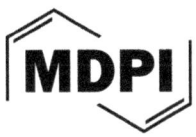

Disclaimer/Publisher's Note: The statements, opinions and data contained in all publications are solely those of the individual author(s) and contributor(s) and not of MDPI and/or the editor(s). MDPI and/or the editor(s) disclaim responsibility for any injury to people or property resulting from any ideas, methods, instructions or products referred to in the content.

www.ingramcontent.com/pod-product-compliance
Lightning Source LLC
LaVergne TN
LVHW070507100526
838202LV00014B/1804